Gerontological Nursing:
A Restorative Approach

Gerontological Nursing:
A Restorative Approach

Joan Fritsch Needham, R.N.C., M.S.Ed.

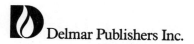 Delmar Publishers Inc.

NOTICE TO THE READER

Cover Design by Caliber Design/Phoenix Color Corp.

Delmar Staff

Executive Editor: David Gordon
Associate Editor: Elisabeth F. Williams
Project Editor: Carol Micheli
Production Supervisor: Larry Main
Design Coordinator: Karen Kemp
Art Supervisor: Judi Orozco

For information, address Delmar Publishers Inc.
3 Columbia Circle, Box 15015
Albany, New York 12212-5015

Copyright © 1993 by Delmar Publishers Inc.

Printed in the United States of America
Published simultaneously in Canada by Nelson Canada, a division of The Thomson Corporation

1 2 3 4 5 6 7 8 9 10 XXX 99 98 97 96 95 94 93

Library of Congress Cataloging-in-Publication Data

Needham, Joan Fritsch.
    Gerontological nursing : a restorative approach / Joan Fritsch Needham.
      p. cm.
    Includes bibliographical references and index.
    ISBN 0-8273-5138-0 (textbook)
    1. Geriatric nursing.   I. Title.
    [DNLM: 1. Geriatric Nursing. WY 152 N374g]
RC954.N34 1993
610.73'65—dc20
DNLM/DLC for Library of Congress
                                      92-10237
                                        CIP

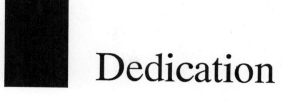

Dedication

This book is dedicated to Sam and Maggie Jo
for giving me the opportunity to experience
one of the greatest pleasures of aging —
being a grandmother.

Contents

**SECTION III
Interdisciplinary Team
Management of Older
Adults with Chronic
Disease Processes**

CHAPTER 8: A RESTORATIVE APPROACH TO CARING FOR THE CLIENT WITH IMPAIRED THOUGHT PROCESSES 157

CHAPTER 9: A RESTORATIVE APPROACH TO CARING FOR THE CLIENT WITH LOWER EXTREMITY AMPUTATION 179

CHAPTER 10: A RESTORATIVE APPROACH TO CARING FOR THE CLIENT WITH JOINT DISEASE 189

CHAPTER 11: A RESTORATIVE APPROACH TO CARING FOR THE CLIENT WITH TERMINAL ILLNESS 205

CHAPTER 12: A RESTORATIVE APPROACH TO CARING FOR THE CLIENT WITH IMPAIRED COMMUNICATION 219

List of Tables

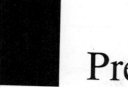

Preface

This is an exciting era for gerontological nurses. It is a time of challenge for professionals committed to improving the quality of life for older adults. As the aging population increases, there is increased demand for knowledgeable and skilled nurses prepared to care for their unique needs.

This book is written for the nurse who is committed to learning the gerontological skills necessary to assist clients to live their final years with dignity. The contents are directed to the nursing care of adults who are dealing with problems associated with chronic disease at the same time they are experiencing the normal changes of aging. Although these adults are not acutely ill, they have a problem for which there is no cure. They require long-term health care, which may be provided in a nursing home, extended care unit of a hospital, clinic, the client's home, or an adult day-care center.

The first section of the book provides a background for subsequent chapters. Demographic data, the aging process, and a summary of current theories of aging are included in chapter 1. A discussion of gerontological nursing and definitions for chronic illness and long-term care are followed with a review of past and present government programs affecting health care of the elderly.

Chapter 2 presents theoretical concepts of restorative nursing and a rationale for practice. Application of the nursing process includes a description of assessment factors based on Maslow's hierarchy of needs and corresponding changes of aging. A list of nursing diagnoses and identification of strengths for each level are included. Directions for developing client goals and nursing interventions are given for the planning process.

The second section contains five chapters providing information specific to the unique health care problems of the elderly. The topics discussed include mobility, skin care, nutrition, and bowel and bladder alterations. These problems are not the result of normal aging but are frequently diagnosed in clients who have a chronic disease process.

Chronic diseases are presented in the third section with an emphasis on restorative aspects of care. A case-study approach is utilized with a brief description of the problem. For each case study, client strengths are identified as an essential aspect of care planning. Interdisciplinary assessment factors and resulting nursing diagnoses are listed. Nursing diagnoses, such as impaired physical mobility, are used repeatedly to differentiate between nursing interventions used to treat the immobility of the individual who has had a stroke, for example, versus the interventions implemented for arthritis. Restorative nursing care focuses on teaching the client to increase functional abilities, maintaining the client's current status, and preventing complications. While taking into account the limitations related to aging, emphasis is placed on ability rather than disability and on independence rather than dependence. Suggestions are given in each case study for collaboration with the interdisciplinary team. The client needing long-term health care has problems that require a holistic approach. Nurses are usually responsible for the case management of the client but cannot expect to be all things to all clients. It is essential that the need for consultation and direction from other health care professionals be recognized and acted upon. Expected client outcomes are described for each intervention.

The term *caregiver* is used frequently throughout the book to include the nurse, the nursing assistant, and the family caregiver. Family refers to all individuals who are significant others for the client. In any case, the nurse is responsible for instruction, supervision, and evaluation of the caregiver and needs a solid understanding of how to implement the appropriate interventions.

Several objectives are presented at the beginning of each chapter; questions and discussion are included at the end. The reader will find this useful for additional self-directed learning. References are listed for each chapter. There are also suggested additional readings for some chapters. The book includes thirty-eight tables as well as numerous figures and nursing procedures. The reader will find specific information for assessing the older adult, for planning care, and for implementing the care. This book is results-oriented and is intended to provide hands-on instruction to the nursing student and to the practicing nurse who is responsible for the delivery of care to older adults. Two appendices are included. Appendix A is a listing of groups that can provide educational literature and audiovisuals for specific subject matter. The second appendix is a summary of residents' rights as legislated by the Omnibus Budget Reconciliation Act of 1987 for clients living in long-term care facilities.

We must move away from a custodial approach to gerontological nursing. The nurses of today are the gerontological nurses of tomorrow. A focus on restorative care will create a foundation for excellence in the provision of care for the elderly. The essence of restorative care is not to increase the length of life, but to assist each client in fulfilling an optimal potential throughout life. It is gerontological nursing at its finest.

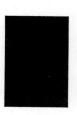

Acknowledgements

I wish to thank the people who have helped make this book possible: my husband, and my daughters and their families for their understanding, caring, and encouragement; my parents and siblings for being family; my friends for their patience and support throughout this endeavor; all of the nurses and nursing assistants who have so willingly shared their creative, caring ideas with me; the residents at the nursing home for teaching me about the process of aging; and Beth Williams from Delmar Publishers Inc. for her patience and kindness.

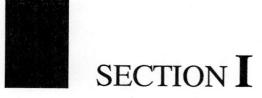

SECTION I

Foundations for Restorative Care

INTRODUCTION

    The first section of this book provides the foundation for sections two and three. Chapter one presents demographic information so the reader will develop an awareness of the numbers of older adults in this country and the effect of these numbers on the nursing profession. The aging process is addressed and includes some of the current biological and psychosocial theories of aging. Although there is no one accepted theory, a general knowledge of the current theories gives the reader the opportunity to formulate a conceptual framework. The influence of government programs is discussed because these programs are rapidly shaping the future of gerontological nursing in long-term care.

    The second chapter presents the nursing process in the context of restorative care with an interdisciplinary approach. The definition, theoretical concepts, and a philosophy for restorative nursing are provided so that the reader can then adapt the nursing process to the needs of the older, disabled adult. The discussion of assessment uses Maslow's hierarchy of needs to systematically identify unmet needs. Each level also identifies possible strengths. Nursing diagnoses are used for the description of both problems and strengths. A discussion of the components of planning, implementation, and evaluation end this section. Staff development is included here because of its significance in correct implementation of the care plan.

CHAPTER 1 Introduction to Nursing Care of the Older Adult

CONTENT OUTLINE

OBJECTIVES

- Describe at least three biological theories of aging.
- Describe at least two psychosocial theories of aging.
- Define the term *gerontological nursing*.
- Summarize the standards of gerontological nursing.
- Discuss the relationship of the nurse to the interdisciplinary health care team.

The people in this country are becoming aware of the changing shift in population as the number of older adults continues to grow. The nursing profession is feeling the impact of this change as the need for health care for older adults also increases. In response to this need, there has been a tremendous growth in home health services, nursing homes, and adult day-care and respite-care programs. Gerontological nurses are offering a wide range of services designed to assist older adults to live longer lives filled with dignity and joy. Myths and stereotypes concerning old age continue to thrive with the perception of old age as synonymous with sickness and helplessness. However, a more positive view is evolving as emphasis is placed on the wellness of aging and the expectation that everyone can live to grow old. Hospitals and other health care agencies are offering educational programs designed to provide instruction on health maintenance and disease prevention. Avoiding the risk factors associated with health problems has extended the number of productive years for many older adults. However, as people get older, the risk of acquiring a chronic disease increases. For those who become ill, the need for skilled care may require in-home services or placement in a nursing home. Both types of health care are providing more diversified services to meet the needs of an aging population. Changes in government funding of hospital care have resulted in earlier discharge of patients, many of whom need further rehabilitation and treatment. Nursing homes and home health agencies are filling this gap by caring for more acutely ill persons than ever before. Gerontological nurses must have the skills to nurse older adults through acute stages of chronic illness, to carry out restorative programs, and to care for the terminally ill. Technology can extend the life span. Now the challenge is to make these years worth living. Nursing research has demonstrated that nurses can increase the quality of life for the clients in their care. Much of this care is extended to clients with chronic health problems who require long-term services.

DEMOGRAPHIC DATA

The term *older adult* is a very subjective one. For purposes of classifying demographic information, the age of sixty-five years and over is used to define the group of people referred to as elderly. There were 3 million people over the age of sixty-five in 1900 (Skinner 1983). By 1987, there were 29.8 million people in this age group, making up 12.3 percent of the population. Growth is expected to continue, with the most rapid increase predicted for the years 2010–2030 when the "baby boom" generation reaches age sixty-five, Figure 1–1.

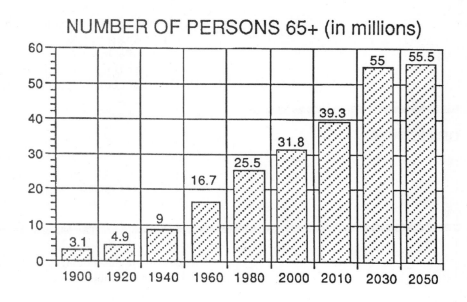

NUMBER OF PERSONS 65+ (in millions)

Figure 1–1 Population growth for persons over sixty-five years of age *(From Illinois Department on Aging)*

By the year 2000, persons age sixty-five and over are expected to represent

13.0 percent of the population; this percentage may climb to 21.8 percent by 2030 (American Association of Retired Persons 1990).

While medical technology is keeping Americans alive longer, this also means that more people are at risk for becoming disabled by chronic illness. Most older adults have at least one chronic condition: arthritis (49%), hypertension (37%), hearing impairments (32%), heart disease (30%), cataracts and sinusitis (17% each), and orthopedic impairments (16%) (American Association of Retired Persons 1990). There are currently over one million people in long-term care facilities needing nursing care. Seven million elderly persons in the community live at home with family and friends as their primary caregivers. These numbers will multiply.

Medicare expenditures are rapidly increasing, but little of this money goes for the payment of long-term care. Most of the cost of long-term care is borne by the client or family. Medicaid pays 44 percent of nursing home care, private insurance plans provide about 1.4 percent of the costs, and clients and families pay 54.6 percent. Most elderly people live in a family setting. Although the number living in nursing homes is large, it represents only 5 percent of all people over age sixty-five. This percentage increases dramatically with age, ranging from 1 percent for persons 65–74 years to 6 percent for persons 75–84 years and 22 percent for persons 85 and older (American Association of Retired Persons 1990). These figures clearly indicate a correlation between the aging process and health related problems.

There is a tremendous need for gerontological nurses who are creative, knowledgeable, and financially astute. The nurse's role extends beyond technology to involvement with the improvement of life for elderly clients.

THE AGING PROCESS

Aging is a complex phenomenon that begins at conception and continues throughout the life span. Alterations in physiology and changes in external characteristics are the most obvious indicators of aging. However, the process must be viewed from a broader perspective with a conceptualization of the psychosocial, cultural, legal, and experiential aspects. Because of its complicated nature, aging is not fully understood. Research has not provided conclusive answers, and at this time, no single theory of aging has been universally accepted by the nursing community. However, an examination of the most frequently reported biological and psychosocial theories will enable the nurse to develop broad concepts on which to base gerontological nursing practice.

BIOLOGICAL THEORIES OF AGING

Programmed Aging

Programmed aging theory is based on heredity. It presumes that the life span of a species is programmed within the genes of body cells. This program or genetic clock sets the speed with which the individual completes the life span and eventually dies (Christ and Hohloch 1988, Eliopoulos 1987, Esberger and Hughes 1989, Matteson and McConnell 1988).

The Immunity Theory

The thymus, a primary organ of the immune system, begins to decrease in size during adulthood. The ability to produce T cell differentiation decreases. Immunological functions then become less effective, resulting in an increased incidence of infections, neoplasms, and autoimmunity. Supporters of the Immunity Theory believe that aging of the immune system influences the aging process of the individual (Christ and Hohloch 1988, Matteson and McConnell 1988).

Somatic Mutation Theory

Some theorists propose a genetic basis for aging. They claim that changes in the DNA occur through radiation or miscoding of enzymes. If not repaired, replicated cells perpetuate the mutation, cellular function diminishes, and organ efficiency decreases, causing the alterations seen with aging (Christ and Hohloch 1988, Eliopoulos 1987).

Cross-Linkage or Collagen Theory

Collagen is the principle component of white fibrous connective tissue and is also found in skin, bone, cartilage, ligaments, muscles, lungs, and heart. The Cross-linkage or Collagen Theory states that chemical reactions between DNA and cross-linking molecules lead to loss of flexibility in connective tissues, impairing functional mobility. This process is also partially responsible for arteriosclerosis (Christ and Hohloch 1988, Eliopoulos 1987, Esberger and Hughes 1989, Matteson and McConnell 1988).

Stress Theory

This theory is based on the premise that throughout the life span, structural and chemical changes occur in the body as a result of stress. The stress reaction causes irreversible tissue damage (Eliopoulos 1987).

Summary

There are many theories that attempt to explain the aging process. The biological theories address the physical changes that appear to be universal in nature. The theories do not agree as to why these changes occur. There is agreement that not all organ systems age at the same time or at the same rate. The uniqueness of each individual suggests that there are many factors that influence the aging process.

PSYCHOLOGICAL THEORIES OF AGING

Psychosocial theories explain the behaviors and social interactions of older adults. These theories do not consider the variables that affect psychosocial aging. Factors such as health history, socioeconomic status, cultural background, and choice of life-style influence the psychosocial aspects of aging.

Disengagement Theory

Disengagement theory describes the withdrawal of the individual from society and society from the individual, resulting in decreased interaction between the aged person and others in his/her social system. Proponents of this theory claim that disengagement is inevitable, mutual, and acceptable to the individual as well as to society (Christ and Hohloch 1988, Eliopoulos 1987, Esberger and Hughes 1989).

Activity Theory

As the individual ages, roles and responsibilities change. The Activity Theory supports the belief that life satisfaction is dependent on the acquisition of new interests, hobbies, roles, and relationships. Maintaining a high level of social activity and involvement with life, promotes a sense of well-being and satisfaction (Christ and Hohloch 1988, Esberger and Hughes 1989).

Continuity Theory

As an individual grows from childhood, personality develops and the individual learns methods for adjusting and adapting to life events. Throughout the aging process, the person tends to repeat those behaviors that were successful in the past. This theory proposes that characteristic traits, habits, values, associations, and goals remain unchanged throughout life, despite life changes (Christ and Hohloch 1988, Esberger and Hughes 1989).

Summary

There is lack of agreement among psychosocial theories of aging as there is between the biological theories. It is evident that neither group of theories can fully explain the aging process. Aging and eventual death are inevitable. At this time, there is nothing that will reverse or prevent aging. It is evident that certain factors can promote healthy aging:

❑ maintaining mental and physical activity
❑ eating a nutritious diet
❑ avoiding known carcinogens
❑ managing stress effectively
❑ preventing diseases and infections
❑ obtaining prompt medical treatment when necessary

GENERAL CONCEPTS OF AGING

Although scientists have been unable to fully explain the phenomenon of aging, the information provided by nurse researchers assists the nurse to develop a rationale for the delivery of care to older adults. Application of the nursing process by a knowledgeable practitioner will improve the health care of each client.

The aging process is very individualized and independent of chronological age. Observation of a group of older adults all of the same age will reveal a great diversity within the group in terms of each person's physical and cognitive skills and psychosocial status. Genetic makeup influences potential for a long life and may determine one's degree of susceptibility to specific health problems. Individual attitudes and the ability to deal with the stresses and strains of living shape one's adaptation to aging. The speed with which one ages may be a reflection of socioeconomic factors and personal choice of life-styles. Regardless of why or how aging occurs, it is universal, progressive, irreversible, and eventually decremental. Most people as they age experience a number of losses. Physical changes resulting in decreased functional capacity, distress associated with loss of loved ones, and socioeconomic deprivations are foci for nursing interventions.

The expected changes of aging are not synonymous with disease. There are no diseases unique to old age and there are few from which the older person is exempt. Throughout life, the total state of health is a continuum — a series of alternating periods of wellness and illness. For most, the periods of illness are infrequent and minor. It is unwise to judge the older adult's state of well-being solely on the lack of actual or potential health problems identified through the nursing assessment. The strengths of the client need to be evaluated for the individual's satisfaction with life, for self-care, and for the ability to function in the home and community. Nursing services may be needed to assist the client to adapt to the changes of aging or during periods of illness.

THE HISTORY OF GERONTOLOGICAL NURSING

For the first half of this century, regulations for health care were loosely defined. In those early years, elderly persons unable to care for themselves were cared for by their families or placed in rest homes, boarding houses, or county poor farms. Little information was available on aging because few people lived beyond middle age. Newton's textbook, published in 1950, gave the first definition for geriatric nursing. During the 1950s and 1960s, there was a growth in nursing research with studies published on chronic illness and the effects of aging. These activities paved the way for the 1962 American Nurses Association first Conference Group on Geriatric Nursing Practice. The association established the Division of Geriatric Nursing Practice four years later, giving nursing of the aged specialty status (Matteson and McConnell 1988). In 1976, the name was changed to the Division on Gerontological Nursing Practice to more accurately reflect emphasis on health rather than on illness. In 1984, the division became the Council on Gerontological Nursing. *Standards and Scope of Gerontological Nursing Practice*, revised in 1987, defines gerontological nursing practice (American Nurses Association 1987).

The American Nurses Association Definition of Gerontological Nursing

Gerontological nursing practice involves assessing the health and functional status of older adults, planning and providing appropriate nursing and other health care services, and evaluating the effectiveness of such care. Emphasis is placed on maximizing functional ability in the activities of daily living; promoting, maintaining, and restoring health, including mental health; preventing and minimizing the disabilities of acute and chronic illness; and maintaining life in dignity and comfort until death.

Gerontological nursing may be practiced in any setting, for example, the nursing home, the hospital, the client's home, the clinic, and the community. Gerontological nursing focuses on the client and family. (In this document, the term family refers to family members and significant others.)

Standards of Gerontological Nursing Practice*

The standards as defined by the American Nurses Association call for quality care at a level beyond that required by minimal regulatory standards. The standards apply to gerontological nurses in all functional areas across all settings. The standards are included here so that gerontological nurses will use them as a model for professional practice.

❑ **Standard I.**   Organization of Gerontological Nursing Services

All gerontological nursing services are planned, organized, and directed by a nurse executive. The nurse executive has baccalaureate or master's prepa-

---

* Reprinted, with permission, from American Nurses Association, *Standards and Scope of Gerontological Nursing Practice,* © 1987.

ration and has experience in gerontological nursing and administration of long-term care services or acute care services for older clients.

❏ **Standard II.** Theory

The nurse participates in the generation and testing of theory as a basis for clinical decisions. The nurse uses theoretical concepts to guide the effective practice of gerontological nursing.

❏ **Standard III.** Data Collection

The health status of the older person is regularly assessed in a comprehensive, accurate, and systematic manner. The information obtained during the health assessment is accessible to and shared with appropriate members of the interdisciplinary health care team, including the older person and family.

❏ **Standard IV.** Nursing Diagnosis

The nurse uses health assessment data to determine nursing diagnoses.

❏ **Standard V.** Planning and Continuity of Care

The nurse develops the plan of care in conjunction with the older person and appropriate others. Mutual goals, priorities, nursing approaches, and measures in the care plan address the therapeutic, preventive, restorative, and rehabilitative needs of the older person. The care plan helps the older person attain and maintain the highest level of health, well-being, and quality of life achievable, as well as a peaceful death. The plan of care facilitates continuity of care over time as the client moves to various care settings, and is revised as necessary.

❏ **Standard VI.** Intervention

The nurse, guided by the plan of care, intervenes to provide care to restore the older person's functional capabilities and to prevent complications and excess disability. Nursing interventions are derived from nursing diagnoses and are based on gerontological nursing theory.

❏ **Standard VII.** Evaluation

The nurse continually evaluates the client's and family's responses to interventions in order to determine progress toward goal attainment and to revise the data base, nursing diagnoses, and plan of care.

❏ **Standard VIII.** Interdisciplinary Collaboration

The nurse collaborates with other members of the health care team in the various settings in which care is given to the older person. The team meets regularly to evaluate the effectiveness of the care plan for the client and family and to adjust the plan of care to accommodate changing needs.

❏ **Standard IX.** Research

The nurse participates in research designed to generate an organized body of gerontological nursing knowledge, disseminates research findings, and uses them in practice.

❏ **Standard X.** Ethics

The nurse uses the code for nurses established by the American Nurses Association as a guide for ethical decision making in practice.

❏ **Standard XI.** Professional Development

The nurse assumes responsibility for professional development and contributes to the professional growth of interdisciplinary team members. The nurse participates in peer review and other means of evaluation to assure the quality of nursing practice.

These standards are the foundation for nursing the elderly.

Nursing the Older Adult with Chronic Illness

As the numbers of elderly people increase, so does the incidence of chronic disease caused by irreversible pathological alteration. There is lack of agreement in the literature on a definition for chronic disease. The Commission of Chronic Diseases (1949) identified the characteristics of chronic disease:

❑ permanency
❑ residual disability
❑ caused by a nonreversible pathological alteration
❑ requires rehabilitation
❑ may require a long period of supervision, observation, or care (Lubkin 1990). This is long-term health care.

The American Nurses Association Committee on Skilled Nursing Care (1975) states

> the individual requiring long-term care is one who suffers from one or more chronic conditions which have resulted in a physical and/or mental impairment of normal activities, and which require prolonged and supervised care or treatment, necessitating at least, but not only, professional nursing assessment, evaluation, monitoring, judgment, and coordination of services and environmental support systems appropriate to the individual's health needs.

Long-term health care is provided in the client's home, nursing homes, clinics, extended care units of hospitals, and adult day-care centers. The client requires either continuous or episodic nursing supervision and assistance. The onset of an acute illness may require additional support and services at least on a temporary basis.

The gerontological nurse in long-term care is concerned not only with the physical aspects of chronic illness but also provides or coordinates services to meet the psychological, social, spiritual, and economic needs of the client. Meeting these needs often requires the expertise of many disciplines because of the complexity of biopsychosocial changes experienced by elderly people.

The Nurse and the Interdisciplinary Health Care Team

The responsibilities of the nurse as a member of the interdisciplinary team are defined in *Standards and Scope of Gerontological Nursing Practice*[*]:

❑ Collaborates and consults with other team members in designing the comprehensive plan of care for the client and family.
❑ Articulates nursing knowledge and demonstrates special nursing skills to other team members.
❑ Participates in or leads regular team conferences to evaluate and revise the plan of care for the client and family.
❑ Acknowledges the special skills and knowledge of other team members in planning and implementing care of the client and family.
❑ Promotes coordination and continuity of care within team meetings.
❑ Participates with interdisciplinary team members in continuing education programs and clinical research.

The membership of the team is dictated by the needs of the client and family and by the setting in which services are rendered. Besides the client, the family, the nurse, nurse assistant, and physician, the team may also include a social

---

[*] Reprinted, with permission, from American Nurses Association, *Standards and Scope of Gerontological Nursing Practice*, © 1987.

worker, physical therapist, occupational therapist, speech/language pathologist, nutritionist or dietician, clergy person, and pharmacist. The services of the podiatrist, dentist, ophthalmologist, and audiologist are required intermittently. Each discipline involved participates in the assessment and interdisciplinary care plan conference. The client and family are encouraged to attend these conferences so that goals can be mutually established and therefore have a greater chance of being attained. Successful collaboration of the team depends upon pre-established protocols that define the responsibilities of each discipline. This prevents gaps in services or overlapping of services. As more services are required to meet the needs of the older adult, continuity of care and coordination of services become more critical.

THE INFLUENCE OF GOVERNMENT PROGRAMS ON GERONTOLOGICAL NURSING

The Omnibus Reconciliation Act (OBRA) of 1987 clearly addresses the issue of interdisciplinary health care. This federal legislation, implemented in 1990, mandates the interdisciplinary approach; it is no longer an option for long-term health services funded by Medicare and/or Medicaid. For several years, the government has shaped and influenced the lives of the country's older citizens through programs designed to improve the quality of life in old age. A summary of these programs provides further understanding of current issues in gerontological nursing.

Social Security and Resulting Title Legislation

The passing of the Social Security Act in 1935 initiated a number of subsequent legislative acts affecting the delivery of health care and social services to the elderly. Amendments to the Social Security Act in 1950 permitted funding to be used for public nursing care facilities (Title XIX). This statute contains the authority of the federal-state Medical Assistance Program (Medicaid). Although the program is financed by federal, state, and local funds, Medicaid is administered at the state level. Thus, the services provided vary from state to state. The Medicaid program is intended to fund medical care for impoverished persons of any age. Because it is often difficult to obtain non-institution-based services, the majority of older recipients are in long-term care facilities. Three-fourths of nursing home care is reimbursed by state Medicaid programs.

In 1965, Social Security Amendments for Medicare and Medicaid were signed into law. Medicare (Title XVIII) contained provisions for nursing home benefits for extended care following hospitalization. Standards established in 1967 mandated the certification of health care institutions receiving funds from Medicare and/or Medicaid. In 1972, Congress directed the establishment of unified standards and regulations so that institutions certified for participation under Medicare and Medicaid had to demonstrate compliance with federal requirements (Illinois Legislative Investigating Commission 1984).

New regulations in 1974 included provisions for residents' rights. In 1981, the Omnibus Budget Reconciliation Act liberalized Medicare home health benefits by removing the limit on the number of visits allowed and the requirement for prior hospitalization. The Tax Equity and Fiscal Responsibility Act of 1983 changed Medicare reimbursement for hospitals from a cost-based system to a prospective payment system.

Omnibus Budget Reconciliation Act of 1987

The Omnibus Reconciliation Act of 1987 includes several directives for Medicare, Medicaid, and other health-related programs. This legislation has tremendous implications for providers of health care. Title IV of this act specifically addresses issues of home health quality and nursing home reform. Criteria for eligibility and benefits for programs for the elderly are set forth. OBRA (1987) emphasizes quality of life for persons receiving long-term health care and attempts to assure the extension of clients' rights. A major requirement of this act is the implementation of restorative services.

Older Americans Act

All aspects of long-term health care have felt the impact of legislation passed in the last two decades. The Older Americans Act (OAA) was enacted in 1965 as a response to problems of older persons without regard to income. Under this act, state units on aging were formed and through the states, area agencies on aging were established. Among several programs offered are home delivered meals and congregate meal programs, transportation services, adult day care, and in-home health care. Funds from this act have been applied to the formation of senior centers that provide information and varied services in the community. Through the Older Americans Act, employment opportunities are developed for those over fifty-five years of age (Matteson and McConnell 1988). The types of services vary in each community based upon the needs and resources of a given locality.

Legislative Initiatives

Providing quality health care has become a very complicated issue for health care professionals in any setting. Throughout history, government has attempted to resolve problems of health care delivery, but legislation alone can really guarantee nothing but paper compliance.

Past studies and investigations have pinpointed staff shortages and lack of education as the causes of many problems in the system. A series of hearings by the Subcommittee on Long Term Care from 1965–1976, chaired by United States Senator Frank E. Moss, resulted in a twelve-volume report, "Nursing Home Care in the United States, Failure in Public Policy." This report found that the use of untrained personnel and a lack of professional nurses educated in gerontology were the major causes of poor care in nursing homes. Fifty-three percent of those applying for jobs as aides and orderlies had no previous training nor were they provided any training as new employees. Ninety percent of the direct care was given by people with no education concerning nursing care or the aging process. While the worst nursing homes were investigated, the best ones were also analyzed during the hearings to determine what it was that made the difference. Facilities providing the finest care were found to be managed by administrators who believed in the need for staff education and were willing to pay for it. Testimony at the hearings was given by experts from the American Nurses Association, the American Association of Nursing Home Physicians, and the American Nursing Home Association (Moss and Halamandaris 1977).

Previous to the OBRA 1987, some states included educational requirements for nursing assistants, aides, and orderlies in the minimum regulatory standards for long-term-care facilities. By 1990, all states were expected to comply with the requirements set forth in the 1987 OBRA. These specify a minimum of seventy-five hours of education and training for unlicensed nursing staff. After completing a formal course of study and clinical training, nursing assistants are required to pass written and manual competency tests. Each state is responsible for implementation of this legislation. Many states exceed these minimum requirements. The quality of these educational programs is dependent on the knowledge and abilities of those who develop and teach them.

A quarter of a century has passed since the hearings by the Subcommittee on Long Term Care were initiated. Legislation enacted in OBRA 1987 for nursing home reform was not published as final regulations by the Health Care Financing Administration until September 1991.

Omnibus Budget Reconciliation Act of 1990

Sections 4206 and 4751 of OBRA 1990 define the *Patient Self-Determination Provisions* (House of Representatives 1990). These assure that Medicare providers implement the patient's right to participate in and direct health care decisions affecting the patient. OBRA 1990 applies to hospitals, skilled nursing facilities, home health agencies, and hospice programs. This act legally requires providers (as defined in the last sentence) to inform patients of their rights to make decisions regarding their health care and to carry out these rights. The Patient Self-Determination Act applies to *all adult patients* and requires that:

❑ all providers maintain written policies and procedures regarding the implementation of this act
❑ the policies must contain information concerning the individual's rights under state law to make decisions concerning medical care and the right to accept or refuse treatment
❑ the policies must explain the patient's right to formulate *advance directives* and how the provider will accommodate those rights
❑ the medical record must indicate whether or not the individual has executed an advance directive
❑ providers cannot discriminate against an individual based on whether or not the individual has executed an advance directive
❑ providers must educate staff and community on issues concerning advance directives

The term *advance directive* means a written instruction, such as a living will or durable power of attorney for health care, recognized under state law and relating to the provision of such care when the individual is incapacitated. Providers must comply with state legislation and case law regarding advance directives. Policies established by providers must provide guidance on DNR (do not resuscitate) orders, appointments of legal guardians, involvement of family members, and philosophical issues such as the removal of nutrition and hydration. In response to these federal requirements, many states have legislated surrogate acts.

Surrogate acts vary from state to state. The intent of the act in each state is to provide a mechanism for decision making in the absence of advance directives when a person is no longer able to make decisions. It is inevitable that nurses will be responsible for the implementation of many aspects of this legislation. Nurses in all health care settings need to be cognizant of the laws in the state in which they are practicing.

THE FUTURE OF GERONTOLOGICAL NURSING

The health care needs of the elderly have changed dramatically over the years and will continue to change as the number of older adults increases. Changing technology and future legislation will present new philosophical and ethical issues. These conditions directly affect the future of gerontological nursing.

The demand for nurses specializing in care of the elderly will be greater than ever. Hospital admission rates for this age group will increase, causing nursing administration to meet the challenge by utilizing the expertise of clinical specialists in gerontology. Long-term-care facilities will employ more nurses with formal preparation in the care of the elderly and restorative nursing. Salaries and benefits will continue to improve in order to recruit qualified nurses. Nursing homes and home health care agencies will be called upon to deliver more sophisticated services as the acuity of admissions increases. Adult day care and respite care will expand to allow families to delay or avoid nursing home placement. All nursing programs will include gerontological nursing in the curricula to meet the demand for qualified professionals.

Nurses will become even more involved in ethical issues concerning do not resuscitate orders and the withdrawing of life-sustaining procedures. The question of quality of life will demand answers as technology continues to lengthen the life span.

The restorative approach will be universally utilized in the care of the elderly in all settings. Assisting clients to attain optimal levels in all aspects of life will be the philosophy of care. Freedom to make informed decisions and freedom from physical and chemical restraints will be a reality.

Nurses will increase their political power with involvement in legislation affecting nursing, health care, and the elderly. Nurses will encourage and assist their clients to become vocal in the political arena.

The use of nursing assistants as direct caregivers in long-term care will continue. The professional nurse will support and accept responsibility for the continuing education, supervision, and evaluation of nursing assistants.

As costs continue to spiral, nurses will be even more creative in the use and distribution of existing funds. They will greatly influence the allocation of financial resources distributed through federal and state governments.

The challenges for gerontological nurses will be greater than ever before. The rewards and satisfactions will also be greater as nurses realize their successes in making a difference in the lives of their elderly clients.

SUMMARY

Gerontological nurses are expected to fill many roles. The planning and implementation of quality care is a priority issue. To provide this care, nurses need to be advocates for clients in need of health care services. In addition, gerontological nurses must be politically astute and work with the legislators of the country in order to have a voice in the future of gerontological nursing.

> You do not know yet what it is to be 70 years old. I will tell you, so that you may not be taken by surprise when your turn comes. It is like climbing the Alps. You reach a snow-covered summit, and see behind you the deep valley stretching miles and miles away, and before you other summits higher and whiter which you may have strength to climb or may not. Then you sit down and meditate, and wonder which it will be. That is the whole story, amplify it as you may. All that one can say is, that life is opportunity.

Henry Wadsworth Longfellow

QUESTIONS AND DISCUSSION

1. Discuss the implications for developing a theory of aging.
2. Trace the effect of legislation on health care for the elderly and project future legislation.
3. What differences, if any, exist between the responsibilities of the gerontological nurse and the responsibilities of nurses in other specialty areas?
4. What do you see as the biggest challenges facing gerontological nurses in the 1990s?

REFERENCES

American Association of Retired Persons. 1990. *A Profile of Older Americans*. Washington, DC: Department of Health and Human Services.

American Nurses Association. 1975. *Nursing and Long-Term Care: Toward Quality Care for the Aging.* Kansas City: American Nurses Association.

———. 1987. *Standards and Scope of Gerontological Nursing Practice.* Kansas City: American Nurses Association.

Christ, M.A. and F.J. Hohloch. 1988. *Gerontologic Nursing.* Springhouse, PA: Springhouse Corporation.

Eliopoulos, C. 1987. *A Guide to the Nursing of the Aging.* Baltimore: Williams & Wilkins.

Esberger, K.K. and S.T. Hughes. 1989. *Nursing Care of the Aged.* Norwalk, CT: Appleton & Lange.

Illinois Legislative Investing Commission. 1984. *Regulation and Funding of Illinois Nursing Homes.* Chicago: State of Illinois.

Lubkin, I.M. 1990. *Chronic Illness.* Boston: Jones and Bartlett Publishers.

Matteson, M.A. and E.S. McConnell. 1988. *Gerontological Nursing.* Philadelphia: W.B. Saunders Company.

Moss, F.E. and V.J. Halamandaris. 1977. *Too Old, Too Sick, Too Bad: Nursing Homes in America.* Germantown, MD: Aspen Systems Corporation.

Newton, K. 1950. *Geriatric Nursing.* St. Louis: C.V. Mosby.

Skinner, B.F. and M.E. Vaughan. 1983. *Enjoy Old Age: Living Fully in Your Later Years.* New York: W.W. Norton and Company, Inc.

U.S. Congress. House. Conference Report. 101st Congress, 1st Session, 1987. *Omnibus Budget Reconciliation Act of 1987.* Washington, DC: U.S. Government Printing Office. Report 100–495.

U.S. Congress. House. Conference Report. 101st Congress, 2nd Session, 1990. *Omnibus Budget Reconciliation Act of 1990.* Washington, DC: U.S. Government Printing Office.

CHAPTER 2   The Restorative Nursing Process

CONTENT OUTLINE

    I. Definition of restorative nursing
   II. Theoretical concepts
      A. Theory of human needs
      B. Learned helplessness
      C. Self-care
  III. Establishing a philosophy for restorative nursing
  IV. Assessment of the older adult
   V. Level I: Physiological needs
      A. Assessment
      B. Changes due to aging
         1. Integumentary system
         2. Musculoskeletal system
         3. Cardiovascular system
         4. Respiratory system
         5. Gastrointestinal system
         6. Urinary system
         7. Neurologic system
         8. Immune system
         9. Endocrine system
       10. Reproductive system — females
       11. Reproductive system — males
      C. Strengths
      D. Associated nursing diagnoses
  VI. Level II: Safety needs
      A. Assessment
      B. Changes due to aging
      C. Strengths
      D. Associated nursing diagnoses
 VII. Level III: Love and belonging needs
      A. Assessment
      B. Changes due to aging
      C. Strengths
      D. Associated nursing diagnoses
VIII. Level IV: Esteem needs from self and others
      A. Assessment
      B. Changes due to aging
      C. Strengths
      D. Associated nursing diagnoses
  IX. Functional assessment
   X. Abilities required to complete activities of daily living
  XI. Description of possible deficits interfering with completion of activities of daily living
 XII. The use of nursing diagnoses
XIII. Planning restorative care
      A. Establishing client goals

OBJECTIVES

- ❏ Define the term *restorative nursing*.
- ❏ Describe the process of learned helplessness.
- ❏ Apply Maslow's theory of human needs to the planning of care for elderly clients.
- ❏ Identify the components of a philosophy for restorative nursing.
- ❏ Recognize the physiological alterations of aging.
- ❏ Recognize the psychosocial alterations of aging.
- ❏ List the sensory/perceptual deficits that affect the activities of daily living.
- ❏ Complete an assessment of an older adult.
- ❏ Identify the nursing diagnoses derived from the assessment data.
- ❏ Initiate an interdisciplinary client care plan.

DEFINITION OF RESTORATIVE NURSING

Restorative nursing is defined as the provision of services designed to enhance psychological adaptation, to increase functional levels in performance of activities of daily living, and to prevent complications associated with inactivity. It is a process of renewing the disabled older adult's self-esteem by placing the client in control, providing opportunities for making decisions, thereby reestablishing and maintaining the individual's sense of dignity and self-worth. The nurse is the pivotal provider of care in a process that requires an interdisciplinary team effort. While the disabilities of the elderly client are recognized, strengths are also identified upon which a satisfying life can be structured — a life which provides the client with gratification, a reason for living, and hope for tomorrow.

THEORETICAL CONCEPTS

The theoretical framework for this definition of restorative nursing is based on the premise that quality of life is dependent on need fulfillment and self-determination. This discussion begins with a presentation of theoretical concepts so that a framework for planning care is established.

Theory of Human Needs

It is logical that Maslow's theory of needs fulfillment, Figure 2–1, serves as the foundation upon which to build a rationale for practice (Maslow 1970).

Basic human needs are universal in nature and not specific to the aged person. However, a person who has lived a long time has developed his/her own unique methods for satisfying these needs. These methods may not be effective if the physiological alterations associated with aging have diminished the individual's independence. In addition, many elderly persons have experienced the loss of loved ones, productive roles, home, personal possessions, and financial resources. Such loss(es) can make adaptation difficult. The combination of these factors has the potential for diminishing one's feelings of usefulness and self-worth. The onset of chronic illness creates additional barriers to need satisfaction. If disruption of health results in a self-care deficit, it may be impossible for the individual to meet even basic survival needs without assistance.

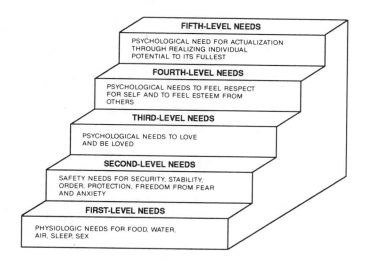

Figure 2–1 Maslow's hierarchy of needs *(From Hegner and Caldwell,* Nursing Assistant, *6th ed. [Albany, NY: Delmar Publishers Inc., 1992].)*

According to Maslow, if physiological needs cannot be met, higher level needs will also go unfulfilled. Nursing staff can effectively meet the physiological requirements for life, but in so doing, may unwittingly reinforce the client's feelings of inadequacy and dependence. The nurse must then intervene for a client who has diminished self-esteem as well as a functional deficit. Our society and many health care professionals tend to encourage the idea of dependency in the aged individual. Nursing staff and families (and often the clients) may feel the client has lived a long life and deserves to take it easy for the remaining years. The presence of a self-care deficit reinforces the myth that capabilities are limited and so the client may be judged incapable of making independent decisions. The problem, then, is not one of physical dependence, but rather one created by nursing staff who assume the client must be dependent on others for all aspects of care and well-being. The client eventually feels totally incompetent, relinquishing all control to others. The lesson has been learned that efforts to maintain control over the environment are futile.

Learned Helplessness

The human reaction to perceived loss of control is explained in the theoretical model of learned helplessness (Seligman 1975). When a person no longer has any decision-making powers, life becomes existence without hope. This phenomenon is manifested by feelings of despair, fatigue, fear, and anxiety. If nursing staff view these manifestations as an inevitable result of aging and illness, care is directed only to meeting the physiological and safety needs required to sustain life. No attempt is made to investigate these psychosocial changes or to intervene. Learned helplessness becomes a chronic state with feelings of hopelessness and uselessness, leading to progressive inactivity and degeneration, possibly culminating in death (Fuller 1978).

The sequence of events is illustrated by this example. An elderly person falls at home and is taken by ambulance to the hospital for assessment of injuries.

After examination in the emergency room, the individual is admitted to the nursing unit for further observation. The client is transferred from stretcher to bed and the side rails are raised. The client has been in a supine position for several hours, seeing little more than the ceiling since the fall several hours ago. Throughout this time, the client has answered several questions asked by strangers. These strangers talk to each other without giving any explanation to the client. The sudden change in environment and the rapidly evolving events result in disorientation. Impaired hearing and a high anxiety level have dulled comprehension. It has been several hours since the client has eaten or voided. The client has a sudden urge to empty the bladder and decides to find the bathroom, but has to maneuver the side rails to get out of bed. The nurse finds the client attempting to crawl over the end of the bed and quickly applies a safety device out of concern for the client's safety. Unable to retain the urine any longer, the client wets the bed, causing feelings of humiliation and frustration. The nurse's documentation describes confusion, disorientation, and incontinence. Completely overwhelmed by the rapid changes, the client struggles to become free of the restraints that have never been explained. The nurse administers medication to decrease the client's anxiety. The client is labeled uncooperative. Finding no major injuries, the client is discharged to a nursing home because of a recent history of falls. This decision is made by the discharge planner and family with a brief explanation given to the client. The transfer information states the client is confused, disoriented, incontinent, uncooperative, and at risk for accidents. The client is introduced to another strange environment with unfamiliar faces asking more questions. The client is treated as a confused, disoriented, incontinent, and uncooperative person.

There is no opportunity to demonstrate competence. Self-care deficit is added to the assessment. Within two or three days, an independent, functioning adult is completely helpless and without feelings of hope. This example may seem dramatic. However, the scene is replayed over and over. It is a result of lack of knowledge of the aging process.

Research suggests that the manifestations of learned helplessness can be reversed and possibly prevented (Fuller 1978; Decker and Kinzel 1985; LeSage, Slimmer, Lopez and Ellor 1989). If this state results from perceived lack of control, then creating opportunities for decision making and directing one's care should help to alleviate the situation. By so doing, the client can be assisted to experience a sense of mastery and competence that can be attained only when the individual feels in control of life. This requires the client's participation and acceptance of responsibility for care.

Self-Care

Self-care refers to the actions taken by an individual to maintain optimal health status. It includes the acquisition of knowledge needed to make informed decisions regarding one's care. There is a relationship between self-care ability and positive self-esteem; the person with feelings of self-worth takes better care of self. As self-care abilities increase, the behaviors of learned helplessness are likely to diminish.

Self-care activities can be utilized by the client throughout the life span, including times of chronic illness and terminal care. If the client can no longer make decisions, a family member or friend acts on behalf of the client. Total independence is not always the major component of self-care. Accepting the care and assistance of others when necessary is also an important ingredient of effective self-care (Hirschfeld 1985).

It is possible, then, for the disabled older adult to experience satisfaction of

Maslow's upper level needs even when total independence is not possible. The culmination of need satisfaction results in the state Maslow identified as self-actualization — the realization of one's full potential. If the client is to be assisted to attain this optimal level of well-being, care must be based on a partnership with the client and family. Provide them with information and create opportunities for decision making. Caregivers need to be aware of the client's capabilities and any restrictions imposed by the environment. To offer choices when there can realistically be no choice is more harmful than no intervention. It is important that nurses distinguish between the client who has accepted and adapted to an irreversible condition and one who has become a victim of learned helplessness. The client who has adapted to an irreversible condition may be functioning at an optimal level and have the characteristics of self-actualization.

McLeish (1976) states that according to Maslow's criteria, self-actualization does not occur in young people. It takes years of living to experience the wonderment of lasting relationships, to weather life's failures and tragedies, and to cherish successes and triumphs. Only through living many years can a sense of values be established with the courage to stand up for one's convictions. These are the components of self-actualization.

To live a long time is to be a survivor. In identifying the problems of the aged client, it is essential to also recognize the strengths that have developed through time and to utilize these strengths in assisting the client to reach an optimal level of well-being. This level is different for each person, depending on the degree of health or illness, the motivation of the individual, and existing family support. Some will be able to regain only minimal functional ability. Although dependence on nursing staff is then necessary, the attitude of staff toward the necessary dependence will oftentimes determine the client's capacity to attain positive self-esteem. The nursing staff needs to continue offering the client opportunities to make decisions regarding care as long as the client's mental competence exists. When the client purposefully relinquishes these responsibilities to others, that decision should be respected by the nursing staff and family.

In summary, quality of life is dependent on fulfillment of physical and psychosocial needs. The opportunity to demonstrate self-care by making informed decisions regarding one's care must exist before psychosocial needs are satisfied. To be denied this opportunity can result in a state of learned helplessness, deterioration, and possibly death. It is imperative that clients be allowed to make decisions regarding their care to prevent this deterioration.

ESTABLISHING A PHILOSOPHY FOR RESTORATIVE NURSING

With a theoretical framework established, a philosophy for restorative nursing can be formulated to facilitate the delivery of care. The following statements reflect this philosophy.

❑ Clients are adults and as such are allowed to make decisions regarding their care insofar as these decisions do not infringe upon the rights of others. This process is initiated by creating a partnership with the client and family in developing the plan of care. The interdisciplinary team accepts responsibility for providing the client with sufficient information to make intelligent choices.

❑ The nurse collaborates with the interdisciplinary team in the client assessment and identification of problems that can be resolved or alleviated by the team interventions. Identifying and utilizing the client's strengths are an important component of this process.

❑ Recognizing that inactivity results in numerous life-threatening complications, the plan of care for all clients includes physical exercise, mental stimulation, and social interaction that are planned within the realm of each client's capabilities. A theme of health promotion and wellness is woven throughout the concept of activity.

☐ Wherever client care is rendered, establishing a homelike setting creates an environment conducive to the restorative philosophy. Efforts are made to establish an environment that is safe and secure, yet stimulating and peaceful. The physiological changes of aging are considered when planning the use of color and design. The need for personal space, privacy, and territory is respected.

☐ Nurses and other caregivers are knowledgeable about the aging process and its ramifications, human needs, the developmental tasks of older adults, and chronic disease. The clients are respected and valued for their uniqueness and individuality which were acquired by surviving a lifetime of experiences.

☐ Nurses accept leadership responsibilities by broadening their own knowledge base and accepting responsibility for providing learning opportunities to other caregivers, the client, and the family.

☐ The restorative philosophy is one in which the element of hope is ever present. To be hopeful is to be realistic yet able to look forward to tomorrow. The nurse can support the client in feeling hopeful by establishing a sense of trust. The client feels secure in the knowledge that the nurse will work with the client to prevent and alleviate physical and mental discomfort.

When the restorative philosophy is implemented, the client finds mental and physical comfort, experiences joy in living, and feels a sense of self-worth. If progressively diminishing health interferes with the client's abilities to direct care, nursing interventions are directed toward palliative measures and prevention of complications. When the time comes, the client is allowed to die with grace and dignity.

ASSESSMENT OF THE OLDER ADULT

Human needs are in a constant state of flux, Figure 2–2. Therefore, it is unlikely that all needs are satisfied for anyone at any given time, especially if they are elderly.

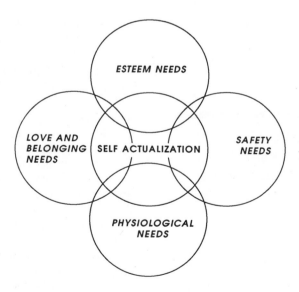

Figure 2–2 Human needs are continually changing.

Needs and the client's ability to satisfy those needs change continually. The older adult often requires assistance in meeting personal needs because of physical health problems and psychosocial losses. Optimal potential may be

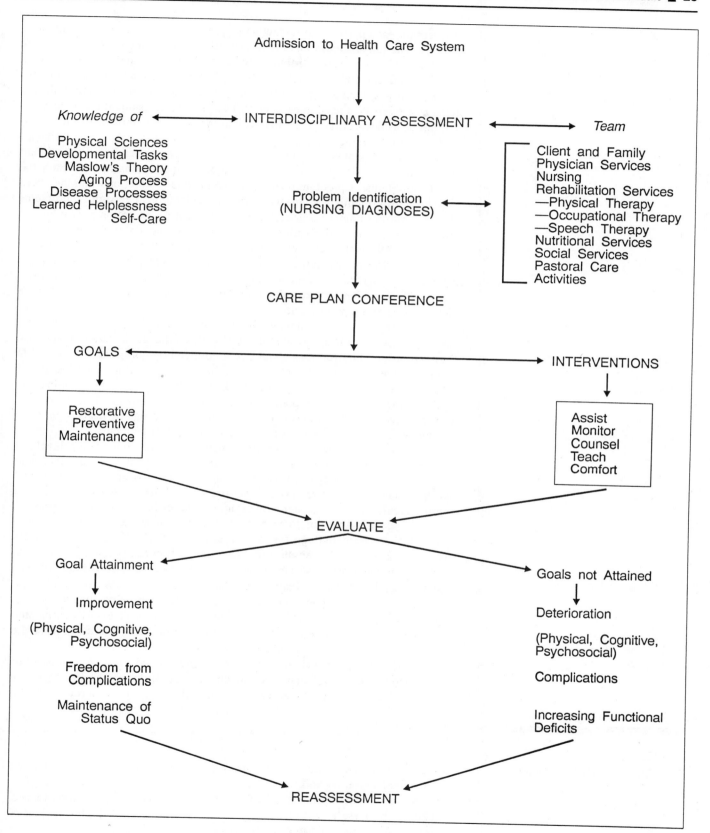

Figure 2–3 The restorative nursing/interdisciplinary health care team process

different for each person, but it results in a joy in living and confidence in one's abilities. The nurse should be able to prioritize and act upon present needs. A need for oxygen, for example, obviously demands attention and supersedes other concerns until the crisis is resolved. Other physical needs may not be so urgent. If the client is grieving over the loss of a loved one, the need to talk with the nurse may override a need to eat dinner. The loss of nourishment from one meal will not be as devastating as the loss of comfort when it is most needed.

Restorative nursing takes into consideration the whole person by assessing all needs in an interrelated method with the use of an interdisciplinary assessment tool, Figure 2–3. The assessment data are documented and used to identify the client's problems. A problem results when a need is not met or when the client uses unhealthy methods to meet the need. Neglecting to recognize problems results in further unmet needs reflected in physical deterioration and/or behavioral problems. The identification of risk factors for potential problems indicates a need for additional assessment. Professionals from all disciplines need a solid knowledge base of the aging process so the expected physiological changes detected in the elderly client are not confused with a pathological process. Conversely, the client may dismiss important symptoms because the changes are viewed as a normal part of aging.

Completing an assessment may take several sessions. The nurse should avoid asking too many questions at one time, especially if the client is tired or anxious. Distractions and interruptions should be minimized by doing the assessment in a quiet, private area. Ask the client or family about glasses and hearing aids if the client has impaired vision or hearing. During the interview and examination, correlate the findings with preadmission information and medical diagnoses. This is a stressful time for the client. Be careful to avoid making hasty, subjective judgments that will affect the perceptions of other staff members.

The following suggestions for assessment items are divided into levels to further clarify the use of Maslow's needs hierarchy in identifying problems and planning care. It is recognized that because of the intertwining of physical and psychosocial aspects of life, it is not wise to attempt to isolate needs into separate compartments without consideration of the affect each has on the other. However, by giving specific attention to each level, it is less likely that essential data will be omitted. Assessment items for each level are listed with the expected changes due to aging. Potential strengths are then listed, followed by nursing diagnoses. Items for the functional assessment are followed by a description of deficit areas that may require further evaluation before the planning process can be initiated.

Aging is a natural phenomenon. The inclusion of nursing diagnoses with changes due to aging does not imply that these changes are necessarily associated with illness. However, the onset of acute illness or personal crises can place the older adult at risk for these problems.

The initial assessment should be reviewed and revised every three months or more often if necessary. Changes in the client's condition may be so subtle they are not noticed unless purposeful investigation is carried out on a regular basis.

LEVEL I: PHYSIOLOGICAL NEEDS

Assessment

- ❑ Take the client's health history and complete a body systems review. Measure the client's vital signs. Listen to breath sounds.
- ❑ Observe the client's appearance for hygiene, grooming, and posture. Inspect skin for bruises, lacerations, scars, moles, pressure areas, skin tears, signs of infection, or any other unusual findings.
- ❑ Study diagnostic data from the client's medical record: laboratory test results, radiology reports, or findings of special tests.

- ❏ Interview the client regarding a medication regime, including the use of nonprescription medications. Ask the client how long each medication has been taken, why the medication is taken, how often it is taken, and whether there have been any side effects.
- ❏ Question the client concerning nutritional habits, including food preferences, number of meals eaten daily, need for special diet, snacking habits, and the location for eating. Measure height and weight. Ask the client whether there has been any variation in the last two years.
- ❏ Question the client about bowel and bladder habits: frequency, incontinence, associated pain or discomfort, the use of laxatives, number of times it is necessary to urinate during the night, and the ability to get to the bathroom.
- ❏ Ask the client about sleep/rest/relaxation habits. Include the time of arising, bedtime, number of hours spent sleeping per day, napping pattern, and bedtime preparation habits.
- ❏ Have the client describe a typical day's activities.
- ❏ Review the client's pattern of past sexual practices and current sexual function.
- ❏ Evaluate cognitive status. (See chapter 8, "Alterations in Thought Processes: Mental Status Examinations.")
- ❏ Evaluate level of comfort. Question client regarding presence of pain, frequency, duration, pattern, and type of pain. Observe facial expressions and body posture for evidence of pain or discomfort.
- ❏ Ask the client for a rating of personal health.
- ❏ Evaluate present living conditions if the client is at home or in the hospital with plans for discharge to home. If the client is in a nursing home, evaluate the potential for discharge and discharge planning that would be required.
- ❏ Ask if the client uses tobacco, alcohol, or recreational drugs.

Changes Due to Aging

Integumentary System:

1. Subcutaneous tissue and elastin fibers diminish, causing the skin to become thinner and less elastic.
2. Eccrine, apocrine, and sebaceous glands decrease, resulting in diminished secretions and moisturization, causing pruritus.
3. Body temperature regulation is impaired due to decreased perspiration.
4. Capillary blood flow decreases resulting in slower wound healing.
5. Blood supply decreases especially to lower extremities.
6. Vascular fragility causes senile purpura.
7. Cutaneous sensitivity to pressure and temperature is diminished.
8. Melanin production is reduced, causing gray-white hair.
9. Scalp, pubic, and axillary hair thins. Females have increased facial hair on the upper lip and chin.
10. Nail growth slows. Nails become more brittle and longitudinal nail ridges form.

Musculoskeletal System:

1. Muscle mass and elasticity diminish, resulting in decreased strength and endurance. This decreases reaction time and coordination.
2. Bone demineralization occurs, causing skeletal instability and shrinkage of intervertebral disks. The spine is less flexible and spinal curvature is often present.
3. Joints undergo degenerative changes, resulting in pain, stiffness, and loss of range of motion.

Cardiovascular System:

1. Cardiac output and recovery time decline. The heart requires more time to return to a normal rate after increasing in response to activity.
2. The heart rate slows with age.
3. Blood flow to all organs decreases. The brain and coronary arteries continue to receive a larger volume of blood than do other organs.
4. Arterial elasticity decreases, causing increased peripheral resistance. This results in a rise in systolic blood pressure and a slight increase in diastolic pressure.
5. Veins dilate and superficial vessels are more prominent.

Respiratory System:

1. The muscles of respiration become more rigid, causing decreased vital capacity and increased residual capacity of the lungs.
2. The cough mechanism is less effective, increasing the potential for lung infection.
3. Decreased functional capacity results in dyspnea with exertion or stress.
4. Alveoli thicken, causing less effective gas exchange.

Gastrointestinal System:

1. Tooth enamel thins.
2. Periodontal disease increases.
3. Taste buds decrease and saliva production is less.
4. The gag reflex is less effective, increasing the danger of choking.
5. Esophageal peristalsis slows and the esophageal sphincter is less efficient. This causes delayed entry of food into the stomach, increasing the risk of aspiration.
6. Hiatal hernia is more common.
7. Gastric emptying is delayed. Food remains in the stomach longer, decreasing the capacity of the stomach.
8. Peristalsis and nerve sensation of the large intestine are decreased, contributing to constipation.
9. Diverticulosis increases with age.
10. Liver size decreases after age seventy.
11. Liver enzymes decrease, slowing drug metabolism and the detoxification process.
12. Gallbladder emptying becomes less efficient. Bile is thicker. Cholesterol content is increased. There is increased incidence of gallstones.

Urinary System:

1. Nephrons decrease, resulting in decreased filtration and gradual decrease in excretory and reabsorptive functions of renal tubules.
2. Glomerular filtration rate decreases, resulting in decreased renal clearance of drugs.
3. Blood urea nitrogen (BUN) increases 20 percent by age seventy. The creatinine clearance test is a better index than the BUN of renal function in the elderly.
4. Sodium-conserving ability is diminished.
5. Bladder capacity decreases, causing increased frequency of urination and nocturia.
6. Renal function increases when lying down, sometimes causing a need to void shortly after going to bed.
7. Bladder and perineal muscles weaken, resulting in inability to empty the bladder. This results in residual urine and predisposes the elderly to cystitis.

8. Incidence of stress incontinence increases in females.
9. The prostate may enlarge, causing frequency or dribbling in males.

Neurological System:

1. Neurons in the brain decrease, resulting in decreased production of neuro-transmitters, causing reduction in synaptic transmission.
2. Cerebral blood flow and oxygen utilization are decreased. These changes result in a need for more time to carry out motor and sensory tasks requiring speed, coordination, balance, and fine motor hand movements. In the absence of pathology, intellect and capacity for learning remain unchanged.
3. Short-term memory may be somewhat diminished without changes in long-term memory.
4. Night sleep decreases due to more frequent and longer wakeful periods.
5. Deep tendon reflexes are decreased.
6. Vision alterations:
   □ The lens is less pliable, causing presbyopia and decreased accommodation. The lens yellows, causing distorted color perception with greens and blues washing out; warm colors are more distinct. Alterations in the lens causes increased incidence of cataracts.
   □ Accommodation of pupil size decreases, requiring more time to adjust to changes in lighting. There is a decrease in the ability to tolerate glare.
   □ Vitreous humor changes in consistency, causing blurring of vision.
   □ Changes in the anterior chamber may cause increased pressure of aqueous humor, resulting in glaucoma.
   □ Lacrimal glands secrete less fluid, causing dryness and itching of the eyes.
7. Hearing alterations:
   □ The pinna is less flexible. The hairs in the inner ear stiffen and atrophy; cerumen increases.
   □ Neurons decrease and the blood supply is less. The tissue in the cochlea deteriorates and the ossicles degenerate.
   □ Presbycusis results from these changes with loss of tone discrimination. Loss of high-frequency tones occurs first.
8. Smell and taste alterations:
   □ Taste buds decrease and atrophy with diminished sensitivity for taste.
   □ Changes in nose receptors cause decreased sensitivity to smell. (Experts do not all agree on this).
9. Touch alterations:
   □ There is less ability to discriminate temperature and pressure; diminished pain sensation.
10. Kinesthesia alterations:
    □ Diminished proprioception causes problems with balance and coordination.

Immune System:

1. Autoantibodies increase, resulting in increased incidence of autoimmune disorders.

Endocrine System:

1. Release of insulin is delayed by the beta cells of the pancreas, causing an increase in blood sugar.
2. Changes in the thyroid may lower the basal metabolic rate.

Reproductive System — Females:

1. Estrogen production decreases with the onset of menopause.

2. Ovaries, uterus, and cervix decrease in size.
3. The vagina shortens, narrows, and becomes less elastic with thinner lining. Secretions decrease and become more alkaline, resulting in increased incidence of atrophic vaginitis. These changes may result in discomfort during coitus.
4. Supporting musculature weakens, increasing risk of uterine prolapse.
5. Breast tissue decreases and nipple erection is diminished during sexual arousal.
6. Libido remains unchanged.

Reproductive System — Males:

1. Testosterone production decreases, resulting in decreased size of testicles.
2. Sperm count and viscosity of seminal fluid decrease.
3. The penis remains softer during erection. More time is required to achieve erection, delaying achievement of orgasm. There is greater control but less intensity of ejaculation.
4. Prostate gland may enlarge.
5. Libido remains unchanged.

Strengths

1. Client is free of deficits or impairments or has successfully adapted to or is adequately compensating for the deficit or impairment.
2. Client is cognitively healthy.
3. Client has history of healthy life-style in regard to diet, sleep, stress management, exercise, and freedom from chemical abuse.
4. Client has adequate functional ability to carry out activities of daily living.
5. Client is free of incapacitating physical discomfort and pain.

Associated Nursing Diagnoses

1. High risk for impaired skin integrity
2. High risk for impaired physical mobility
3. High risk for activity intolerance
4. High risk for alterations in nutrition
5. High risk for alterations in bowel elimination (constipation)
6. High risk for alterations in urinary elimination
7. Fatigue
8. Sleep pattern disturbance
9. High risk for ineffective thermoregulation
10. High risk for disuse syndrome
11. Self-care deficit
12. Pain
13. Sensory perceptual alterations
14. Altered patterns of sexuality

LEVEL II: SAFETY NEEDS

Assessment

❑ Review Level I for cognitive status and presence of sensory deficits.
❑ Question client regarding past accidents and resulting injuries.
❑ Question client regarding history of seizures or unconsciousness.
❑ Question client regarding ability to ambulate.
❑ Identify behaviors of client that threaten personal safety.

- ❑ Evaluate safety of client's place of residence.
- ❑ Evaluate client's communication skills.
- ❑ Observe for evidence of abuse or neglect.

Changes Due to Aging

1. Sensory/perceptual alterations result in absence of the stimuli that provide warnings of danger. The risk for suffocation, poisoning, and burns is increased.
2. Musculoskeletal, neurological, and sensory changes increase the risk for falls.
3. Lack of knowledge, equipment, finances, or a support system can result in unsafe behaviors and conditions.
4. Impaired communication increases the risk for injury.
5. Physical, mental, or financial abuse results in fear.

Strengths

1. Client lives in physically safe environment.
2. Client feels secure in present environment.
3. Client is knowledgeable and realistic about capabilities.
4. Client avoids dangerous situations and does not take unnecessary chances.
5. Client is compliant with health care regime.
6. Client is capable of managing own environment.

Associated Nursing Diagnoses

1. High risk for suffocation
2. High risk for trauma
3. Fear
4. Knowledge deficit
5. Noncompliance
6. Health maintenance alteration
7. Impaired verbal communication

LEVEL III: LOVE AND BELONGING NEEDS

Assessment

- ❑ Ask the client about losses and changes in life that have occurred and how these have been managed.
- ❑ Question client about current relationships and the availability of significant others in the client's life. Note comments about feelings of loneliness.
- ❑ Ask the client about past or present pet ownership.
- ❑ Review, from Level I, sexual history and practices.
- ❑ Review, from Level II, current living conditions/arrangements.
- ❑ Question the client about past and present affiliation with groups associated with church, community, or occupation.
- ❑ Question the client about past and present volunteer activities.
- ❑ Evaluate client's access to transportation.

Changes Due to Aging

1. Client has experienced the loss of loved ones through death, relocation, divorce, or estrangement.
2. Client participates in few meaningful activities because of diminished health status, lack of transportation, disrupted relationships, or retirement.
3. Client experiences loss of identity, resulting from a change in living environment.
4. Client has difficulty socializing because of sensory deficits.
5. Client may be doubtful of sexuality in absence of loving partner for reaffirmation of sexuality.
6. Client finds usual coping mechanisms ineffective.
7. Client experiences frequent demands to adapt to changing situations as a result of health status, relationships, and financial status.
8. Client's adult children are unable or unwilling to accept increasing dependency of parent.

Strengths

1. Client has an intact support system.
2. Client has satisfying relationships with others.
3. Client has opportunities for sexual expression.
4. Client has access to transportation.
5. Client has adequate functional mobility.
6. Client has successfully adjusted to past changes and crises in life.
7. Client has relinquished roles as phases of life require and has replaced them with satisfying new roles.
8. Client has a pattern of successful mourning for losses.
9. Client participates in groups — church, community, hobbies.
10. Client's family members respect each other and are willing to give and receive help when necessary.
11. Client utilizes successful problem-solving skills.

Associated Nursing Diagnoses

1. Anticipatory grieving
2. Disturbance in role performance
3. Diversional activity deficit
4. Social isolation
5. Altered sexual patterns
6. Ineffective coping
7. Impaired adjustment
8. Alterations in family processes
9. Ineffective family coping

LEVEL IV: ESTEEM NEEDS FROM SELF AND OTHERS

Assessment

☐ Question client concerning changes in health status. (Review Level I.)
☐ Note changes in the client's appearance related to physical aspects of aging.
☐ Observe the client's personal grooming and hygiene.
☐ Observe the client's posture and eye contact.
☐ Note self-deprecating statements.

❏ Question client concerning history of past accomplishments and activities that were sources of pleasure. Ask about special skills, talents, and hobbies.

❏ Ask client if other activities have been developed to utilize the time acquired through retirement.

❏ Evaluate the presence of unresolved issues in the client's life related to past acts and relationships.

❏ Note the client's conversation expressing a lack of control over current situation.

❏ Observe the client for evidence of passivity or apathy.

❏ Listen for expressions of frustration related to lack of abilities to function independently.

❏ Ask the client about changes in eating and sleeping habits in the last year.

❏ Ask the client what makes life meaningful.

❏ Listen for verbalizations of inner conflict about beliefs.

❏ Note the client's ability to make decisions when given the opportunity.

❏ Note expressions of fear of alienating caregivers.

Changes Due to Aging

1. Client may experience negative feelings about self, related to changes of aging and health status.
2. Client may have feelings of worthlessness related to loss of roles.
3. Client may question the meaning of life.
4. Client may perceive a lack of opportunity for making choices and feels little control over personal life.
5. Client may have difficulty making decisions due to lack of information or inadequate support system.

Strengths

1. Client seeks information to improve situation.
2. Client gives evidence of initiative and self-confidence in abilities and judgment.
3. Client participates in self-care by making decisions and accepting responsibility for decisions.
4. Client has developed a well-defined value system.
5. Client accepts what cannot be changed.
6. Client uses assertive skills successfully.
7. Client has strong spiritual beliefs and finds comfort and strength in spiritual and religious practices.
8. Client embraces aging and takes advantage of the positive aspects and adapts to the negative aspects.
9. Client participates in healthy reminiscing and has few regrets for past life.
10. Client finds meaning and enjoyment in hobbies and activities.
11. Client experiences joy in nature, art, and music and has a well-developed sense of humor.

Associated Nursing Diagnoses

1. Disturbance in body image
2. Disturbance in self-esteem
3. Spiritual distress

4. Powerlessness
5. Hopelessness

FUNCTIONAL ASSESSMENT

A number of tools have been developed for measuring the client's ability to complete activities of daily living. These activities include personal hygiene and grooming, feeding oneself, toileting, dressing, and mobility. Some tools also evaluate the client's level of independence in carrying out more complex skills, such as household management tasks, money management, using the telephone, writing, and shopping. These are referred to as instrumental activities of daily living.

A task analysis breaks down each activity of daily living into the individual steps that must be carried out in order to accomplish that specific activity. Completing this analysis is helpful in establishing restorative programs.

Visit the client during the time these activities are normally scheduled. The use of a task analysis list will indicate which steps in the activity the client is able to complete. This is not a scoring process. It only indicates what steps in the task the client is unable to complete. Interventions and goals are based on this data. (See section on planning.) This information also allows the caregivers to give the client the opportunity to do the steps of an activity that the client is capable of performing.

TABLE 2–1	Functional Assessment
BATHING	❑ Gets to tub/sink/shower ❑ Regulates water ❑ Washes/rinses upper body ❑ Washes/rinses lower body ❑ Dries body
DRESSING/UNDRESSING	❑ Obtains/selects clothing ❑ Puts on/takes off slipover top ❑ Puts on/takes off cardigan style top ❑ Manages buttons, snaps, ties, zippers ❑ Puts on/takes off skirt/pants ❑ Buckles belt ❑ Puts on shoes/socks
EATING	❑ Gets to table ❑ Uses spoon, fork, knife appropriately ❑ Opens/pours ❑ Brings food to mouth ❑ Chews, swallows ❑ Uses napkin
TOILETING	❑ Gets to commode/toilet ❑ Manipulates clothing ❑ Sits on toilet ❑ Eliminates in toilet ❑ Cleans self ❑ Flushes toilet ❑ Gets clothing in place ❑ Washes hands
MOBILITY	❑ Gets self to side of bed ❑ Maintains upright position ❑ Comes to standing position

Continues

- Places self in position to sit in chair
- Locks wheelchair brakes
- Turns body to sit
- Lowers self into chair
- Propels wheelchair
- Repositions self in chair
- Raises self from chair
- Places self in position to sit on edge of bed
- Walks alone/with assistance
- Uses assistive device

ABILITIES REQUIRED TO COMPLETE ACTIVITIES OF DAILY LIVING

In order to carry out daily activities, the client must have sufficient range of motion, strength, and endurance. Full range of motion is not necessary for most tasks and compensation for limited strength and endurance can be made by appropriately timing activities. Adequate trunk control and balance are required to allow the client to remain in an upright position for the duration of the activity. Coordination is needed to carry out purposeful movements. Before planning a restorative program, review the assessment data to determine:

- the client's ability to communicate: Can the client comprehend verbal instructions? Can the caregiver understand the client?
- presence of visual or hearing impairments: Do deficits in either sense hinder the ability to complete an activity?
- the ability to solve problems: For example, can the client determine how to bring a pair of slacks up over the feet?
- the length of attention span: Does the client lose interest or wander off before completing a task?
- judgment and memory: Does poor judgment cause safety problems? Does the client have the ability to remember simple instructions?

The presence of deficits in any of these areas does not necessarily preclude a restorative program but adaptations need to be incorporated into the plan. Additional deficit areas may be present in persons with central nervous system disease or trauma. Developing a restorative program requires the nurse to collaborate with the physical therapist and occupational therapist to utilize an interdisciplinary approach to the client's problems. Correlating activities planned by the therapists further increases the client's ability to master the task.

DESCRIPTION OF POSSIBLE DEFICITS INTERFERING WITH COMPLETION OF ACTIVITIES OF DAILY LIVING

- *Agnosia*: This may be a visual, auditory, or somatosensory deficit in which an individual with normal visual perception does not recognize a common item such as a comb or toothbrush. The stimulus has no meaning or the meaning is distorted. There are several forms of agnosia.
- *Alexia*: The ability to read words or sentences is impaired. The client may be unable to identify even individual letters.
- *Apraxia*: The client cannot carry out a familiar motor act despite the absence of paralysis. This can occur in the client who is willing and able to comprehend. For example, the individual may recognize a pencil and know what it is used for, but is unable to actually pick up the pencil and use it. There are several forms of apraxia.
- *Latency*: The client is unable to initiate a planned action. Once the action is started, the individual is usually able to continue the action.
- *Perseveration*: The client is unable to switch from one movement to another or to discontinue an activity once it is initiated, even though the stimulus has been removed.

❏ *Loss of proprioception*: The client has impaired kinesthetic sense and is unable to determine where all body parts are and in what position without visualizing the body parts. For example, the client cannot tell the position of the legs and feet without looking down at them.

❏ *Sequencing disorder*: The client is unable to carry out specific components or steps in a task in the correct order or sequence.

❏ *Spatial analysis deficits*: The client has impaired depth perception and cannot judge distances.

❏ *Unilateral neglect*: The hemiplegic client does not attend to the impaired side of the body.

❏ *Body scheme/image disturbance*: The client has altered mental perceptions of the self and body parts.

❏ *Figure-ground impairment*: The client is unable to distinguish foreground from background. For example, the client is unable to find mashed potatoes on a white plate or to find the sleeve of a jacket if it is lying on top of the rest of the jacket.

THE USE OF NURSING DIAGNOSIS

After the assessments are completed, the data are analyzed, actual and high-risk problems are identified, and nursing diagnoses are developed. The nursing diagnoses, etiologies, or relating factors are further defined at the client's care plan conference. Each problem may involve intervention by more than one discipline. For example, both nursing and rehabilitation staff may be working with the client on impaired physical mobility. It is redundant to enter this problem twice on the care plan, even though each discipline will have a specific intervention.

Each diagnosis has two parts: the problem statement and the etiology. Knowing the etiology or the probable cause of the problem provides the information needed to establish effective interventions. The two-part statement reflects a problem that can be alleviated, resolved, or changed by the interdisciplinary team. Each nursing diagnosis must be validated by the presence of signs and symptoms (defining characteristics). This information is documented in the client's record and may also be entered in the care plan.

PLANNING RESTORATIVE CARE

The plan of care serves as a communication tool for all shifts and disciplines so that the care provided is consistent and continuous twenty-four hours a day, seven days a week. The formulation of a plan based on an accurate and comprehensive assessment is the single most important task undertaken for an individual client. It will affect every aspect of the client's life as well as his/her perception of the quality of life. Regulatory agencies are placing more and more emphasis on care plans for state licensing surveys and reimbursement procedures from Medicare and Medicaid. The guidelines for the Federal Survey Process resulting from the Omnibus Reconciliation Act (OBRA) of 1987 address this issue. The purpose of the "Quality of Care Assessment" portion of the survey is to determine whether the care provided has enabled the client to reach or maintain his/her highest practicable physical, mental and psychosocial well-being. The determination is based on implementation of the care plan and the degree to which the plan is reflective of the client's condition. Emphasis is placed not solely on the written plan, but on outcomes: Are the objectives or goals being met? The guidelines further state that the plan must be prepared by an interdisciplinary team that includes the attending physician, a registered nurse with responsibility for the client, representatives from other disciplines as determined by the client's needs, the client, and the family or legal representative, if possible. The interdisciplinary care plan conference is the most effective method for completing the care plan. This communication among team members at the conference enhances understanding of the client and the client's problems.

Establishing Client Goals

After the problems are identified, goals or expected outcomes are set and agreed upon by the team, including the client and the family. There are different types of goals.

Restorative (improvement) goals attempt to increase the level of physical, cognitive, or psychosocial functioning. Goals associated with nursing interventions are stated in functional terms — for example, "will walk to the bathroom with assistance of one at least b.i.d." instead of "will walk twenty feet twice a day." Refer to the task analyses completed during assessment when setting restorative goals. Goals are formulated based on the parts of the task the client cannot complete but has potential for completing. Cognitive goals include outcomes for client teaching. Verbal expressions, acceptance, or evidence of decreased anxiety are examples of psychosocial goals.

Preventive goals are established in response to high-risk problems such as pressure ulcers, injuries, infections, contractures, agitation, confusion, pain, and negative behaviors. For example, the client will "remain free of impaired skin integrity" or will "remain free of a urinary tract infection."

Maintenance goals are aimed at keeping the client at the current status or slowing the rate of deterioration. Maintenance goals are set after the client has reached optimal levels for improvement goals. For example, the client may have reached a goal of putting on upper body clothing. Assessment may reveal that it is unrealistic to expect the client to do more than this. A maintenance goal may state that the client will "continue to put on upper body clothing" or "maintain current level of range of motion in all joints." By keeping a maintenance goal on the care plan, it is more likely that staff and client will continue to carry out the actions necessary to maintain the skill.

When the nursing diagnoses indicate a need for interventions from more than one discipline, there may be one goal with a specific intervention for each discipline, or there may be a goal for each intervention. Communication at the care plan conference ensures that the goals and interventions are interrelated and coordinated.

Each goal should meet these criteria:

❏ The goal is the outcome the client will achieve as a result of the interventions.
❏ Each goal is specific, realistic, measurable, and time limited.
❏ The goal statement is client centered and states what the client will do.
❏ Restorative (improvement) goals are achievable within a three-month time frame. (This correlates with federal regulations for reassessment.)
❏ Action verbs are used to describe the expected outcome. *Examples*: walk, transfer, eat, reduce, lose, gain, increase, decrease, talk, nod head, and blink eyes. For example, the client will "transfer from wheelchair to bed with the assistance of one."
❏ The goal indicates what help (number of assistants needed) or devices are needed by the client (cane, walker, adapted utensils, dressing aids). It states when and where the activity will take place — for example, at meal time, in the dining room.
❏ Avoid meaningless, ambiguous terms such as normal, better, more, less, good, bad, and average.

Developing Interventions

Interventions are actions designed to help the client achieve mutually agreed upon goals. The care plan indicates who is responsible for the action and when, where, and how the action is carried out. Utilize the documented strengths of the client to select the most effective interventions. There are several types of interventions.

Assisting interventions are designed to help the client accomplish a task. The level of assistance may decrease as the client's goals are met. The client will "walk to the bathroom with the assistance of one."

Monitoring interventions require observation or inspection for signs of complications or side effects of medication. They are generally used with preventive goals. For example, a goal for maintaining intact skin may include an intervention for a skin check twice daily to observe for signs of skin breakdown.

Counseling interventions assist the client to work out problems of adjustment and adaptation. This may include such interventions as individual sessions with a social worker.

Teaching interventions provide information and instruction, enabling the client to acquire new skills and abilities. This may include teaching a skill as complicated as self-administration of insulin or as simple as locking a wheelchair before getting up.

TABLE 2–2	**Guidelines for Client Teaching**
	❑ Clients learn only if they perceive a need for learning and are willing to invest the time and energy required. For the elderly, disabled client, energy resources are limited so appropriate timing is essential.
	❑ The nurse must believe in the program and have the knowledge and skills to effectively deliver the instruction and evaluate client progress.
	❑ Attend to the client's physical and safety needs before initiating the teaching/learning process. Physical discomfort related to hunger, elimination needs, or pain makes learning impossible.
	❑ For the elderly, disabled client, energy resources are limited so appropriate timing is essential. The person in a nursing home who views the placement as preparation for death may see no need for learning. Occasionally a client and family feel that staff members are getting paid to provide services that the client is capable of performing independently. The nurse is a key factor in altering these beliefs.
	❑ Arrange an environment with a comfortable temperature, free from distractions and noise.
	❑ The client's trust and respect for the nurse enhance the learning progress. Build on the client's higher level needs. The person who is learning feels increased esteem, and in turn this increases the desire to learn and succeed. Offer feedback, encouragement, and praise.

Comforting interventions are designed to alleviate physical or emotional distress. Examples may include moving an agitated client to a quiet environment, changing the client's position to alleviate discomfort, or listening to a client verbalize fears.

Families are often included in counseling, teaching, and comforting interventions.

Implementation

Considerable time and effort are required to develop an effective care plan. However, the time and effort will result in a well-designed plan that increases the chance of success. Clients, families, and staff will be encouraged when the client reaches even the smallest of goals. However, the entire process will fail if those responsible for its implementation neglect to carry out their duties of assisting, monitoring, counseling, teaching, and comforting.

The planning and implementation of restorative care will succeed only if the philosophy of restorative care is accepted by the entire staff. Support for restorative nursing begins with administration. The facility administrator and director of nursing must be committed to the philosophy and goals of restorative nursing if the process is to succeed. Administrative support is needed for developing a system that promotes the utilization of the interdisciplinary approach. This means allowing time in the budget for care plan conferences. Professional nurses are role models and have the visibility and power to influence the entire staff. The attitude of the nurses can make the difference between failure and success for the care plan.

Successful implementation of the care plan depends on communication. All team members need a clear understanding of their responsibilities and must be committed to fulfilling assignments to the best of their abilities. The written plan must be accessible and may need to be interpreted to nonprofessional staff. Staff development serves to increase the knowledge and skills needed by staff to effectively implement the plan.

STAFF DEVELOPMENT

Each member of the interdisciplinary team needs to understand the restorative process. (See Figure 2–3.) Without a similar frame of reference, the team will not function in a cohesive manner.

The educational process begins with orientation. During this period, the philosophy and goals of restorative nursing are reviewed and demonstrated by staff as the new employees participate in classroom and clinical orientation. Implementing the restorative process when caring for the elderly may be a new experience for health care staff. Professional nurses often receive little clinical or theoretical background in gerontology. To many nurses, the term *restorative* is synonymous with rehabilitation and implies the treatments and procedures implemented by therapists in the room designated "physical therapy" or "rehab." However, in some long-term care settings, therapists may be available only for consultation. They must rely on the nursing staff to implement restorative procedures. Restorative nursing is the responsibility of nursing and is implemented twenty-four hours a day, seven days a week.

The nursing skills required for the restorative process are generally learned by students early in the educational program. Instruction for positioning, range-of-motion exercises, transfers, and ambulation is usually very basic. The nurse who then chooses to work with chronically ill, elderly clients must acquire advanced skills and instruction. For example, the restorative nurse needs to know that the client with Parkinson's disease is taught different ambulation techniques than the client with a hip prosthesis or the client who has had a stroke.

Nursing assistants in long-term-care settings are often the primary direct caregivers. They work under the supervision of the professional nursing staff and deliver much of the "hands on" care. The quality of care that is rendered by the nursing assistant may depend on the effectiveness of the supervision provided by professional nurses. The nurses themselves must be confident of their skills before they can successfully educate and evaluate nursing assistants.

The nurse may also be a teacher for the family. Caregivers for the client at home can learn many of the procedures and techniques that will prevent complications.

Learning and applying restorative skills is not enough. The implementation of the restorative nursing process is based on the belief that all clients are allowed and encouraged to do for themselves as much as they are capable of doing. This includes the physical activities of daily living and making decisions regarding one's care.

Continuing education for all levels of staff reinforces restorative philosophy and procedures. Specific client problems, unusual diagnoses, new procedures, and new information provide topics for ongoing staff development programs. Well-educated employees are creative employees who have the motivation and skill to provide more than custodial care to their clients. They have the ability and the talent to implement the restorative approach, thereby increasing the quality of life for all clients in their care.

EVALUATION

Ongoing evaluation determines whether the client is meeting the goals of the care plan. Observation and consultation with the client and direct caregivers provide the data for this portion of the restorative process. The actions taken at this time depend on the types of goals that were set and whether or not the goals were attained.

When restorative (improvement) goals are reached, extend or increase the goals. If this is not realistic or necessary, then consider converting the goal to a maintenance goal. Establishing maintenance goals ensures that staff will continue with the appropriate intervention, thereby preventing the loss of progress that was attained by meeting the restorative goal. For example, if the client has met the goal of self-feeding and the correlating problem is deleted from the care plan, the staff may unintentionally foster dependence by feeding the client when perhaps all that is needed are verbal reminders to the client to eat. If a restorative goal is reached and it is not necessary to replace it with a maintenance goal, delete the problem from the care plan.

Preventive goals are met when the high-risk problem fails to occur. If the client remains at risk for the complications that prompted the goal, then the problem, goal, and intervention need to remain on the plan. If the client's condition has improved and the risk is no longer present, delete it from the care plan.

Maintenance goals are met when the client continues a specific level of performance. If the client is likely to continue at this level of performance without staff intervention, delete the problem. Consider the motivation and cognitive status of the client in making this decision.

If the goals have not been attained, analyze the situation so the plan can be revised. Review the assessment data for accuracy, completeness, and notation of any changes in the client's condition. Additional assessments may be required which will result in changing the nursing diagnoses and etiologies. Find out if the client and family participated in the planning process. Consult with them to determine whether they understand and agree with their responsibilities in the implementation of the plan. Were the client's strengths utilized in planning the interventions? If not, they should be. If they were, consider the possibility that the strengths identified initially may no longer be available to the client due to changes in health, financial status, or relationships.

Were the appropriate caregivers designated to carry out the interventions? Perhaps they do not understand their responsibilities or they lack the skills and knowledge needed to fulfill their assignment.

Reconsider the goal statement. It may be unrealistic for the client. Or the problem may lie in the statement itself if it is not stated in objective and measurable terms.

SUMMARY

With a revised care plan in hand, renewed enthusiasm, and fresh ideas, success is imminent. Care given to the client must have a purpose and be individualized if quality of life is to be extended to elderly individuals with chronic health problems. For some clients, the time will come when it is no longer realistic or kind to expect continued improvement. Goals are then directed to preventing complications and maintaining the comfort and dignity of the client.

QUESTIONS AND DISCUSSION

1. Review the changes related to aging listed in this chapter. Select one system and discuss the implications of these changes for the delivery of nursing care to older adults.
2. Interview or study the medical record of an older adult. Review the problems of the client. To what degree do the expected alterations of aging affect this individual's health problems?
3. How well do you think most older adults are able to meet their higher level needs? What do you think influences the ability to meet one's higher level needs during the last years of life?
4. What can professional nurses do to increase the quality of life for older adults?

REFERENCES

Decker, S.D. and S.L. Kinzel. 1985. Learned Helplessness and Decreased Social Interaction in Elderly Disabled Persons. *Rehabilitation Nursing* 10(2): 31–32.

Department of Health and Human Services. 1988. *State Operation Manual*. Health Care Financing Administration. Publication 7.

Fuller, S. 1978. Inhibiting Helplessness in Elderly People. *Journal of Gerontological Nursing* 4(4): 18–21.

Hirschfeld, M. 1985. Self-Care Potential: Is It Present? *Journal of Gerontological Nursing* 11(8): 29–34.

LeSage, J., L.W. Slimmer, M. Lopez, and J. Ellor. 1989. Learned Helplessness. *Journal of Gerontological Nursing* 15(5): 9–15.

Maslow, A.H. 1970. *Motivation and Personality*. 2d ed. New York: Harper and Row.

McLeish, J.A.B. 1976. *The Ulyssean Adult*. New York: McGraw-Hill Ryerson Ltd.

Seligman, M. 1975. *Helplessness: On Depression, Development and Death*. San Francisco: W.H. Freeman.

SUGGESTED READINGS

Carpenito, L.J. 1989. *Handbook of Nursing Diagnosis 1989–1990*. Philadelphia: J.B. Lippincott Company.

Clark, J.B., S.F. Queener, and V.B. Karb. 1986. *Pocket Guide to Drugs*. St. Louis: The C.V. Mosby Company.

Gordon, Marjory. 1991. *Manual of Nursing Diagnosis 1991–1992*. St. Louis: Mosby-Year Book, Inc.

Marrelli, T.M. 1988. *Handbook of Home Health Standards*. St. Louis: The C.V. Mosby Company.

Mitchell, P.H., L.C. Hodges, M. Muwaswes, and C.A. Walleck. 1988. *AANN's Neurologic Nursing*. Norwalk, CT: Appleton and Lange.

Newman, D.K. and D.A.J. Smith. 1991. *Geriatric Care Plans*. Springhouse, PA: Springhouse Corporation.

Pagana, K.D. and T.J. Pagana. 1986. *Pocket Guide To Laboratory and Diagnostic Tests*. St. Louis: The C.V. Mosby Company.

Saxon, S.V. and M.J. Etten. 1987. *Physical Change and Aging*. New York: The Tiresias Press, Inc.

Thompson, J.M., G.K. McFarland, J.E. Hirsch, S.M. Tucker, and A.C. Bowers. 1989. *Mosby's Manual of Clinical Nursing*. 2d ed. St. Louis: The C.V. Mosby Company.

Walz, T.H. and N.S. Blum. 1987. *Sexual Health In Later Life*. Lexington, MA: D.C. Heath and Co.

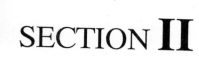

SECTION **II**

Interdisciplinary Health Care Team Issues Related to the Older Adult

INTRODUCTION

The five chapters in section II contain information on problems frequently seen in the practice of gerontological nursing. The problems that are presented are not normal and expected changes of aging. However, elderly clients are predisposed to these problems because of aging changes. These problems are: impaired physical mobility, impaired skin integrity, alterations in nutrition, alterations in bowel elimination, and alterations in bladder elimination.

Each chapter follows the nursing process approach with suggestions for assessment and interventions. The contributions of the appropriate interdisciplinary health care team members are considered in each chapter. In many facilities, physical therapists, occupational therapists, dieticians, and other health care professionals are available only on a consultation basis. These chapters are presented with the understanding that the nurse in a long-term care facility frequently is expected to initiate and carry out the interventions that are suggested. In any situation, it is still the responsibility of the nursing staff to coordinate and manage the care of the clients on a twenty-four-hour basis, seven days a week. The suggestions given in the chapters must be implemented consistently if the client is to be successful in reaching the mutually established goals.

Interdisciplinary Health Care from Issues Related to the Older Adult

INTRODUCTION

CHAPTER 3 Exercise and Activity

CONTENT OUTLINE

I. Complications associated with inactivity
   A. Pressure ulcers
   B. Contractures
   C. Disuse osteoporosis
   D. Nutritional concerns
   E. Respiratory changes
   F. Cardiovascular changes
   G. Urinary tract complications
   H. Psychosocial changes
II. The benefits of exercise
III. Planning exercise programs
IV. Types of exercise
   A. Range-of-motion exercises/Procedures for passive and self range-of-motion exercises
   B. Stretching exercises/Procedure
   C. Aerobics
   D. Isotonic exercises
   E. Isometric exercises/Procedure
   F. Isokinetic exercises
   G. Yoga
   H. Sexual activity
V. Opportunities for exercise
VI. Impaired physical mobility
   A. Impaired mobility related to body restraints or safety devices
   B. Identifying clients at risk for falling
VII. Avoiding the need for restraints
   A. Attend to physical and psychosocial needs
   B. Clothing
   C. Environment
   D. Family
   E. Staff and administration
VIII. Policies for the use of restraints
   A. Documentation for the use of restraints
IX. Levels of immobility
X. Progressive mobilization
XI. Moving the client in bed/Procedures for moving and turning the dependent client with a turning sheet
XII. Positioning
   A. Principles of positioning
   B. Use of supportive equipment
XIII. Independent bed movement/Procedure for teaching the client to move independently in bed
XIV. Transfer techniques
   A. Determining the method of transfer
   B. Preparation for transfer
   C. Guidelines for safe transfers/Procedure for using a transfer (gait) belt
   D. Coming to a sitting position on the edge of the bed/Procedure

E. Pivot (standing) transfers/Procedures for two- and one-person transfer with transfer belt and independent transfer, standby assist

F. Sliding board transfers/Procedures for passive transfer with sliding board alone and with two assistants and active transfer with sliding board

G. Toilet transfers/Procedure

H. Tub transfers/Procedure

I. Car transfers/Procedure

XV. Ambulation

A. Guidelines for ambulation

B. Normal gait pattern

C. Assistive devices

D. Gaits to use with assistive devices/Procedures for crutch, cane, and walker gaits

XVI. Using a wheelchair

A. Fitting the wheelchair to the client

B. Wheelchair safety/Procedures for tilting a wheelchair backward, using ramps and inclines, manipulating curbs, and going up and down stairs

C. Positioning the dependent client in a wheelchair/Procedures

D. Wheelchair activity/Procedures for push-ups and leaning

OBJECTIVES

❑ Describe the complications associated with inactivity.

❑ Implement nursing interventions to prevent the complications associated with inactivity.

❑ Identify the benefits of the different types of exercise.

❑ Describe the assessment findings that may contribute to impaired physical mobility.

❑ Demonstrate each procedure in this chapter.

❑ Identify the factors that effect positioning procedures.

❑ List the factors that determine an appropriate method of transfer.

❑ List the factors that influence the selection of assistive devices and ambulatory gait.

❑ Describe the relationship of the physical therapist and occupational therapist to the professional nurse for planning programs for progressive mobilization.

Restorative nursing is based on the concept of activity. Anticipated (or normal) age-related changes that affect the musculoskeletal, cardiovascular, and respiratory systems tend to contribute to loss of strength, flexibility, and endurance, even in healthy individuals. Levels of physical activity decrease through the years as a result of these losses. The work capacity of the average sedentary person declines by 30 percent between the ages of thirty and seventy. Many researchers believe that disuse or inactivity accounts for half this change (Webster 1988). While remaining strong and fit is a goal for many elderly people, there are still a large number who believe that exercise is not necessary in later years. These individuals feel that problems such as joint stiffness and fatigue are best treated by increasing periods of rest. Thus, the vicious cycle of disuse becomes fixed. Inactivity creates more lethargy, fatigue, weakness, and boredom. This in turn convinces the individual that more rest is needed. The hazards of inactivity and the dangers of prolonged rest are well documented. A study of the effects of three weeks of bed rest on healthy, well-conditioned young men revealed decreases in cardiac output, ventilatory capacity, maximal oxygen consumption, and amount of total muscle mass. These changes were equivalent to thirty years of physiological aging (Dwyer and Bottomley 1988).

In the elderly person, these changes would very likely be irreversible, resulting in permanent functional limitations. The individual would then be at risk for a number of life-threatening complications. The presence of a disease process often contributes to immobility and may preclude the individual's participation in extended forms of activity. The interdisciplinary team is responsible for planning and implementing a program of exercise appropriate for each client in an effort to prevent the complications resulting from inactivity.

COMPLICATIONS ASSOCIATED WITH INACTIVITY

Immobility resulting from sitting in a chair can present many of the same risks as bed rest for the dependent person. For example, pressure is greater on the ischial tuberosities and coccyx while seated than when lying in bed. The client with poor trunk stability may slump in the chair, hampering the breathing process. Sitting in an inappropriate chair can cause the legs to adduct and internally rotate, leading to contractures of the hip. To transfer the dependent client from bed to chair serves little purpose unless an exercise program is incorporated into the daily plan of care, the chair is suitable for the client, and the client's position is altered at frequent intervals. Without these interventions, some of the complications presented here can occur just as readily in the chairbound person.

Pressure Ulcers

(See chapter 4, "Maintaining Skin Integrity.")

Contractures

As people age, the tendons, ligaments, and joints tend to lose elasticity. Range of motion decreases and mobility is impaired (Steinberg 1988). This increases the risk of contracture.

A contracture is a painful and disabling complication of muscle disuse. A contracture can effect any joint that is not moved sufficiently. It is caused by the shortening and tightening of a set of muscles and stretching of the opposing group of muscles (Loeper 1985). Flexor muscles are stronger than extensor muscles, so contractures usually follow a pattern of flexion (Knight and Scott 1990).

Any time range of motion is restricted, changes in the connective tissue develop, further restricting movement. Collagen is a protein that makes up white fibrous connective tissue found in the subcutaneous tissue around the joint capsule. This normally allows for motion of the joint. But when motion is inhibited, the tissue becomes dense, further limiting movement. The presence of edema in a joint increases the risk of contracture formation by inhibiting motion and speeding up the process of fibrosis (Talbot, Pearson, and Loeper 1978). Spasticity resulting from central nervous system disorders or trauma also increases the risk of contractures. Decreased range-of-joint motion can occur within three or four days of immobility (Knight and Scott 1990).

Ankle flexion contractures occur most often. This is not only from disuse but also from the weight of bed covers on the feet and the force of gravity. If the client sits in a chair and the feet do not reach the floor, the foot dangles in a position of plantar flexion.

After a period of time, the immobility caused by contracture results in ankylosis. This is the fusion of bones across the joint space. Once ankylosis develops, weight bearing on that extremity and ambulation become impossible.

Contracture often precedes formation of pressure ulcers. The flexed joint results in increased pressure of the joint against the mattress and in skin surfaces rubbing together. Circulation is impeded in the soft tissues under a bony prominence (Knight and Scott 1990).

Contractures can be prevented with proper positioning and range-of-motion exercises. Splinting may be necessary in some cases (Steinberg 1988). Whether in bed or in a chair, repositioning the immobile client at least every two hours further reduces the risk of contractures. Supportive devices must be used correctly to avoid facilitating the onset of contractures. In most situations, the client's body should be supported so that joints are in a neutral position with minimal degrees of flexion. In addition, *avoid these joint positions*: retraction and adduction of the shoulders, adduction and internal and external rotation of the hips.

Passive range-of-motion exercises done twice a day will not increase strength, but will maintain joint flexibility. Muscle strength can be maintained by exertion of maximal tension carried out frequently throughout the day. Isometric and isotonic exercises carried out with the physician's order and in consultation with the physical therapist will accomplish this.

Disuse Osteoporosis

Bone loss in postmenopausal women may reach 30 percent by age seventy (Dwyer and Bottomley 1988). The combination of immobility and the lack of pressure that is normally associated with standing and walking causes additional loss of calcium from the bones. The bones become fragile and prone to pathological fractures. These occur because of alterations in the bone rather than because of injury.

Exercise slows bone loss and decreases the risk of fractures. Chair exercises done thirty minutes a day, three days a week can prevent bone loss (Dwyer and Bottomley 1988).

Nutritional Concerns

Decreased activity reduces the body's energy requirements and this affects the body's use of nutrients. Negative nitrogen balance can occur within a few days of immobilization. In this state, cells are breaking down more rapidly than new cells are being produced. This leads to protein deficiency and results in changes in body tissue. The loss of protein increases the risk of pressure ulcer formation and delays wound healing. The lack of physical activity and associated anorexia contributes to the problem of constipation (Talbot, Pearson, and Loeper 1978).

(See chapter 5, "Alterations in Nutritional Status," and chapter 6, "Alterations in Bowel Elimination.")

Respiratory Changes

In the absence of physical activity, the lungs do not completely expand, inhibiting the normal flow of air in and out of the lungs. Sitting or lying too long in one position impedes chest expansion due to the counterresistance of the bed or chair. The presence of abdominal distention also limits chest expansion. Sedatives depress the respiratory center in the medulla and decrease the rate and depth of respirations. Because of muscle weakness, the ability to cough is diminished. Secretions pool in the lungs, providing a medium for the growth of bacteria. Secretions build up in the alveoli, causing inflammation and resulting in hypostatic pneumonia (Thompson 1990).

Frequent repositioning and exercises prescribed for the client's ability aid in preventing complications of the respiratory system. Increase fluid intake to 2000 ml unless contraindicated. Regular deep breathing and coughing routines are additional preventive measures. Pneumonia vaccine is usually recommended for individuals with chronic health problems. This decreases the risk of pneumonia.

Cardiovascular Changes

The heart has to work harder to circulate the blood when the body is lying in bed. To accomplish this, cardiac output and stroke volume increase. As the heart rate increases, the heart has less time to recover between beats, causing the heart muscle to become fatigued.

Orthostatic hypotension is another complication associated with immobility. When a person who has been lying down for a long time stands up, the autonomic nervous system cannot balance the blood supply. This results in a rapid fall in blood pressure when there is a change from a sitting or lying position to a standing position.

When the person in bed tries to move about, the upper trunk and arm muscles are usually used while the individual tends not to breathe as movement is attempted. This results in the Valsalva maneuver which increases the intrathoracic pressure. When the breath is exhaled, the pressure decreases rapidly and a large amount of blood is sent to the heart. For the person with compromised cardiovascular status, this poses a risk for tachycardia and cardiac arrest (Johnson 1990).

Immobility diminishes the muscle contractions in the legs. These contractions normally promote venous return of the blood to the heart. The resulting venous stasis causes edema of the lower extremities. The pressure of the legs against the bed or chair further impedes circulation. This combination of factors can cause a thrombus to form.

Wearing elastic stockings and elevating the feet while sitting can reduce the possibility of venous stasis. The back of the chair should not press against the client's legs. Avoid the use of the knee gatch or pillows under the client's knees. Check extremities frequently to be sure that the circulation is not impaired due to inappropriate positioning.

Instruct the client to concentrate on exhaling rather than holding the breath when moving in bed to prevent the Valsalva maneuver.

Urinary Tract Complications

The urinary system too is subject to the adverse effects of inactivity. Lying prone increases retention of urine. Retention of urine in the bladder can lead to urinary tract infections. (See chapter 7, "Alterations in Bladder Elimination.") The loss of minerals from the bones contributes to formation of renal or bladder stones. (Talbot et al. 1978)

Psychosocial Changes

The person confined to bed suffers mental and emotional changes. Continued sensory deprivation may cause hallucinations, resulting in further anxiety and feelings of hopelessness. Time perception is distorted and seems to go very slowly. This causes the person to feel more tired and bored. Without cues from the environment, disorientation occurs. The client may appear mentally incompetent and not be allowed to make decisions. A sense of powerlessness diminishes self-esteem. Feelings of anger, depression, guilt, and fear have all been associated with inactivity, compounding the medical problems of the client.

Allow the client to verbalize experiences and to ventilate feelings. Accept these statements without judgment. The client needs reassurance of mental and emotional stability.

Provide a clock and calendar to maintain orientation. After the acute phase of illness, resume socialization, with individual counseling or group activities. If there is a medical reason why the client cannot get out of bed, moving the bed out of the room for certain periods of time provides sensory stimulation.

Assist the client with dressing and grooming. Encourage clients who can be out of bed to be dressed in attractive clothing. Remaining in night clothes all day increases feelings of dependence and sickness.

It is evident that inactivity places the client at risk for many complications that are especially dangerous for the elderly person. Incorporating exercise into the plan of care can increase the quality of life for the elderly client.

THE BENEFITS OF EXERCISE

People of all ages benefit from regular exercise. Participation in vigorous activity produces more energy, increases resistance to fatigue, enhances relaxation, and helps counter anxiety and depression. Sleep habits may improve and the ability to deal with stress is greater. Exercise can refresh, invigorate, and strengthen, thus improving self-image. Several studies have demonstrated the positive effects of exercise for the elderly. Improved cardiovascular status and lung status, decreased blood pressure, increased muscle strength, and joint flexibility have been documented (Benison and Hogstel 1986). Exercises planned for the abilities and limitations of the individual can prevent complications, maintain current levels of ability, and increase functional capacity.

Clients in any setting need the opportunity to participate in appropriate exercises on a regular basis. Nursing homes, extended care facilities, and retirement centers can establish programs at minimal cost. Consultation with the client at home can assist in planning a program to meet individual needs and resources. Senior centers, YMCAs, and hospital outpatient departments often have programs designed for older adults with chronic health problems. Shopping malls across the country are offering their facilities for walking before opening hours. Many of these are marked for distance with resting places located at strategic points. Videotapes are available with low-impact aerobics, some with exercises that can be carried out while sitting in a chair. These can be used with groups or in the privacy of one's home.

Maintaining or increasing strength, endurance, flexibility, and range of motion and improving balance are long-range goals for the client. These changes will not occur as quickly in the elderly as they do in younger persons. Because it is difficult to determine what is considered normal performance or even desired performance for the elderly client, evaluation of functional capacity is more indicative of goal attainment.

PLANNING EXERCISE PROGRAMS

Include the client in planning activities that are enjoyable as well as beneficial. Explain the reasons for participation and, more specifically, what improvements the individual may expect to see as a result of the program. Encouraging competition between group members may subject them to unnecessary stress and is not advised. Consider the physiological changes of aging, the client's current functional status and any limitations imposed by the physician on the basis of current medical diagnoses.

Equipment provides opportunities for a variety of activities, but is not required for an effective program. Space is needed to allow participants room to stretch out. A minimum of five hundred square feet for every fifteen to twenty people is recommended. Exercise mats or a carpeted floor decrease the risk of injury.

Lightweight, loose-fitting clothing, and well-fitting, cushioned shoes with safe soles enhance the comfort of the client (Harrison 1988).

A leader for every eight people enables each person to receive assistance if necessary and to be monitored for ill effects. Avoid strenuous programs when starting out. Gradually increase the length and intensity of the exercise. Three to five sessions of twenty-five to forty minutes each, spread throughout the week, are recommended. If sessions are missed, the client must resume activity at a lower level. Motions for all exercises should be steady, smooth, rhythmical, and repetitive. Use of correct body mechanics will prevent injuries due to improper use of back muscles.

The group leader should explain the term *target heart rate* (THR) and determine the optimum heart rate for each person. Maximum heart rate is the fastest the heart can beat and is usually 220 minus the person's age. Target zone is 60–75 percent of the maximum heart rate and generally occurs about ten minutes after warm-up exercises (National Institutes of Health 1981). For elderly persons, the lower end of the zone — 60 percent — may be considered maximum. Thus, a seventy-year-old person would have a THR of ninety beats per minute. The physician may recommend gradually increasing the THR as the client progresses, if the physical condition permits. Cardiovascular medications, such as beta blockers and calcium channel blockers, can affect heart rate, so this formula would not be appropriate. For individuals taking these medications, the rate can be based on an exercise treadmill test ordered by the physician (Webster 1988).

It is advisable to monitor resting pulse rate and cool-down rate at the end of the session. It is usually not necessary to take blood pressure during each class, but if blood pressure exceeds 140/90 or resting pulse exceeds ninety-five, consult the physician before beginning (Harrison 1988).

The body needs to limber up and get ready for more vigorous exercise by starting each session with a five- to ten-minute warm-up. Slow stretching movements during warm-up decrease the risk for musculoskeletal injuries (Webster 1988).

TYPES OF EXERCISE

Each type of exercise provides specific benefits. Ideally, a program includes each type of activity, carried out for a specific length of time on a regular basis. Frail elderly persons may be able to participate in only the less strenuous forms of exercise.

Range-of-Motion Exercises

The range of motion for any joint is the extent to which the joint can be moved. A loss of range occurs when a joint is immobile over a period of time. Contractures, spasticity, arthritic joint changes, and rigidity limit the range. Passive range-of-motion exercises are carried out by the nurse or other caregiver without any assistance from the client. All dependent clients need to receive passive range-of-motion exercises at least twice daily. All joints are passively moved through the client's available range of motion.

Passive exercises greatly reduce the risk of contractures but have little effect on muscle mass and strength or on cardiovascular and respiratory performance (Loeper 1985). However, for some clients, these are the only exercises that are appropriate.

TABLE 3–1	**Guidelines for Passive Range-of-Motion Exercises**

- ❑ Tell the client what you are doing and why. Assist the client to lie in good body alignment before starting. Cover the client with a bath blanket.
- ❑ Assess the abilities of the client so you do not do passive motions that the client can do actively.
- ❑ Know whether or not an exercise is contraindicated for any joint.
- ❑ With the palm of your hand, hold the extremity above and below the joint being moved. Do not use your fingertips. Support the limb from underneath.
- ❑ Support painful joints to feel for limitations in movement. Avoid causing pain. For a comatose or cognitively impaired client, watch the client's face for signs of discomfort.
- ❑ Carry out all motions slowly and smoothly. Come to a complete stop before continuing with the next movement.
- ❑ If a muscle spasm occurs, stop the action and maintain slow, gentle pressure until the muscle relaxes. Then continue the motions through the pain-free range.
- ❑ Rapid, jerky movements may trigger clonus. To control this, restart the movement slowly and gently with firm pressure.
- ❑ Rigidity may be noted in a person with extrapyramidal dysfunction. Move against the pressure of the rigidity and slowly continue the movement.
- ❑ Never passively exercise a client's neck. Cervical arthritis increases the risk for damage to the neck and spinal cord. Teach the responsive client to actively carry out neck movements within existing limitations.

During *active assistive range-of-motion exercises*, the nurse provides support and direction with the client performing some of the activity. *Active range-of-motion exercises* are carried out by the client without assistance. These are often combined with other forms of exercise, such as stretching. *Self range-of-motion exercises* are performed by the client on immobile limbs. A person with hemiplegia, for example, uses the strong extremities to passively move the paralyzed extremities. These exercises are completed at least two times a day, moving each joint through its available range from five to ten times. The benefits of these forms of range-of-motion exercises depend on the capabilities of the client. Active exercises may have aerobic benefits if carried out under the appropriate conditions.

Procedure: Passive Range-of-Motion Exercises

Shoulder

1. Flexion and extension
   - ❑ Start with arm lying parallel to body.
   - ❑ Support wrist and elbow. (Elbow may be extended or flexed.) Raise arm over client's head (flexion), Figure 3–1.
   - ❑ Return arm to starting position (extension).
2. Abduction and adduction
   - ❑ Start with arm lying parallel to body.
   - ❑ Support wrist and elbow. (Elbow may be extended or flexed.) Bring entire arm out at right angle from body (abduction), Figure 3–2.
   - ❑ Move arm back to body, crossing over body (adduction).
3. External and internal rotation
   - ❑ Start with arm lying parallel to body.

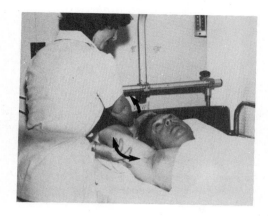

Figure 3–1 Shoulder flexion *(From Hegner and Caldwell,* Assisting in Long-Term Care *[Albany, NY: Delmar Publishers Inc., 1988], 266.)*

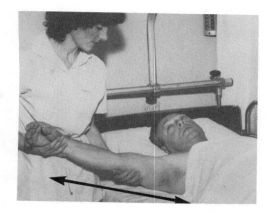

Figure 3–2 Shoulder abduction *(From Hegner and Caldwell,* Assisting in Long-Term Care *[Albany, NY: Delmar Publishers Inc., 1988], 266.)*

    ❏ Move arm so elbow is parallel with shoulder. Hand is pointing upward with palm facing outward (external rotation).

    ❏ Maintain shoulder and elbow positions with one hand. Use your other hand to move client's forearm down so hand is pointing downward and palm is against bed. (internal rotation).

  4. Hyperextension[*]

    ❏ Client must be in prone position.

    ❏ Start with arm lying parallel to body. Support wrist and elbow.

    ❏ Raise arm gently and return to original position.

  5. Protraction and retraction[**]

    ❏ Client must be in prone position with arms lying parallel to body.

    ❏ Place one hand under client's shoulder. Raise client's shoulder (retraction) and then return to original position (protraction).

Elbow

  1. Flexion and extension

    ❏ Start with arm lying parallel to body.

    ❏ Support shoulder and wrist.

    ❏ Bring forearm toward upper arm with palm facing client (flexion), Figure 3–3.

    ❏ Return forearm to starting position (extension).

  2. Pronation and supination

    ❏ Start with arm lying parallel to body.

    ❏ Grasp client's hand as if to shake hands. Allow elbow to rest on bed.

    ❏ Move your hand and client's hand so client's hand is palm down (pronation), Figure 3–4.

    ❏ Then move your hand and client's hand so client's hand is palm upward (supination).

---

[*] Many elderly clients cannot lie in prone position. These exercises may be omitted.

[**] Many elderly clients cannot lie in prone position. These exercises may be omitted.

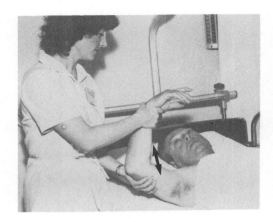

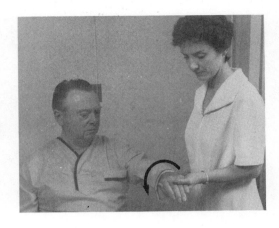

Figure 3–3 Elbow flexion *(From Hegner and Caldwell, Assisting in Long-Term Care [Albany, NY: Delmar Publishers Inc., 1988], 266.)*

Figure 3–4 Elbow pronation *(From Hegner and Caldwell, Assisting in Long-Term Care [Albany, NY: Delmar Publishers Inc., 1988], 266.)*

Wrist

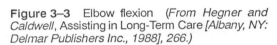

1. Flexion, extension, hyperextension
   - ❑ Support client's arm with elbow slightly flexed and palm of hand in supination.
   - ❑ Bend client's wrist forward (flexion), Figure 3–5.
   - ❑ Straighten wrist out (extension), Figure 3–6.
   - ❑ Bend wrist back, carefully (hyperextension).
2. Ulnar and radial deviation
   - ❑ Allow client's elbow to rest on bed. Support wrist.
   - ❑ With client's wrist in extension, move client's hand to ulnar side (ulnar deviation).
   - ❑ Then move client's hand to radial side (radial deviation), Figure 3–7.

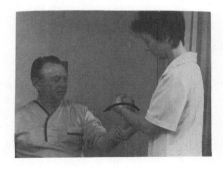

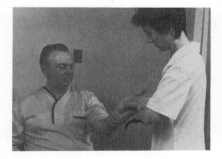

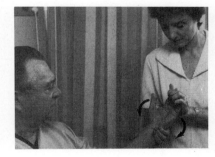

Figure 3–5 Wrist flexion *(From Hegner and Caldwell, Assisting in Long-Term Care [Albany, NY: Delmar Publishers Inc., 1988], 267.)*

Figure 3–6 Wrist hyperextension *(From Hegner and Caldwell, Assisting in Long-Term Care [Albany, NY: Delmar Publishers Inc., 1988], 267.)*

Figure 3–7 Wrist-ulnar and radial deviation *(From Hegner and Caldwell, Assisting in Long-Term Care [Albany, NY: Delmar Publishers Inc., 1988], 267.)*

Fingers and Thumb

1. Flexion and extension
   - ❏ Allow client's elbow to rest on bed. Support wrist.
   - ❏ With your other hand, bend client's fingers toward palm of hand (flexion), Figure 3–8.
   - ❏ Straighten client's fingers out (extension), Figure 3–9.
   - ❏ Repeat actions with client's thumb.
2. Abduction and adduction
   - ❏ Support wrist as above.
   - ❏ Separate fingers (abduction) and return to original position (adduction), Figure 3–10.
   - ❏ Repeat actions with client's thumb.

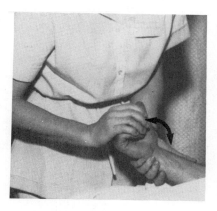 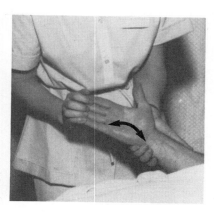

Figure 3–8 Finger flexion *(From Hegner and Caldwell, Assisting in Long-Term Care [Albany, NY: Delmar Publishers Inc., 1988], 267.)*

Figure 3–9 Finger extension *(From Hegner and Caldwell, Assisting in Long-Term Care [Albany, NY: Delmar Publishers Inc., 1988], 267.)*

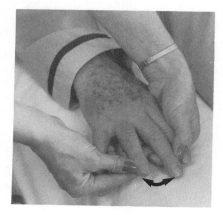

Figure 3–10 Finger abduction and adduction *(From Hegner and Caldwell, Assisting in Long-Term Care [Albany, NY: Delmar Publishers Inc., 1988], 267.)*

3. Opposition
   ❑ Support wrist as above.
   ❑ Move client's thumb to base of each finger.

Hip

1. Flexion and extension
   Note: This exercise also includes knee hip and flexion at the same time.
   ❑ Start with client's leg parallel to other leg, resting on bed. Support client's knee and ankle.
   ❑ Bend knee and hip (flexion), Figure 3–11.
   ❑ Straighten knee and hip (extension).
2. Abduction and adduction
   ❑ Start with client's leg parallel to other leg, resting on bed. Support client's knee and ankle.
   ❑ Move entire leg away from body (abduction), Figure 3–12.
   ❑ Return leg to starting position (adduction).

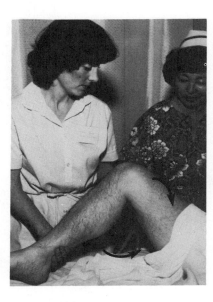 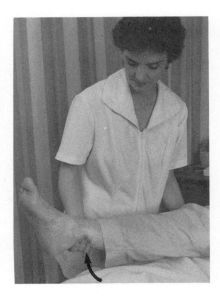

Figure 3–11 Hip and knee flexion *(From Hegner and Caldwell,* Assisting in Long-Term Care *[Albany, NY: Delmar Publishers Inc., 1988], 268.)*

Figure 3–12 Hip abduction *(From Hegner and Caldwell,* Assisting in Long-Term Care *[Albany, NY: Delmar Publishers Inc., 1988], 268.)*

3. Internal and external rotation
   ❑ Start with client's leg parallel to other leg, resting on bed. Supporting ankle and thigh, flex knee and bring leg toward midline (internal rotation), Figure 3–13.
   ❑ Supporting ankle and thigh, rotate hip outward, turning leg away from midline (external rotation), Figure 3–14.

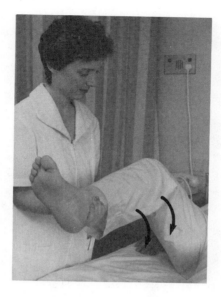

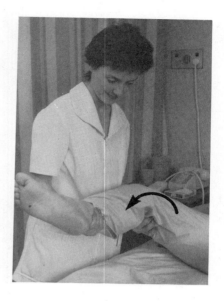

Figure 3–13 Hip internal rotation *(From Hegner and Caldwell, Assisting in Long-Term Care [Albany, NY: Delmar Publishers Inc., 1988], 268.)*

Figure 3–14 Hip external rotation *(From Hegner and Caldwell, Assisting in Long-Term Care [Albany, NY: Delmar Publishers Inc., 1988], 268.)*

4. Hyperextension*
   - ❏ Client must be lying in prone position.
   - ❏ Start with client's leg parallel to other leg. Support ankle and knee.
   - ❏ Gently raise client's leg and then return to starting position.

Ankle

1. Plantar flexion and dorsiflexion
   - ❏ Support ankle.
   - ❏ With client's knee slightly flexed, bend foot forward toward bed (plantar flexion), Figure 3–15.
   - ❏ Then gently bend foot back toward client's body (dorsiflexion), Figure 3–16.
2. Inversion and eversion
   - ❏ Support ankle. Allow leg to rest on bed.
   - ❏ Move client's foot so sole is facing inward (inversion), Figure 3–17.
   - ❏ Move client's foot so sole is facing outward (eversion), Figure 3–18.

---

* Omit this exercise if client cannot lie in prone position.

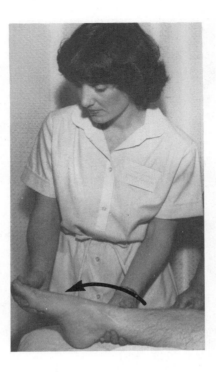

Figure 3–15 Ankle plantar flexion *(From Hegner and Caldwell,* Assisting in Long-Term Care *[Albany, NY: Delmar Publishers Inc., 1988], 269.)*

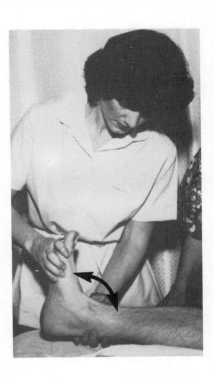

Figure 3–16 Ankle dorsiflexion *(From Hegner and Caldwell,* Assisting in Long-Term Care *[Albany, NY: Delmar Publishers Inc., 1988], 269.)*

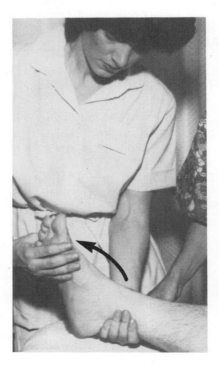

Figure 3–17 Ankle inversion *(From Hegner and Caldwell,* Assisting in Long-Term Care *[Albany, NY: Delmar Publishers Inc., 1988], 269.)*

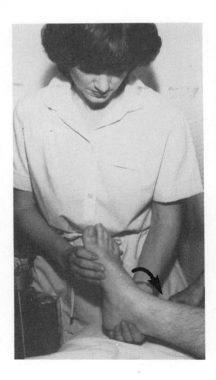

Figure 3–18 Ankle eversion *(From Hegner and Caldwell,* Assisting in Long-Term Care *[Albany, NY: Delmar Publishers Inc., 1988], 269.)*

Toes

1. Flexion and extension
   ❏ Allow client's leg to rest on bed.
   ❏ Bend (flexion), Figure 3–19, and straighten (extension) each toe, Figure 3–20.

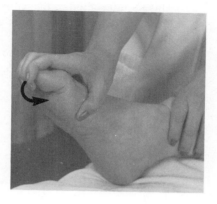

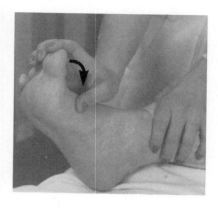

Figure 3–19 Toe flexion *(From Hegner and Caldwell,* Assisting in Long-Term Care *[Albany, NY: Delmar Publishers Inc., 1988], 270.)*

Figure 3–20 Toe extension *(From Hegner and Caldwell,* Assisting in Long-Term Care *[Albany, NY: Delmar Publishers Inc., 1988], 270.)*

2. Abduction and adduction
   ❏ Move each toe away from the one next to it (abduction), Figure 3–21, and then return to position (adduction), Figure 3–22.

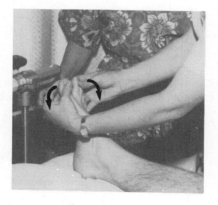

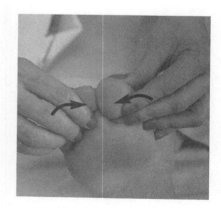

Figure 3–21 Toe abduction *(From Hegner and Caldwell,* Assisting in Long-Term Care *[Albany, NY: Delmar Publishers Inc., 1988], 270.)*

Figure 3–22 Toe adduction *(From Hegner and Caldwell,* Assisting in Long-Term Care *[Albany, NY: Delmar Publishers Inc., 1988], 270.)*

Procedure: Self Range-of-Motion Exercises

The client can use the strong arm to exercise the affected arm. The strong arm is actively exercised while the affected arm is receiving passive exercise. These can be done with the client seated or in bed. Repeat each exercise five to ten times.

Instruct the client:

1. Shoulder flexion and extension
   - ❑ This requires good trunk stability.
   - ❑ Clasp hands in lap, reach forward and down to the floor with the elbows straight, Figure 3–23.
   - ❑ Raise hands directly above the head, Figure 3–24.
   - ❑ Bring hands back down to lap, Figure 3–25.

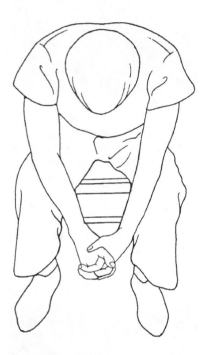

Figure 3–23 Shoulder extension *(Adapted from* Range of Motion Exercises, *J. Loeper, 1985, courtesy of the Sister Kenny Institute, Minneapolis, MN)*

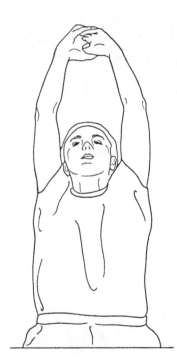

Figure 3–24 Shoulder flexion *(Adapted from* Range of Motion Exercises, *J. Loeper, 1985, courtesy of the Sister Kenny Institute, Minneapolis, MN)*

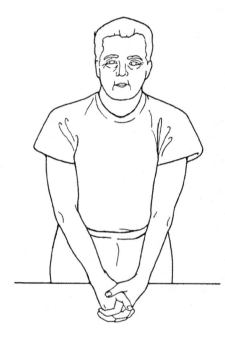

Figure 3–25 Shoulder extension *(Adapted from* Range of Motion Exercises, *J. Loeper, 1985, courtesy of the Sister Kenny Institute, Minneapolis, MN)*

2. Shoulder abduction and adduction
   ❑ Fold arms on chest with affected arm on top. Move arms to right, lifting arms away from the chest.
   ❑ Move arms to left, lifting arms off chest, Figure 3–26.
   ❑ Return to starting position.

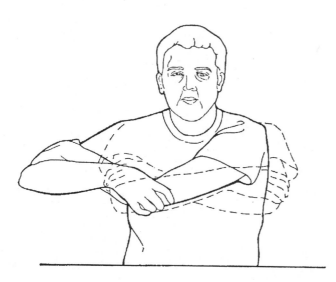

Figure 3–26 Shoulder adduction (dotted line) and abduction *(Adapted from* Range of Motion Exercises, *J. Loeper, 1985, courtesy of the Sister Kenny Institute, Minneapolis, MN)*

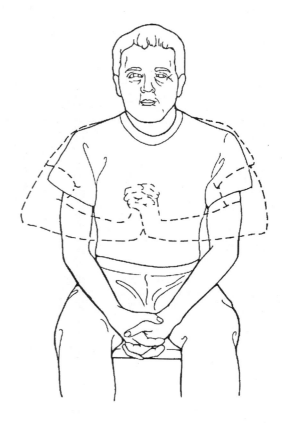

Figure 3–27 Elbow flexion (dotted line) and extension *(Adapted from* Range of Motion Exercises, *J. Loeper, 1985, courtesy of the Sister Kenny Institute, Minneapolis, MN)*

3. Elbow extension and flexion
   ❑ Clasp hands in lap. Bend elbows and bring the hands to the chest.
   ❑ Straighten elbows and touch hands to knees, straightening elbows completely, Figure 3–27.
4. Pronation and supination
   ❑ Grasp the wrist with the stronger hand and bend the elbows. Turn the forearms so that the back of the hand is facing the ceiling.
   ❑ Then turn the forearms so that the palm of the hand is facing the ceiling. Return to starting position, Figure 3–28.
5. Wrist extension and flexion
   ❑ Clasp hands by interlacing fingers with thumbs up.
   ❑ Bend wrist to far left, then far right, Figure 3–29.
6. Radial and ulnar deviation
   ❑ Clasp hands by interlacing fingers with thumbs up, weaker thumb on top.
   ❑ Bend wrist toward ceiling. Then bend wrist toward floor.

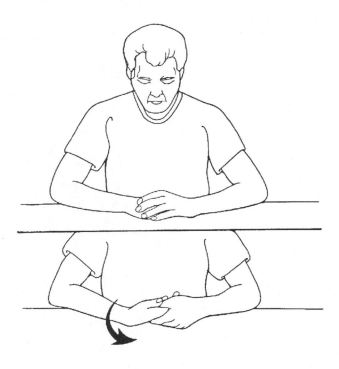

Figure 3–28 Elbow pronation and supination *(Adapted from Range of Motion Exercises, J. Loeper, 1985, courtesy of the Sister Kenny Institute, Minneapolis, MN)*

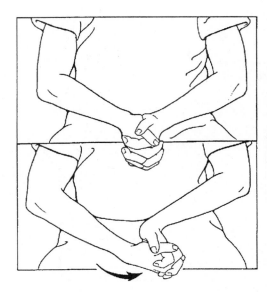

Figure 3–29 Fingers and thumb — flexion and extension; wrists — flexion, extension, hyperextension, and radial and ulnar deviation *(Adapted from Range of Motion Exercises, J. Loeper, 1985, courtesy of the Sister Kenny Institute, Minneapolis, MN)*

7. Thumb extension
   ❑ Place involved hand on lap.
   ❑ Grasp thumb with uninvolved hand and move thumb gently in large circle.
8. Finger extension and flexion
   ❑ Place involved arm on lap. With uninvolved hand, straighten the fingers of the involved hand.
   ❑ Curl fingers of involved hand into a fist.

(Loeper 1985)

Stretching Exercises

Stretching increases body temperature, circulation, and oxygen delivery to muscles, making muscle contraction more efficient. The body needs to limber up and get ready for more vigorous exercise by starting each session with a five- to ten-minute warm-up session. Slow stretching during the warm-up decreases the risk of musculoskeletal injuries if movements are carried out in a relaxed, sustained, and slow manner. Both the primary movers and antagonist muscles on all extremities are involved in the stretching routine. Effective and regular stretching maintains and increases flexibility (Webster 1988).

Begin the stretch in a slow, steady manner until mild tension is felt and then relax. Move slowly, a fraction of an inch further until mild tension is again felt and hold the stretch for a few seconds. Individuals with impaired balance and limited mobility can do stretching exercises while seated in a chair (Webster

1988). Stretching exercises should always precede vigorous routines. They can also be done alone without other exercises. Selection of stretching exercises can be made from the suggestions listed, based on the client's abilities.

Procedure: Stretching Exercises

Pectoral Stretch

1. Grasp your hands behind your neck and press your elbows back as far as you can.
2. Return to starting position, then drop your arms and relax.

Back Stretch

1. Raise your right arm and grasp it below the elbow with your left hand.
2. Gently pull your right elbow toward your left shoulder as you look over your right shoulder.
3. Hold for five seconds. Repeat with the other side.

Side Stretch

1. Interlace your fingers and lift your arms over your head with elbows straight.
2. Press your arms backward as far as you can.
3. Slowly lean to the left and then to the right until you feel the stretching.

Shoulder Stretch

1. Put your hands together behind your back.
2. Lift your arms up and hold for a few seconds. Stretch gently.

Hamstring Stretch (Standing)

1. Stand with your feet at shoulders' width apart and pointed straight ahead.
2. Bend slowly forward.
3. With your knees slightly bent, stretch gently. Relax your neck and arms. Hold for a few seconds.

Hamstring Stretch (Sitting)

1. Do this one in sitting position.
2. Place your extended right leg level on another chair. Keep your other foot on the floor.
3. Lean forward and slowly try to touch your right toe with right hand ten times and then with left hand ten times.
4. Switch legs and repeat with each hand.

Calf Stretch

1. Face a wall. Rest your forearms on the wall with your forehead on the back of your hands.
2. Bend one knee and move it toward the wall. Your back leg should be straight with the foot flat and pointed straight ahead.

3. Move your hips forward until you feel the stretch.
4. Stretch gently and slowly. Hold for thirty seconds and switch legs.

Buttocks

1. Lie on your back.
2. If you can, keep your head on the floor and pull your right leg toward your chest.
3. Hold for a few seconds and switch legs.

Aerobics

The word *aerobics* is a term coined by Dr. Kenneth H. Cooper, the medical authority on exercise programs for health and fitness. The sustained, repetitive movements of aerobic exercise improve cardiovascular and respiratory function. To condition the heart and lungs, the exercises must be brisk enough to raise the heart and breathing rates — must be done for twenty minutes four times a week or for thirty minutes three times a week. Aerobic exercise causes the lungs to expand, taking in more oxygen. More oxygen is carried throughout the body, the heart has to work less and the resting heart rate and recovery rate after exercise decrease (Cooper 1982).

Always precede aerobic routines with a five- to ten-minute warm-up session including stretching exercises and follow with a five- to ten-minute cool-down session (Webster 1988). Strenuous aerobic activities are not recommended for persons sixty years of age and over who are totally inactive or for individuals with a chronic disease (Cooper 1982).

Low-impact aerobics produces cardiovascular benefits but place less strain on the joints because one foot is always on the floor. The large muscles of the arms and legs are involved in repetitive, rhythmical movements of ten counts or more. Low-impact aerobics should be done five times per week.

Isotonic Exercises

Weight lifting and calisthenics are examples of isotonic exercises. These require the contraction of a muscle and movement of a joint in the process of the contraction. Isotonic exercises build up muscle mass and increase flexibility, thereby improving agility, coordination, and muscle strength. Including calisthenics in the exercise routine can help avoid injuries during more strenuous activity (Cooper 1982). Isotonic activities can be carried out in the bed, while seated in a chair, or while standing. Using a trapeze to lift the body off the bed, and pushing the body to a sitting position are examples of isotonic exercise (Milde 1988). (See Wheelchair Activity.)

Avoid isotonics or use with caution for persons with compromised cardiovascular status. There is a rise in systolic blood pressure and there may be possible inadvertent use of the Valsalva maneuver (Milde 1988).

Isometric Exercises

Isometric exercises are performed by contracting muscles against resistance but without movement of the joints of extremities. Despite the increase in tension, the muscle fibers do not shorten in length. Isometric exercises increase and strengthen muscle tone (Milde 1988). During the exercise period, the contractions may increase diastolic and systolic blood pressures. Persons with cardiovascular problems are advised not to engage in isometric activity (Cooper 1982). There is a possibility of doing the Valsalva maneuver as well as a risk of inducing cardiac arrhythmias. Isometrics can be done while sitting, standing, or lying down.

Procedure: Isometric Exercises

Instruct the client:

1. For arms and shoulders
   - ❑ Sit up straight.
   - ❑ Grasp sides of chair with both hands and pull up.
2. For the back
   - ❑ Keep the back straight and clasp hands behind the head.
   - ❑ Hold your elbows forward. Pull forward with your hands and press your head backward, Figure 3–30.
3. For the shoulders, arms, and abdomen
   - ❑ Keep the back straight and lean forward.
   - ❑ Place both hands, palm sides down against the sides of the chair.
   - ❑ Hold the legs straight out and attempt to raise the body off the chair, Figure 3–31.

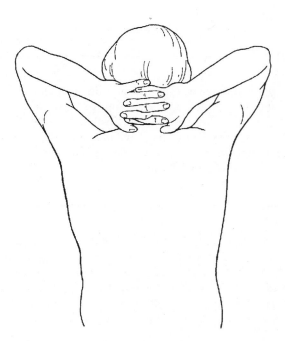

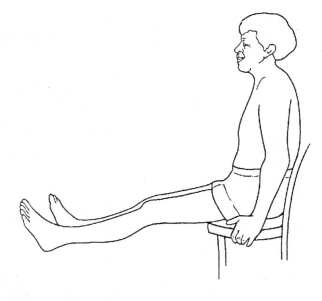

Figure 3–31 Shoulders, arms, and abdomen: keep back straight, place both hands with palms down against sides of chair, hold legs straight out, try to raise body off the chair.

Figure 3–30 Back: keep back straight, clasp hands behind head, hold elbows forward, pull forward with hands, press head backwards.

4. For the legs
   - ❑ Place feet four inches apart. Bend forward and place hands against the inside of opposite knees.
   - ❑ Try to press your knees together while you hold them apart with your hands, Figure 3–32.

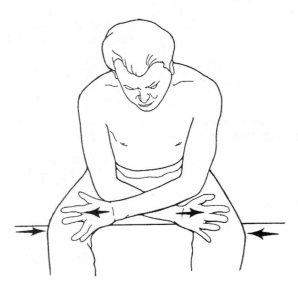

Figure 3–32 Legs: place feet four inches apart, bend forward, place hands against inside of opposite knees, try to press knees together while holding them apart with your hands.

Isokinetic Exercises

Isokinetic exercises involve weight lifting through an entire range of motion, requiring effort not only to pick up the weight, but also to take it back to the starting point. Exercise machinery promotes isokinetic activity. Studies at the Institute for Aerobic Research in Dallas have indicated that isokinetic exercise, if done properly, strengthens muscles and produces endurance training similar to that of aerobic exercise (Cooper 1982).

Yoga

Yoga began in northern India five thousand years ago as a philosophy of living that leads to physical and spiritual health and well-being. There are different training methods, but the elderly can benefit greatly from the assistance of a qualified instructor. The deep breathing and stretching increase oxygen intake, release tension, and limber up the entire body. Yoga meditation can assist in achieving harmony, inner growth, and peace of mind.

Sexual Activity

There are many components to sexuality, each of which can be beneficial to older adults. Intimacy fulfills upper level needs of love and belonging and can be expressed by emotional or physical means. Sexual activity is included here because it is beneficial exercise and helps maintain fitness. The heart and breathing rates are increased by stimulation of the adrenal glands and pain and stress can be relieved (Rankin 1989). Clients may need instruction on adapting the activity to their abilities. (This topic is addressed in the chapters on case studies.)

OPPORTUNITIES FOR EXERCISE

The opportunities for exercise are endless. Walking requires no equipment (clients may need walkers or canes) and provides many benefits. Nursing homes can provide safe areas for walking, with distance marked off. Walking outdoors in mild weather allows clients to interact with nature and may also provide socialization opportunities.

A swimming pool would provide useful exercise for clients in a nursing home or in group living facilities. The benefits of water exercise are worth the cost of transportation if arrangements can be made to use a pool in the community. Park districts sometimes offer pool programs specifically designed for older adults.

Nursing homes and other group living facilities can set up health and fitness trails indoors or outdoors. A variety of exercises located throughout the trail with simple, easy to read directions at eye level can be completed independently or with the assistance of staff or family members, Figures 3–33 and 3–34. When the trail is set up permanently, clients have the flexibility of using it at the time of their choice.

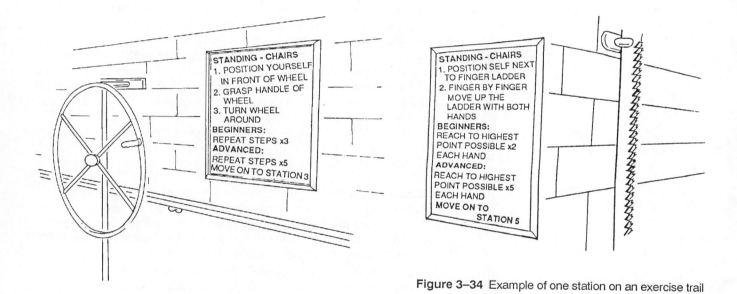

Figure 3–34 Example of one station on an exercise trail

Figure 3–33 Example of one station on an exercise trail

Most recreational activities can be adapted to the abilities of the client. Volleyball, basketball, bowling, and shuffleboard are games that can increase range of motion and endurance. Bowling centers frequently have leagues for older adults and will often reserve specific times for nursing home residents.

IMPAIRED PHYSICAL MOBILITY

Older adults, particularly in the presence of a chronic health problem, may experience some degree of impaired mobility. Joint pain and stiffness can discourage the client from moving about. Clients with cardiovascular or pulmonary disease may not have the endurance to participate in extended forms of activity. Paralysis, spasticity, and cognitive and sensory impairments also effect mobility.

Impaired Mobility Related to Body Restraints or Safety Devices _____

Restraints are a major cause of immobility in nursing homes and hospitals. It has been estimated that in hospitals, one in five patients over age seventy is restrained. In skilled nursing homes, over 41 percent of residents are restrained (Strumpf, Evans, and Schwartz 1990). The application of physical restraints can impede circulation, inhibit breathing, and predispose to pressure ulcers and incontinence. Disorientation, memory impairment, and emotional distress are common psychosocial reactions to being restrained.

A physical restraint is defined in the *Federal Register* as "any manual method or physical or mechanical device, material or equipment attached or adjacent to the client's (patient's) body that the individual cannot remove easily which restricts freedom of movement or normal access to one's body" (Department of Health and Human Services 1991). This definition includes vests, jackets, safety belts, mitts, limb holders, bed sheets, and geriatric and cardiac chairs. Chemical restraints are drugs administered to inhibit movement. Unfortunately, the client who reacts with anger and hostility to being restrained is often treated with a psychotropic medication to increase attempts at altering behavior.

Fear of injury to self or others is the reason used most often to justify the use of restraints. The elderly are at risk for falls even when healthy. Wanderers are restrained to prevent them from entering other clients' rooms. In some cases, mobility is impaired for the sake of carrying out a treatment or procedure. The threat of litigation over failure to restrain and consequent injury is a justifiable concern of health care providers.

In December 1989, the U.S. Senate Special Committee on Aging sponsored a national symposium entitled "Untie the Elderly: Quality Care Without Restraints." A statement by Alan R. Hunt, Esq. addresses the issue of liability.

> Health care institutions may abandon the use of physical restraints without incurring a significant risk of being sued for malpractice. There are few precedents supporting successful malpractice claims against long-term care facilities based upon a failure to restrain. In fact, the striking conclusion from an examination of cases involving restraints both in nursing homes and hospitals is that the use of restraints has produced more successful lawsuits than nonuse.

The use of restraints does not prevent falling and injury. Death by strangulation has occurred as a result of improper use of restraints.

It is clear that to be restrained severely diminishes quality of life. Certainly it contradicts the philosophy of restorative care. How can independence be attained or maintained when one is only allowed to ambulate at the whim of the staff, or not at all? Staff time is a necessary concern. However, implementing interventions to prevent complications resulting from immobility is just as time-consuming as is monitoring clients who are not restrained. In addition, each client who is restrained must have the device released every two hours for ten minutes (per federal regulation). This would utilize two hours of staff time per restrained resident per day. It requires time to locate the device, put the devices on and take them off, and tie them and untie them for each transfer and position change. Documentation related to the use of restraints is also a time factor.

The federal government is prepared to support the reduction or elimination of the use of restraints in long-term care facilities. The Omnibus Budget Reconciliation Act of 1987 addressed this issue in the strengthening of residents' rights. Several nursing homes across the country have made significant progress in this endeavor.

Initiating a program for reduction or elimination of restraints is preceded by planning and forethought. It is truly an interdisciplinary project, requiring the cooperation of all staff.

Identifying Clients at Risk for Falling

Persons at risk for falling need to be identified at the time of admission. Clients with any of these problems may be at risk:
- disorientation, deficits in short-term memory, lack of judgment
- inability to follow simple directions and answer simple questions, impaired communication skills
- inability to use call light
- impaired mobility
- alterations in bowel or bladder control
- fluid deficit
- sensory and perceptual deficits
- medications affecting mental status

If the evaluation indicates that the client is at risk for falling, interventions need to be implemented that will either correct or compensate for the underlying risk factor.

AVOIDING THE NEED FOR RESTRAINTS

Attend to Physical and Psychosocial Needs

- Attend to unmet physiological needs promptly: thirst, hunger, sleep, rest, exercise, elimination.
- Correct underlying physiological problems: infections, dehydration, urinary retention, fecal impaction, hypoxia, blood sugar imbalance.
- Alert staff if client has taken a laxative or is on diuretics. Monitor client's reaction to other drugs affecting behavior.
- Provide measures to relieve fear and anxiety. Avoid situations that can trigger emotional outbursts. (See chapter 8.)
- Correct sensory deficits with glasses and hearing aids. Assist or teach the client to compensate for sensory or spatial-perceptual deficits. (See chapters 20 and 21.)
- Establish communication methods for the verbally impaired client. (See chapter 12.)
- Instruct client on slow transfer techniques and to obtain balance before transferring. Instruct client on the correct use of assistive ambulation devices and gaits.
- Plan varied activities appropriate for client's abilities and interests to avoid boredom.
- Give encouragement and positive reinforcement to client at every opportunity.

Clothing

- Instruct client to wear well-fitting shoes with nonslip soles. Shufflers need nonslip shoes that glide well on the floor. Avoid shoelaces if possible.
- Check pants for length and shorten if necessary. Check socks and nylons for proper fit. Instruct client to avoid ambulating in a long robe.

Environment

- Orient the client to the environment: unit and room number, location of call light, location of bathroom and telephone.
- Avoid an overstimulating environment to prevent agitation. Minimize noise and commotion. Television can be disorienting to clients who cannot distinguish between the television and reality.
- Provide bright, diffuse lighting without glare.
- Remove wheels on beds, chairs, and tables. Use wheelchairs for transport, not continued seating. Instruct client on safe wheelchair techniques. Keep bed in lowest position. Avoid moving furniture in the client's immediate environment.
- Set up strategically placed seating areas around the facility that are attractive and inviting so clients can sit down when they become fatigued.
- Provide safe, attractive, outdoor areas for walking and visiting. An area such as a courtyard offers freedom to wander.
- Maintain an obstacle-free environment. Wipe up spills and pick up items off the floor immediately.
- Install safety systems that alert staff if a wanderer goes outdoors.

Family

- Discuss with the family and client the facility philosophy regarding the use of restraints. Explain that the nonuse of restraints is a decision based on a consideration of independence and mobility versus the risk of incidents. Seek the family's support and cooperation to avoid the use of restraints. Discuss with the family the interventions that will be implemented to maintain the safety of the client.
- Seek assistance of families, friends, and volunteers to provide companionship to the client.

Staff and Administration

- Educate all staff in the rationale for a restraint-free environment and assist them to implement interventions to prevent falls.
- Consider flexible scheduling to maintain staffing levels high enough to meet clients' mental, physical, and psychosocial needs.
- Seek staff input from all departments in identifying and meeting the needs of all clients. Employees from all departments should be aware of which residents are at risk for falls. All employees must share the responsibility for monitoring clients at risk as the clients move about the building.
- Develop a facility protocol for a restraint-free environment and policies for the use of restraints in emergency or temporary situations. If a restraint is the only alternative, implement the following measures.

POLICIES FOR THE USE OF RESTRAINTS

- If all alternatives to the use of restraints have been ineffective and a restraint must be used, consider the use temporary.
- Assess the need for the device regularly and frequently. Use the least restrictive device. Apply any device only as recommended by the manufacturer.
- Clients with restraints need to be checked every thirty minutes. The device should be released at least every two hours. Exercise the client for ten minutes during this time. This can include walking the client to the bathroom. If the

client is nonambulatory, provide range-of-motion exercises. Clean incontinent clients and give skin care.

Documentation for the Use of Restraints

These items must be included in the client's medical record:
- ❏ A physician's order
- ❏ The date and time of application
- ❏ The type of restraint applied
- ❏ The conditions that justify the use of the restraint
- ❏ All alternatives that were tried first and why they were not effective
- ❏ The explanation given to the client
- ❏ The client's response after application of the restraint

LEVELS OF IMMOBILITY

A client's level of mobility may change throughout the day or from one day to the next. An individual may ambulate independently within a personal environment but require a cane, walker, or wheelchair for greater distances. Others find their abilities are greater in the morning than later in the day. For some, a disease such as arthritis may create fluctuations in ability from one day to the next. Wheelchair-bound clients are often able to transfer independently but are unable to walk.

Instruct the client to be aware of these changes and to adapt a personal routine accordingly. In long-term care or other group living facilities, the staff needs to be alerted to the changing needs of clients.

PROGRESSIVE MOBILIZATION

A stair-step approach is used to increase the client's mobility level and thus facilitate independence. The use of correct positioning techniques and passive range-of-motion exercises carried out twice daily helps prevent complications due to immobility. Each client's abilities should be evaluated and documented before implementing a mobility program. Not all clients need to start with the first step. For example, some may be able to move about in bed, but be unable to transfer independently. The first step of progressive mobilization is teaching the client to move independently in bed. This activity begins to increase strength and endurance. It encourages the client to progress to transfer techniques and then ambulation. Include interventions on the care plan that will maintain current abilities as well as build to the next level. Some clients will never reach the last step of independent ambulation. Again, continuing evaluation and setting very small goals will assist the client to reach an optimal level. In performing the following procedures, follow all principles of infection control, safety, and privacy. As the client gains skill and self-confidence, gradually decrease the amount of assistance.

Monitor the client during periods of activity. Take the resting pulse rate before initiating the activity. It is normal for the pulse to increase twenty beats per minute during mild exercise. With strenuous activity (climbing stairs, for example) the pulse may increase up to fifty beats more. The pulse should return to within ten beats of the resting pulse within two minutes after the activity has ceased. If this does not occur or if the pulse increases by more than what would be expected for the type of activity, stop the activity. Consult the physician and reevaluate the client (Wilson 1988). Monitor the client for other signs of intolerance, such as disorientation, shortness of breath, and chest pain.

It is imperative that all persons working with the client understand the mobility program. They need to know the client's goals and how these will be attained. The care plan should include specific instructions for the approach that will be used. Inexperienced staff or family members (for clients at home) may need a demonstration on how to carry out the procedures. They should be evaluated through a return demonstration before attempting to work with the client.

Back injuries are a major concern for individuals working with dependent, older adults. Many of these could be prevented with the use of appropriate body mechanics. Remind caregivers to always follow these basic rules.

1. Keep the back straight at all times.
2. Bend the knees, flex the hips, and assume a broad base of support.
3. Get as close as possible to the client.

MOVING THE CLIENT IN BED

Procedure: Moving the Dependent Client with a Turning Sheet

When the client is unable to move independently in bed, the staff needs to carry out this procedure in a safe manner. Using a turning sheet prevents friction and shearing between the skin and the sheets. It allows caregivers to utilize better body mechanics, reducing the risk of injury. Without the sheet, caregivers must use their arms and hands to move the client's body. This can cause the client much discomfort and places the caregivers at risk for back injuries.

Moving the Client Toward the Head of the Bed

1. Use a turning sheet long enough to extend from the client's shoulders to the knees and wide enough to enable the movers to get a secure hold on the sheet. A flat bed sheet can be used by folding it in half from top to bottom. Place it on the bed crosswise when the sheets are changed. Keep it wrinkle free and in place.
2. To move the client up in bed, one assistant is on each side of the bed. If the person is very heavy or lacks head control, a third and fourth person may be necessary. Move the pillow and place it against the headboard. Cross the client's arms over the chest or abdomen to reduce drag.
3. Roll the ends of the sheet toward the client until your hands touch the body. Use an overhand grasp for better control, with one hand at the level of the client's shoulders and the other at the hip.
4. To move the client up in bed, face the foot of the bed with your outer leg forward and your weight on this leg. Assuming this position allows you to utilize the stronger muscles of flexion instead of the weaker extensors.
5. Bend your knees, assume a wide base of support, and keep your back straight. On the count of three, shift weight to the back leg. At the same time, flex your elbows and move the client toward the head of the bed.

Moving the Client Toward the Foot of the Bed

1. To move the client down in bed reverse the procedure, with both care providers facing the head of the bed.

Moving the Client Toward the Side of the Bed

1. To move the client to the side of the bed, the person on the side to which the client is moved is doing most of the work. That person gives the signals to move.

2. First, move the client's legs to the side of the bed and cross the arms over the chest or abdomen. Roll the sheet as before.
3. The person on the side toward which the client will move places one foot forward with the weight on this foot. On the count of three, that person bends the knees, assumes a wide base of support, and pulls the sheet toward that side of the bed, while the other person guides the move.
4. The person on the other side of the bed assists the move by grasping the sheet and lifting it to avoid friction while the client is moved.

Procedure: Turning the Dependent Client with a Turning Sheet

Turning the Client to the Side

These directions are for moving the client onto the right side.

1. Move client to the left side of the bed with the turning sheet.
2. Place the client's right arm in a position of external rotation. Place the left arm over the client's abdomen and cross the left leg over the right leg. The person on the client's right side reaches across, grasps the turning sheet, and gently rolls the client onto the side.

Reverse the procedure to turn the client to the left side.

Turning the Client to the Prone Position

Most older adults prefer not to lie in the prone position or are unable to because of hip and knee flexion. For cognitively impaired clients, this position imposes the risk of suffocation. There are many benefits if it is deemed safe for a client. It relieves pressure sustained from supine and lateral positions and stretches the muscles used for walking. In some facilities, a physician's order is required for placing a dependent person in the prone position. Begin with a five- or ten-minute session, gradually increasing the time to twenty or thirty minutes, observing the client throughout the period. Provide caregivers with thorough instructions and supervision in this procedure before implementing it because of the potential risks involved.

The following directions describe how to move the client onto the left side and then over into the prone position.

1. Move the client down in bed so the heels are at the end of the mattress. When the client is turned, the feet will lie between the end of the bed and the mattress, preventing plantar flexion of the ankle. If there is no space for this, place a small pillow under the ankles after the client is turned.
2. Move the client to the right side of the bed, using the procedure described previously. Tuck the left arm, with palm up, under the hip.
3. Place the right arm at the client's side and cross the right leg over the left leg.
4. The person on the left side of the bed grasps the turning sheet as instructed previously. The person on the right side of the bed places one hand on the client's right hip and the other on the right arm.
5. On the count of three, the client is moved from the left side over onto the abdomen. Watch the client's arms throughout the procedure to avoid injury. Adjust the client's position.

POSITIONING

Positioning is a basic nursing skill, but the importance of the procedure is often overlooked. For the client with minimal independent movement, a positioning program can make a crucial difference in regaining mobility and preventing complications. The client's comfort is a major concern. To be dependent on others for all movement is frustrating and demeaning.

TABLE 3–2	**Principles of Positioning Dependent Clients**
	❑ Assess the client's condition for the presence of: — Contractures or other joint problems — Pressure ulcers — Loss of sensation in any part of the body — Vision or hearing impairments — Spasticity and paralysis — Indwelling catheter or other tubes — Impaired mental status — Amputation or missing body part ❑ Always strive for normal body alignment in bed and in the chair. ❑ Incorporate range-of-motion exercises into the positioning procedure. Do not use these exercises to replace regular range-of-motion exercises. ❑ Use a turning sheet to move the client in bed. This prevents friction and shearing. ❑ Avoid tight bedding over the toes. ❑ Provide adequate support for all extremities. ❑ Adapt positioning procedures to the individual's specific problems, needs, and wishes. ❑ It is generally advised to work against what the client's body tends to do. If spasticity flexes an extremity, position in extension. If a joint tends toward extension, flex the joint. ❑ Assess the client's comfort. ❑ Instruct staff on the purpose and correct use of supportive devices or special mattresses.

Use of Supportive Equipment

Footboards are not recommended in the presence of spasticity (Alexander 1990). Pressure on the plantar surface of the foot increases spasticity, which in turn increases the risk of contracture. A pillow may be placed between the feet and the foot of the bed. Avoiding pressure on the feet from the covers and doing range of motion at least twice a day will prevent contractures of the ankles. There are also several types of boots and splints available that may be worn in bed to maintain the feet in correct alignment.

Any equipment placed in the hand should promote functional position and preserve the movement of opposition. The habit of placing folded washcloths in the hand is detrimental as the rough surface increases spasticity. In the presence of a fixed contracture of the fingers, give special attention to the fingernails and cleanliness of the hand to prevent odors and infection. A thin, absorbent pad placed in the palm of the hand will absorb moisture. Functional resting splints promote normal hand position and prevent formation of contractures, Figure 3–35.

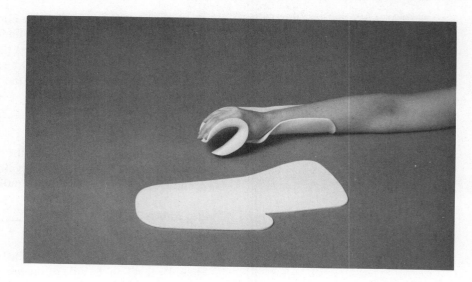

Figure 3–35 Functional position splint *(Provided by Fred Sammons Inc. © 1991 by Bissell Health Care Company)*

If hand rolls are used, they should be smooth, firm, and large enough to avoid complete finger flexion.

Use pillows, folded sheets, towels, and bath blankets as positioning devices to elevate extremities. (Additional information on specific positioning procedures is included in the chapters in section III).

In every step of progressive mobilization, monitor the client for signs of cardiovascular distress or other ill effects. Consider the client's ability and tolerance for bed movement and plan accordingly. Avoid carrying out several activities in a row if the client is easily fatigued. Performance may not always be consistent.

INDEPENDENT BED MOVEMENT

Procedure: Teaching the Client to Move Independently in Bed

Moving to the Head of the Bed

The next step is teaching the client to move independently in bed — up, down, and to the side. Once this is accomplished, the client can turn onto either side.

1. Raise both side rails and roll the bed flat. Fold the top covers to the foot of the bed, giving the client freedom to move. Remove the pillow and place it against the head of the bed.
2. Instruct the client to bend the knees and reach for the headboard with both arms. If there is insufficient range of motion available for this, the client can grasp the side rails at shoulder level.

Note: A trapeze may be used for this procedure. However, the consistent use of a trapeze for all bed activities may be detrimental because it does not promote conditioning of the triceps muscles. Strong triceps muscles will be needed when the client learns to push off the bed during transfer and standing activities.

3. Tell the client to push the feet into the bed and to push toward the head of the bed. Instruct the client with hemiplegia to place the affected arm over the abdomen to prevent dragging. You can support the affected leg while the client is moving.

4. As an alternative method, have the client slide the strong foot under the weak leg, moving the strong foot down under the ankle of the weak leg. The weak leg is resting on the strong one as the strong foot is used to push into the mattress.
5. Replace the pillow and complete the positioning procedure.

Moving to the Foot of the Bed

1. To move the client down in bed, the procedure is reversed, with the client's hands on the side rails at hip level. Instruct the client to flex the knees, pushing the feet into the bed and pulling toward the foot of the bed.

Moving to the Side of the Bed

1. To move to the side of the bed, instruct the client to grasp the side rail at shoulder level on the side of the move.
2. Tell the client to bend the knees and lift the hips off the bed and to the side of the move. Have the client move both legs to the same side and, while grasping the side rail, pull the shoulders to that side.
3. Instruct the client with hemiplegia to slide the strong foot under the ankle of the affected leg before moving the hips and legs. To move toward the affected side, the client will need to place the affected arm on the abdomen and use the strong arm to push the upper body toward the affected side.

Once these activities are accomplished, the client can learn to roll onto the side.

Rolling Onto the Left Side

1. Have the client move to the right side of the bed. Then instruct the client to cross the right leg over the left leg.
2. Tell the client to reach across the chest and grasp the left side rail with the right hand, pulling onto the side. The client with hemiplegia may need assistance when turning onto the strong side.
3. Reverse these steps for rolling onto the right side.

Provide the client with the assistance needed to avoid frustration and discouragement. Remember, the stairs of progressive mobilization are climbed one step at a time. Consult with the physical therapist to determine the need for additional bed exercises to strengthen and stretch the muscles. Teaching transfer techniques is the next step.

TRANSFER TECHNIQUES

In preparation for transferring, evaluate the client to determine existing abilities and readiness for this step. This information is used to select the most appropriate technique.

Determining the Method of Transfer

In preparation for transferring, evaluate the client's physiological condition, strength, and endurance. Test the ability to maintain trunk control and to bear weight on one or both legs. Consider the presence of paralysis in any limb, spasticity, or any condition causing unexpected, involuntary movement of the extremities. The client's height, weight, comprehension, and motivation also influence the selection of method. In the home setting, the number and abilities of the caregivers will also determine the type of transfer. Use the least dependent method possible, Figure 3–36.

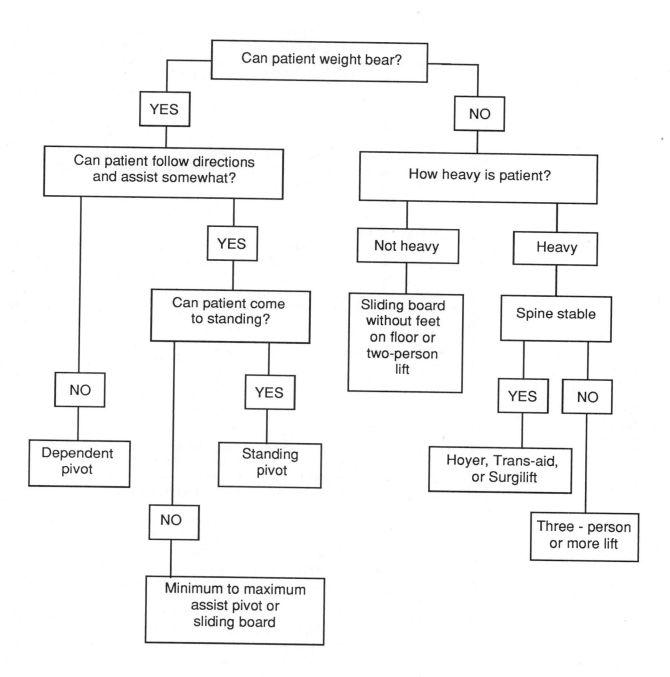

Figure 3–36 Steps for determining the best transfer method *(Reprinted, with permission, from C. Carlson, W. Griggs, and R. King, Rehabilitation Nursing Procedures Manual, page 40. © 1990 by Aspen Publishers, Inc.)*

Preparation for Transfer

In order to prepare the client for transfer activities, the client needs to develop tolerance for the standing position by gradually increasing upright activity. This can be accomplished by elevating the head of the bed, placing the bed in reverse Trendelenburg position at intervals, or using a tilt table.

Once this is achieved, have the client practice sitting on the edge of the bed. Weight should be even on both buttocks, with feet flat on the floor and shoes on. Stand in front of the client and assess static balance. Can the client maintain an upright position while sitting still on the edge of the bed? Evaluate the client's ability to move the arms up, down, and sideways. Then add resistance to check dynamic balance. With the client still sitting on the edge of the bed, use your hand to gently push the client to one side, to the back, or to the front. Protect the client by using your other hand and arm to stop the client in case balance is lost. Note the presence of spasticity or involuntary movements that may cause a sudden loss of balance. Consult with the physical therapist for additional exercises to facilitate balance, if necessary.

Consider any weight-bearing limitations due to hemiplegia, fractures, or contractures when selecting the appropriate transfer technique. A standing transfer requires weight-bearing ability in at least one leg.

When the transfer technique has been selected, give the client step-by-step instructions along with praise and encouragement. Even with minimal potential for ambulation, many individuals can be taught to successfully transfer independently in a safe manner. The wheelchair-bound person who can get in and out of bed or on and off the toilet without assistance experiences freedom and increased self-esteem.

Guidelines for Safe Transfers (Table 3–3)

TABLE 3–3

- ❏ Assess the client to determine the appropriate transfer technique.
- ❏ Explain the procedure and tell the client how to help.
- ❏ Place the bed in lowest position and lock the wheels.
- ❏ Place a transfer belt (gait belt) snugly around the client's waist for standing transfers.
- ❏ Never place your hands or arms under the client's shoulders. An elderly person's shoulders are frail. This practice can cause injury and pain.
- ❏ Never allow the client's hands to be placed on your body. If the client suddenly loses balance or is disoriented, the client can inadvertently grab your neck. This can cause you to lose your balance or could cause severe injury to your neck.
- ❏ Instruct the client to wear well-fitting shoes with nonskid soles. Make sure these are on correctly before attempting to move the client.
- ❏ Allow the client to sit on the edge of the bed for five minutes before standing to avoid orthostatic hypotension.
- ❏ Instruct the client before standing to separate the knees for a wide base of support, to lean forward ("nose over toes"), and to move the feet back.
- ❏ When possible, transfer to the client's stronger side.

Transfer Procedures

Procedure: Using a Transfer (Gait) Belt

A transfer belt is 1½" to 4" wide and 54" to 60" long. It is an assistive and safety device used to transfer clients from one surface to another. When used to ambulate clients, it is called a gait belt.

1. Explain the transfer or ambulation procedure to the client.
2. Explain that the belt is a safety device and will be removed as soon as the transfer is completed.
3. Always apply the belt over the client's clothing.
4. Apply the belt around the client's waist. Buckle the belt in front. Thread it through the teeth side first and place the belt through both openings to double lock.
5. Use an underhand grasp when holding the belt to provide greater safety.
6. The belt should be snug enough to just get your fingers underneath.
7. Check female clients to be sure the breasts are not under the belt.
8. Do not overuse the belt by pulling the client up and down with too much force.

The transfer belt may be contraindicated for a client with:

- ❑ a colostomy located in the upper abdomen
- ❑ an abdominal pacemaker
- ❑ recent abdominal surgery
- ❑ back or rib fractures
- ❑ advanced cardiac or lung disease
- ❑ abdominal aneurysm

Coming to a Sitting Position on the Edge of the Bed

Before transferring, the client has to get to a sitting position on the edge of the bed. Remind the client to use the skills that have been previously learned about moving in bed. Place the chair in position first, parallel to the bed at a slight angle, either at the foot or the head of the bed, moving to the client's stronger side. If you are using a wheelchair, put on the brakes and remove the foot pedals or move them out of the way.

Procedure: Sitting Position on the Edge of the Bed

These instructions are for getting out of the right side of the bed.

1. Roll the bed flat. Assist the client to put on shoes.
2. Instruct the client to move toward the right side of the bed. (Stand against the right side of the bed.) Have the client roll over onto the right side, flexing the knees and bending the right arm so it can be used for propping. Bend the elbow of the top arm so this hand can be used to push off the bed.
3. Instruct the client to use the elbow of the right arm to raise the upper body and to push with the hand of the left arm to raise up to an upright position.
4. At the same time, instruct the client to let the legs slide off the bed.
5. If assistance is needed, place one arm under the client's shoulders (not the neck) and one arm over and around the knees. Bring the legs off the bed at the same time the shoulders are being raised off the bed.
6. Allow the client to sit on the edge of the bed. Monitor for signs of intolerance. Stand in front of the client in case the client loses balance. The client's weight should be distributed equally on both buttocks, with the knees apart for a

broad base of support, feet flat on the floor, and arms at the sides. Always protect a paralyzed arm and prevent it from dangling during the transfer. Subluxation of the shoulder can occur in this manner. To avoid dangling, place the arm in a sling or place the hand in the client's pocket. If neither of these is possible, carefully tuck the client's fingers in the transfer belt until the client is seated.

7. Apply the transfer belt to the client's waist.
8. Proceed with a one- or two-person transfer as described below.

Pivot Transfers

Procedure: Two-Person Transfer with Transfer Belt

Individuals with moderate weight-bearing ability, general weakness, potential for sudden movement, or only moderate balance may need the assistance of two people for transfers.

Directions are given for transferring toward the client's right side.

1. Place the chair on the right side of the bed, parallel to the head of the bed. Remove the left arm of the wheelchair if possible. Remove or raise the foot pedals. Lock the wheels.
2. Complete pretransfer activities as described earlier.
3. The care providers stand one on each side of the client. Each one places the hand closer to the client through the belt with an underhand grasp in back of the client and the other hand in the belt in front of the client.
4. The care provider closer to the chair (on the client's right side) stands in a position to step or pivot around in a smooth manner to allow the client access to the chair. This person stands with the left leg further back than the right leg.
5. The other care provider uses the left knee to brace the client's weaker left leg. This person's right leg is further back than the left one.
6. Instruct the client to bend forward (nose over toes) and to place the palms of the hands on the edge of the mattress in order to "push off." The client's knees should be spread apart. Have the client put both feet back, with the stronger foot slightly in back of the weaker foot. The caregivers bend their knees, "squat," and assume a broad base of support.
7. On the count of three, the client stands. Tell the client to keep the head up. The caregivers help the client pivot by slowly and smoothly pivoting the feet, legs, and hips to the left. Allow the client to stand for a moment and bear weight (if not contraindicated).
8. To sit, have the client bend forward slightly, bend the knees, and lower into the chair. At the same time, the client reaches for the arms of the chair with both hands.
9. Remove the transfer belt.

Procedure: One-Person Transfer with Transfer Belt

This method is used for the person who can bear weight in one or both legs and has good trunk stability and adequate balance. Remember to provide only the help that is necessary. Instructions are given for moving toward the client's right side.

1. Follow instructions 1 and 2 above.
2. The client's hands should be grasping the edge of the bed. Bend your knees and assume a broad base of support. If the client has a weak leg, use your leg and foot to brace the weak foot and knee. Place your hands in the transfer belt as directed in Figure 3–37.

3. Instruct the client to bend forward and spread the knees apart. Both feet should be back, with the stronger foot slightly in back of the weaker foot.
4. Instruct the client to push off the bed on the count of three and to stand up as you provide the necessary assistance, Figure 3–38.

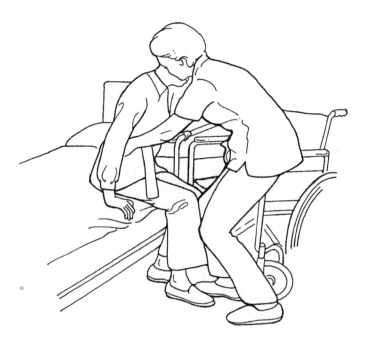

Figure 3–37 Step 1 — pivot transfer (*Adapted from* Transfers for Patients with Acute and Chronic Conditions, *P.T. Flaherty and S.J. Jurkovitch, 1970, used with permission, Sister Kenny Institute, Minneapolis, MN)*

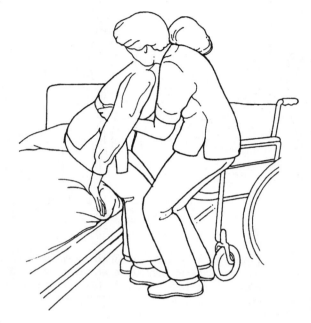

Figure 3–38 Step 2 — pivot transfer (*Adapted from* Transfers for Patients with Acute and Chronic Conditions, *P.T. Flaherty and S.J. Jurkovitch, 1970, used with permission, Sister Kenny Institute, Minneapolis, MN)*

5. Allow the client to remain standing for a time to give opportunity for weight bearing. Maintain your hands on the transfer belt and continue to brace the weak leg if necessary, Figure 3–39.
6. To complete the transfer, instruct the client to step or pivot around to stand in front of the chair. Tell the client to sit when the edge of the chair is touching the back of the legs.
7. To sit, have the client bend forward slightly, bend the knees, and lower into the chair. At the same time, the client reaches for the arms of the chair with both hands, Figure 3–40.
8. When the client is safely positioned in the chair, remove the transfer belt.

Procedure: Independent Transfer, Standby Assist

This method is appropriate for the person who has good balance, bears full weight on at least one leg, and comprehends instructions. Put a transfer belt on the client the first time this is attempted.

1. Follow the instructions for coming to a sitting position on the side of the bed. For an independent transfer, the client should be able to do this without help.
2. Now have the client place the stronger foot slightly in back of the other foot. The client's knees should be spread slightly apart.
3. Instruct the client to place the palms of the hands at the edge of the bed, and to lean slightly forward. Tell the client to press hands into the bed to push off at the same time the legs straighten to assume a standing position.

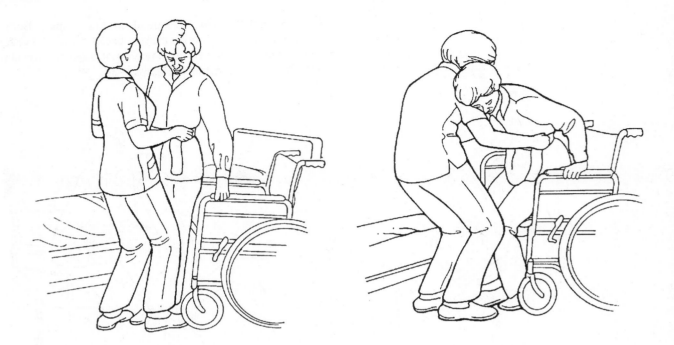

Figure 3–39 Step 3 — pivot transfer *(Adapted from* Transfers for Patients with Acute and Chronic Conditions, *P.T. Flaherty and S.J. Jurkovitch, 1970, used with permission, Sister Kenny Institute, Minneapolis, MN)*

Figure 3–40 Step 4 — pivot transfer *(Adapted from* Transfers for Patients with Acute and Chronic Conditions, *P.T. Flaherty and S.J. Jurkovitch, 1970, used with permission, Sister Kenny Institute, Minneapolis, MN)*

4. Once standing, have the client reach for the far arm of the chair and then step or pivot to stand in front of the chair. Instruct the client to sit when the edge of the seat is felt against the back of the legs.

Sliding-Board Transfers

This procedure is used for individuals who cannot bear weight; paraplegia and lower extremity amputation are two examples. Clients with good upper body strength can learn to perform this procedure independently. A sliding (transfer) board is constructed from ¾" lightweight pine wood. The size is usually 28" by 9". The ends are beveled on the top surface of the board. The board has a smooth finish and should be kept waxed (paste wax) to facilitate the client's move.

Procedure: Passive Transfer with Sliding Board

1. The client should wear slacks to avoid skin contact with the board. Keeping the board waxed facilitates the move.
2. For this method, you need a wheelchair with a removable side. Position the chair at a slight angle parallel to the bed. Lock the brakes. Apply the transfer belt around the client's waist.
3. Have the client sit up and move to the side of the bed. Place one end of the board, with beveled side up, under the client's buttocks. Place the other end of the board on the seat of the wheelchair.
4. Stand in front of the wheelchair and place both your hands through the transfer belt to give any needed assistance. Instruct the client to reach for the arm of the far side of the chair and to slide over the board into the chair using the other arm to push toward the chair, Figure 3–41.
5. Remove the board and transfer belt and replace the side of the wheelchair.

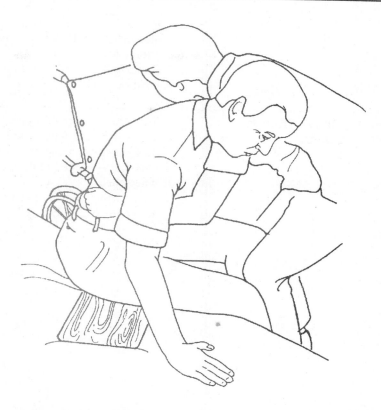

Figure 3–41 Passive transfer with sliding board (Adapted from Transfers for Patients with Acute and Chronic Conditions, P.T. Flaherty and S.J. Jurkovitch, 1970, used with permission, Sister Kenny Institute, Minneapolis, MN)

6. To return to bed, reverse the procedure.

Procedure: Passive Sliding-Board Transfer with Two Assistants

This method is used when the wheelchair does not have a removable side.

1. Place the chair against the bed, with the front edge of the chair seat against the edge of the bed. Lock the brakes.
2. Apply transfer belt to the client's waist. Have the client sit up in bed and turn to face the side opposite the wheelchair with the back toward the wheelchair. A third assistant may need to stand on that side of the bed to help the client assume this position.
3. Instruct the client to lean forward so that the end of the sliding board can be placed, beveled side up, under the buttocks.
4. Two care providers stand one on each side of the client's back, placing their outer knees on the bed, assuming a broad base of support and bending the other knee. With both hands in place on the transfer belt, count to three and slide the client backward into the chair. Instruct the client to use the hands to push against the bed to facilitate the move. If the client is unable to do this, the arms can be folded across the chest.
5. Remove the transfer belt and sliding board from under the client and adjust position as needed.
6. To return to bed, wheel the client up to the bed with the chair in position as before. Lift the client's legs while the other care provider places the board

in position. Place the other end of the board on the bed with the client's legs also on the bed. Care providers assume positions as described previously, sliding the client into bed.

7. Remove the board and transfer belt and assist the client to the appropriate position.

Procedure: Active Transfer with Sliding Board

1. This procedure requires a wheelchair with removable arms. Be sure the bed and wheelchair wheels are all locked. The sliding board bridges the gap between the bed and wheelchair.
2. One end is tucked under the client's buttocks and the other end is on the wheelchair.
3. Instruct the client to push up with the hands, shift the buttocks, and slide across the board, Figure 3–42.

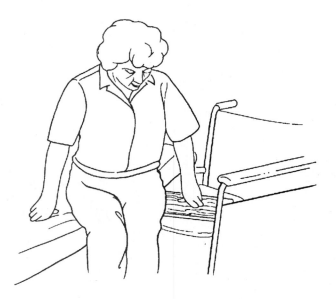

Figure 3–42 Active transfer with sliding board *(Adapted from Transfers for Patients with Acute and Chronic Conditions, P.T. Flaherty and S.J. Jurkovitch, 1970, used with permission, Sister Kenny Institute, Minneapolis, MN)*

Toilet Transfers

To toilet independently, the client must possess transfer skills, be able to manipulate clothing, and clean the genitals after using the toilet. Unless the client has full weight bearing on both legs and good balance, a wall rail is needed for support while transferring. Towel racks are not safe for this purpose.

Procedure: Toilet Transfer

1. Instruct the client to position the wheelchair at a right angle to the toilet to face the wall rail.
2. Teach the male client with slacks/pants to open the pants zipper while still seated. Tell the client to lean forward slightly with the stronger foot slightly behind the other foot and to come to a standing position by pushing off from the wheelchair, Figure 3–43.

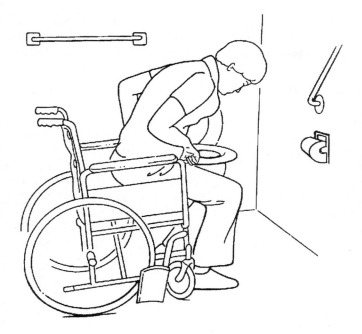

Figure 3–43 Transfer from wheelchair to toilet *(Adapted from* Transfers for Patients with Acute and Chronic Conditions, *P.T. Flaherty and S.J. Jurkovitch, 1970, used with permission, Sister Kenny Institute, Minneapolis, MN)*

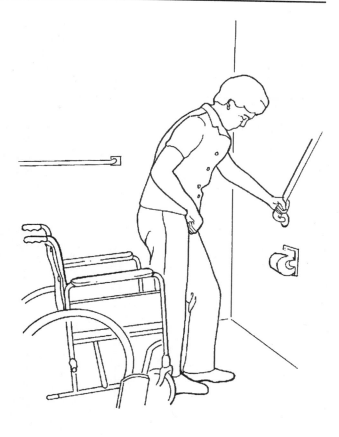

Figure 3–44 Instruct the client to use the grab bar to maintain balance. *(Adapted from* Transfers for Patients with Acute and Chronic Conditions, *P.T. Flaherty and S.J. Jurkovitch, 1970, used with permission, Sister Kenny Institute, Minneapolis, MN)*

3. While the client is standing and has one hand on the wall rail, tell him/her to use his/her other hand to open his/her pants, letting them fall to his/her knees, Figure 3–44. With one hand on the wall rail, he/she can pivot or step around until he/she feels the toilet against the back of his/her legs.

4. The female client in a dress or skirt pulls her panties down and then holds her dress up before sitting.

5. Place the toilet paper within reach. After the client has wiped the genital area, instruct the client to stand, reach for the wall rail, and then pull the pants/panties up. Adaptations in clothing can be made to allow for more independence since it is very difficult to manipulate buckles and buttons with one hand.

6. If the sink is close enough, the client can pivot or step to the sink to wash hands before sitting down in the wheelchair. Otherwise this step can be completed while seated.

Tub Transfers

In the institutional setting, a shower with chair or tub with hydraulic lift is available. If client discharge to home is contemplated, it is important to practice in a setting similar to what the client will be using at home. A rail on the wall beside the tub and slip-proof mats in the tub are needed to provide safety. Add water to the tub after the client has safely transferred, with cold water turned on first and off last. A hand-held shower attached to the faucet of the tub is safer and easier for self-bathing.

Procedure: Transferring into the Bathtub

1. Place a sturdy tub chair in the tub facing the faucets.
2. If the wheelchair does not have removable arms, it is safer to place another armless, sturdy chair parallel to the tub. Have the client transfer from the wheelchair to this chair and then into the tub.
3. Once the client is seated in the chair beside the tub, instruct the client to place the leg closer to the tub into the tub. If this is the weaker leg, the strong arm can be used to lift the leg over the side of the tub, Figure 3–45.
4. Tell the client to use the stronger arm to reach for the wall rail. Sliding across onto the tub chair, have the client bring the other leg over the side of the tub, Figure 3–46.

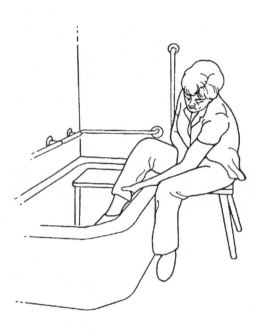

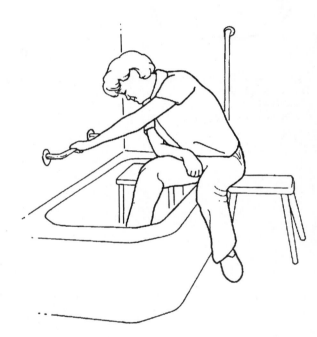

Figure 3–45 Instruct the client to transfer the affected leg into the tub first. *(Adapted from* Transfers for Patients with Acute and Chronic Conditions, *P.T. Flaherty and S.J. Jurkovitch, 1970, used with permission, Sister Kenny Institute, Minneapolis, MN)*

Figure 3–46 Instruct the client to grab the wall rail with the strong hand to transfer over onto the tub chair/bench. *(Adapted from* Transfers for Patients with Acute and Chronic Conditions, *P.T. Flaherty and S.J. Jurkovitch, 1970, used with permission, Sister Kenny Institute, Minneapolis, MN)*

Note: For this procedure, it is safer to have the weaker side toward the tub if possible. The strong arm can be brought around to the wall rail. When the client gets out of the tub, the strong side will be next to the outer chair, allowing the client to get the strong leg out of the tub and use the strong arm for support moving onto the chair. Then the client can use the strong arm to get the weaker leg out of the tub.

Car Transfers

Once the client can transfer independently or with minimal assistance, learning a car transfer opens up additional opportunities for socialization and change of environment. A two-door car makes the transfer easier because the door is wider, allowing more room for moving in and out of the car. With either a two-door or four-door car, the client should always transfer onto the front seat. The front door is usually wider and opens wider.

Procedure: Car Transfer

1. Place the wheelchair at a 45-degree angle, parallel to the car, with brakes set. Have the client come to a standing position in the usual manner.
2. If transferring to the stronger side, the back of the car seat can be used for support. If moving toward the weaker side, instruct the client to use the strong arm and the door with the window open for support. Another person should hold the door for stability.
3. Tell the client to pivot or step around so the side of the car seat is touching the back of the legs. After the client is seated, have the client raise one leg at a time into the car to face forward.
4. To get out of the car, reverse the procedure. Car seats are usually lower than other sitting surfaces. The client may need help in getting to a standing position.
5. A car transfer can be accomplished with the assistance of one person and use of a transfer belt if it is needed. For the client who cannot stand, a sliding board transfer can be used if the wheelchair has removable arms. After the board is in place, the client slides across onto the car seat and then places legs, one at a time, into the car, Figure 3–47. The board is then removed.

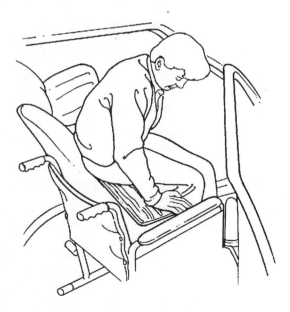

Figure 3–47 Transfer from wheelchair to car with sliding board *(Adapted from* Transfers for Patients with Acute and Chronic Conditions, *P.T. Flaherty and S.J. Jurkovitch, 1970, used with permission, Sister Kenny Institute, Minneapolis, MN)*

The client who is able to complete a standing transfer is now ready for the next step of progressive mobilization.

AMBULATION

Ambulation is the last step of progressive mobilization. Consider the following factors before initiating an ambulation program.

1. The client's tolerance to movement in bed
2. The client's ability to participate in active (as opposed to passive) exercise
3. The client's ability to safely transfer with minimal assistance
4. The client's ability to stand and bear weight
5. The client's strength, endurance, and balance should be evaluated
6. Determine if the client's cognitive state affects ambulatory ability
7. Will the client be able to walk alone or will the assistance of a person or equipment be needed?
8. Consult with the physician and physical therapist for the use of assistive devices and gait patterns. The therapist may prescribe the device and gait but the nursing staff is responsible for monitoring the client.

TABLE 3–4

Guidelines for Ambulation

❏ Instruct the client to wear well-fitting shoes with flat heels and nonslip soles.
❏ Use a transfer belt (gait belt) until the client exhibits consistent ability to maintain balance while ambulating. Stand behind the client on the affected side, with one hand on the transfer belt and the other hand near the shoulder.
❏ After the client has risen from the chair, have the client stand for a few minutes before walking, until balance is established. Instruct the client to look straight ahead, keeping the head up while walking.
❏ Use a well-lighted, dry, level walking surface free of litter and obstructions. The cognitively impaired client will do better in an area that is quiet and without distractions.
❏ Monitor the client throughout the procedure. Another assistant may need to walk behind with a wheelchair in case the client becomes dizzy or weak. Establish small goals, extending them gradually as the client is able to tolerate.

Normal Gait Pattern

There are two phases to a normal gait. The leg is on the floor during the stance phase and the leg is brought forward during the swing phase. Walking begins with the ankle in dorsiflexion and the heel striking the floor first, rolling onto the ball of the foot. The client must be able to stand straight on this leg while bringing the other leg forward. As walking occurs, the arms are normally in a slight swinging movement, each arm moving in the same direction as the opposite leg. To attain a normal gait, the client needs the ability to flex and extend the hips and knees, to slightly abduct the hips, and to push off onto the toes and balls of the feet (Wilson 1988). Strong quadriceps and gluteal muscles facilitate ambulation. The physical therapist can recommend specific exercises for strengthening. For the older adult, the use of an assistive device can be substituted for the inability to perform certain movements.

Assistive Devices

There are several types of devices that facilitate ambulation. These are selected according to the needs of the client and the cause of the impairment. Adjust the device to fit the client and inspect it for safety. The gait is determined by the client's abilities, the cause of the impairment, and the type of assistive device that is used.

Lifts are attached to the shoe worn on the stronger leg. This leg is longer than the weaker one, thus compensating for the functional longer length of the weaker leg. This leg can then swing past the strong leg to establish a more efficient movement (Wilson 1988).

An ankle-foot orthosis is a brace that is used when muscle weakness causes the toes to drag as the client walks. The brace stabilizes the ankle, preventing unwanted movements. Two types of short leg braces are available. One type is metal and is attached to the shoe. The other type is plastic and is molded to the shape of the client's calf, ankle, and foot. It fits over the sock, into the shoe, and under the pant leg. Either type is fitted and obtained through a certified orthotist. Orthoses compensate for but do not improve muscle strength, sensation, or coordination.

The knee immobilizer allows proper swing of the leg for the client who cannot maintain extension of the other knee during the stance phase. The immobilizer is considered a temporary device during early gait training (Wilson 1988).

There are a wide variety of canes, crutches, and walkers available to facilitate ambulation. All have rubber tips on the bottoms and rubber handgrips. Replace the tips if the ridges are cracked, loose, or worn down. If the ridges are filled with debris, use alcohol and cotton swabs to clean them. Replace handgrips when loose or cracked and check the axillary pads of crutches. Check screws, nuts, and bolts for tightness.

Standard wooden or steel adjustable axillary crutches are seldom recommended for older adults. They can be cumbersome to handle and require considerable balance and two strong arms. For situations when they are appropriate, the nurse may be responsible for fitting the crutches and providing gait training.

To measure for crutches, have the client stand, wearing the shoes that will be worn when walking with the crutches. Position the crutch tips two inches in front of and six inches to the side of the feet. The tops of the crutches should be about two to three finger widths below the axillae. To check placement of the handgrips, have the client grasp them. The elbows should be flexed about thirty degrees, with the wrists at the level of the hip joint.

Standard crutches are used for partial or no weight bearing on one foot, or general weakness of both legs. Any of the gaits can be used with standard crutches. Remind the client to support body weight on the hands and not the axillae. Tingling or numbness in the upper torso may indicate incorrect use of the crutches.

Metal forearm or Canadian crutches require upper extremity strength, trunk strength, and balance. In addition, there is no axillary bar to brace against the rib. The cuff of the crutch encloses the forearm so the client can release that hand without dropping the crutch. Correct measurement of handgrip placement is determined as with standard crutches. The cuff of the crutch should fit comfortably around the forearm. The distance from the handgrip to the top of the forearm cuff is determined by measuring from the fist to one inch above the elbow. Forearm crutches are used with general weakness of one or both legs with a four-point or two-point gait.

Forearm crutches with platforms permit weight bearing on the forearms, providing stability. During use, the elbows are in a constant ninety-degree angle to the shoulder. This may be a detriment to the use of forearm crutches with some clients. The client may need assistance in attaching the arm straps of the platforms. A four- or two-point gait is used.

Gaits to Use with Assistive Devices (Figure 3–48)

The client needs supervised, assisted practice before attempting to use any of these devices independently. Once the client has learned the appropriate gait and has gained self-confidence, supervise the independent use until you are sure the client can safely ambulate without your help.

Procedure: Crutch Gaits

1. Apply the gait belt (transfer belt) and stand in back and to the affected side of the client, with one hand in the belt and the other on the client's shoulder.

Instruct the client:

2. Stand with your weight distributed between both legs and the crutches.
3. Always advance the strongest leg first. If there is no difference, either leg may advance first. (Directions here are given for advancing the right leg first.)

Four-Point Gait

1. This is the slowest gait but one of the safest. It requires concentration to learn it correctly.
2. Apply the gait belt and assume your position.

Instruct the client:

3. Move the left crutch first, then the right leg. Then move the right crutch, then the left leg.
4. As you move, shift your weight so it is distributed evenly to both legs and the stationary crutch as the other crutch is moved.

Two-Point Gait

1. This is faster than the four-point but requires more balance since there are only two points in contact with the floor at any one time. The two-point gait resembles a normal walking gait.
2. Apply the gait belt and assume your position.

Instruct the client:

3. Move your right leg and left crutch together and then left leg and right crutch together.
4. As you move, shift your weight to the stationary crutch and leg as the other crutch and leg are moved.

Three-Point Gait: Non-Weight Bearing

1. This gait is used for lower extremity amputation before the prosthesis is applied, for a sprained ankle, or casted foot. Good balance, upper body strength, and one strong weight-bearing leg are required.
2. Apply the gait belt and assume your position.

CRUTCH GAITS

4 point gait

1 4 2 3

2 point gait

1 2 1

3 point partial weight bearing gait

1 2 1 1

swing to gait

1 2 2 1

swing through gait

1 2 2 1

2 point gait

1 2 1 2

CANE GAITS

3 point gait

1 3 2

2 point gait

1 2 1

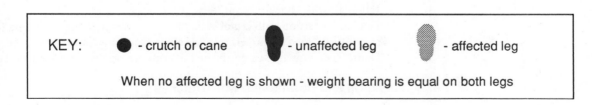

KEY: ● - crutch or cane ⬤ - unaffected leg ⬤ - affected leg

When no affected leg is shown - weight bearing is equal on both legs

Figure 3–48 Ambulation gaits to use with crutches and canes

Instruct the client:

3. Distribute your body weight evenly on the crutches and strong leg with your pelvis forward. Bend at the ankle rather than the hips so your balance is maintained.
4. Shift your weight to the strong leg and bring both crutches ahead four to six inches. Shift your weight onto the crutches and swing ahead with the strong leg so the foot is just behind the crutches.
5. Shift your weight to the strong leg and move the crutches ahead again.
6. Move both crutches, swing to the crutches with the strong leg, and move both crutches.

Three Point and One Gait: Partial Weight Bearing _____

1. This gait is recommended for use after a fracture or surgery of the hips or knees, for arthritis, or when the client is beginning to wear a prosthesis after an amputation.
2. Apply the gait belt and assume your position.

Instruct the client:

3. Distribute most of your body weight on the crutches and strong leg with some weight on your affected leg.
4. Shift your weight to the strong leg. Now move both crutches and your affected leg forward.
5. Shift most of your weight onto the crutches with partial weight on the affected leg. Step ahead with the strong leg.
6. Move both crutches and the involved leg and step through with strong leg.

Getting In and Out of a Chair with Crutches _____

Instruct the client:

1. Getting out of the chair: (if one leg is weaker or non-weight bearing) hold the crutches in one hand (at the handgrip), on your affected side.
2. Place the tips of the crutches on the floor, slightly ahead of and to the side of your feet, with the axillary bars away from your body.
3. While the one hand grasps the handgrip of the crutches, put your other hand on the chair arm or seat. Push off the chair to a standing position.
4. Remember, your stronger foot should be slightly behind the affected foot. Bending forward helps in getting up.
5. Take the outermost crutch and place it under your opposite arm and then turn the other crutch so it is in place under the other arm.
6. Sitting down: Approach the chair and turn or pivot so the front of the seat is felt against the back of your legs.
7. Hold and position both crutches as they were when getting up. Bend forward slightly and lower yourself into the chair, reaching for the arm or seat of the chair. Once you are seated, place the crutches on the floor next to the chair.

Going Up and Down Stairs with Crutches _____

1. A handrail and two assistants are recommended, with a gait belt on the client. One assistant stands on the step above, facing the client. The other assistant stands on the step below, facing the client with one hand through the transfer belt and the other hand on the rail. The assistants move with the client.

Instruct the client:

2. Going upstairs: Hold both crutches on your strong side under the axillae with your hand grasping both handgrips. Place your other hand on the rail.
3. Move your strong leg up to the first step. Then lift the crutches up to the first step. Then lift the weaker leg up to the same step.
4. Going downstairs: (the assistants position themselves in the same manner.)
5. Move the crutches down one step. Then bring the weaker leg down to the same step. Then move your strongest leg down.

There are several styles of canes, so choose the type that will best serve the needs of the client. For correct measurement, with the cane tip four inches to the side of the foot, the top of the cane should reach to the hip joint. In this position, the elbow should be flexed at a thirty-degree angle. If one side is stronger than the other, canes are generally held on the stronger side.

The walkcane has four legs and provides the most stability. It is often recommended for the client with balance problems or for persons with hemiplegia. These can be purchased with glider tips so the client can push the cane instead of lifting it.

Quad canes and tripod canes also provide a wide base of support and are used for clients with the same problems but who are less impaired than those requiring walkcanes. Pyramid canes are four-pronged devices with a broad base and are narrower at the top.

The single-prong cane with a T-handle or a J-handle has a straight handle with a handgrip and is easier to hold than the half-circle handled cane. Canes are recommended for improving balance rather than for providing support.

Procedure: Cane Gaits

Three-Point Gait

1. Place the gait belt on the client and position yourself slightly behind on the weaker side.

Instruct the client:

2. Hold the cane on your stronger side, with the tip about four inches to the side of the stronger foot. Your weight should be distributed evenly between your feet and the cane.
3. Shift your body weight to the strong leg and advance the cane about four inches.
4. Support your weight on the strong leg and the cane. Move the weak leg forward so it is even with the cane.
5. Shift your weight to the weak leg and the cane, moving the strong leg forward, ahead of the cane.

Two-Point Gait

1. Follow numbers 1 and 2 above.

Instruct the client:

2. Move the cane and weaker leg forward at the same time, while your weight is on the stronger leg.
3. Shift your weight to the weak leg and cane, and move the stronger leg forward.

Getting In and Out of a Chair with a Cane

Getting Up:

Instruct the client:

1. Hold the cane in your strong hand and use both hands to grasp the armrests of the chair.
2. Lean slightly forward and put your strong foot slightly forward. Push off against the armrests to a standing position.
3. Place the cane four inches to the side of your strong foot before beginning to walk.

Sitting Down:

Instruct the client:

1. Stand so the front of the chair seat touches the back of your legs.
2. Keep the cane in the strong hand. Reach back with both hands and grasp the armrests. Now lower yourself into the chair. Once you are seated, you can hook the cane over the back of the chair. (A multipronged cane can be placed on the floor beside the chair.)

Going Up and Down Stairs with a Cane

1. If the client has equal strength in both hands, follow directions for going up and down stairs with crutches.

The Person with Hemiplegia Going Up Stairs:

Instruct the client:

1. Stand with your strong side next to the handrail, with your feet about six inches apart.
2. Grasp the rail with your strong hand about four inches ahead of your body.
3. (Have the client hook the cane in a belt or place it over the affected arm if the arm can remain flexed. A broad-based cane can be placed on the step above as the client goes up and on the step below when going down.)
4. Continue to move the strong foot up and follow with the weaker foot.

Going Down:

1. Follow the same procedure, lowering the weak leg first and following with the strong leg.

Walkers also come in a variety of styles. Walkers are recommended for individuals who have general weakness of both legs, partial weight bearing on one leg, or mild balance problems. The client needs strength in both arms to pick up the walker. Select a walker that is wide enough to allow the client to walk into it. For proper fit, the elbow is flexed thirty degrees when the hands are on the handgrips and the top of the walker reaches the hip joint.

Gliding walkers have metal plates on the tips instead of rubber and can be pushed or slid. These are used for individuals who lose their balance when picking up a regular walker. Roller walkers have wheels on the front legs that lock when pressure is applied. Reciprocal walkers have a hinge mechanism, allowing one side to be advanced ahead of the other. This type is more stable than a stationary walker.

Most walkers are adjustable. There are many additional features available from most manufacturers.

Procedure: Walker Gaits

Reciprocal Walker: Two-Point Gait

1. Follow previous instructions for gait belt and assistant's position.

Instruct the client:

2. Stand with your weight evenly distributed between the walker and both legs.
3. Move the walker's right side and your left leg at the same time.
4. Now move the walker's left side and your right leg at the same time.

Reciprocal Walker: Four-Point Gait

1. Follow previous instructions for gait belt and assistant's position.

Instruct the client:

2. Move the right side of the walker forward, then your left foot. Then move the left side of walker, then your right foot.

Stationary Walker: Three-Point Gait: Non-Weight Bearing

1. Follow previous instructions for gait belt and assistant's position.

Instruct the client:

2. Shift your weight to the walker and your strong leg.
3. Shift your weight to the right leg as you lift and move the walker ahead about six to eight inches.
4. Now with your weight supported on the walker, swing your strong foot forward.

Stationary Walker: Three-Point Gait: Partial Weight Bearing

1. Follow previous instructions for gait belt and assistant's position.

Instruct the client:

2. Stand with the walker slightly in front of you. Shift your weight to the strong leg as you lift and move the walker and the weak leg six to eight inches ahead.
3. Now shift your weight to the weaker leg and the walker (with most of the weight on the walker).
4. Move your strong leg six to eight inches ahead.

Getting In and Out of a Chair with a Walker

Getting Up:

1. Position the walker in front of the chair.

Instruct the client:

2. Slide forward in the chair and sit with your strong foot slightly in back of the weaker foot.
3. Push off the seat or armrests with your hands and come to a standing position.

Support yourself with your strong leg and opposite hand. Grasp the walker with your other hand and then position both hands on the walker.

Sitting Down:

Instruct the client:

1. Stand in front of the chair with the front of the seat touching the back of your legs. Your weaker foot should be slightly off the floor. Place your weight on the strong leg.
2. Grasp the opposite armrest and then the armrest on your strong side. Lower yourself into the chair and slide back on the seat. You can then place the walker beside the chair.

Going up and down stairs with a walker is dangerous and not recommended.

USING A WHEELCHAIR

Staff, clients (if possible), and other caregivers should be familiar with the wheelchair, Figure 3–49.

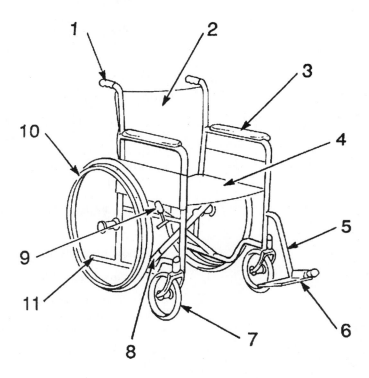

1. Handgrips/Push Handles
2. Back Upholstery
3. Armrests
4. Seat Upholstery
5. Front Rigging
6. Footplate
7. Casters
8. Crossbraces (Serial No.)
9. Wheel Locks
10. Wheel and Handrim
11. Tipping Lever

Figure 3–49 Wheelchair terminology *(Courtesy Everest and Jennings 1979)*

The options available for wheelchair selection are far too numerous to describe here. The reader is advised to research a manufacturer's catalogue for more specific details.

There are three basic sizes: standard adult, intermediate or junior, and child, with variations for each size. Outdoor wheelchairs can be used inside as well. Large wheels are in the rear. Tipping levers in the back help the assistant to balance the chair on the rear wheels when negotiating stairs, ramps, and curbs. It is easier to self-propel an outdoor wheelchair. Indoor wheelchairs have the large wheels in front. Because of this, lateral transfers are difficult or impossible. This style requires a smaller turning radius but is difficult to maneuver outside. The third style is the amputee wheelchair. The large wheels are set further back to compensate for the loss of forward weight.

There are choices for construction: standard, lightweight, active duty lightweight, or heavy duty. There are also many variations in seats, backs, arms, footrests, wheel types, handrim types, cushions, wheel lock types, caster types, and special use chairs. A multitude of accessories are available to meet the needs of the client. Power-driven wheelchairs provide more independence for the client who cannot self-propel a standard chair.

Fitting the Wheelchair to the Client

1. Assist the client to maintain body alignment and good position in the wheelchair so contractures and deformities are prevented. Measure the client so the wheelchair fits, checking the following points.
2. There are about four inches between the top of the back upholstery and the client's axillae.
3. The armrests support the arms without pushing the shoulders up or forcing them to hang.
4. There is a two- to three-inch clearance between the front edge of the seat and the back of the client's knee.
5. You can slide your hand between the client's hips on each side and the side of the wheelchair. The right amount of space avoids internal or external rotation of hips.
6. There are two inches between the bottom of the footrests and the floor.
7. The feet are at ninety-degree angles to the legs whether they are on the footrests or on the floor (when the footrests have been removed).

Wheelchair Safety

1. Instruct the client regarding safe use of the wheelchair. Place the casters in forward position for balance and stability. To do this, go forward and then back up so the casters swing to the forward position. Remind the client to keep the wheelchair locked when not moving. Remind the client to lift footrests out of the way when getting in or out of the wheelchair.
2. It is usually not a safe practice for the client in a wheelchair to attempt picking up an object off the floor. If there are satisfactory trunk stability and balance, the client may be taught to do so, but instruct client to
   ❏ remember to avoid shifting weight in the direction of the reach
   ❏ not move forward in the seat
   ❏ not reach down between the knees

The safest method is to position the chair alongside the object, with casters in the forward position. Lock the chair and reach only as far as the arm will extend (Safety and Handling 1983).

Note: The following procedures would rarely be implemented in a long-term care facility. However, clients may go out or be discharged, necessitating the use of these skills. The caregiver should be evaluated on the ability to carry them out.

Procedure: Tilting a Wheelchair Backward

1. This procedure is used for negotiating curbs, single steps, ramps, and doorsills. Do not use this procedure with an indoor wheelchair.
2. Before proceeding, make sure the client understands what you are doing. Check to see that arms, hands, fingers, and legs are in safe position. Use good body mechanics to avoid injury. Have an assistant with you the first few times you do this.
3. The purpose of the procedure is to rotate the wheelchair around the axles of the rear wheels until it reaches the balance point.
4. With your foot on the tipping lever, apply a pushing force down and under the chair while pulling back and down on the handgrips, Figure 3–50.
5. Tilt back until little or no effort is required to stabilize the chair. This is the balance point, about thirty degrees, Figure 3–51. You can now maneuver the chair on the rear wheels.

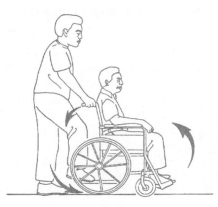

Figure 3–50 Tilting a wheelchair backward. *(Courtesy Everest and Jennings 1983)*

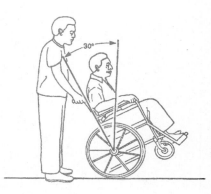

Figure 3–51 The wheelchair is at the balance point. *(Courtesy Everest and Jennings 1983)*

6. To return the wheelchair to the upright position, keep your foot on the tipping lever. Lower the chair, reversing the procedure. Do this slowly and smoothly and do not let the chair drop.

Procedure: Using Ramps and Inclines

1. The client goes up a ramp or incline facing forward, with the trunk slightly forward, with or without an attendant.
2. To go down, the client faces forward but does not lean forward.
3. It is safer if you help the client going down the ramp. Position yourself behind the chair, place it in balance position, and slowly move it down the ramp.
4. Keep your back straight and knees bent throughout the procedure.

Procedure: Manipulating Curbs

1. To go up, place the chair in balance position. Move forward until the front casters are on top of the curb and the rear wheels are touching the curb.

2. Lower the front of the chair to the sidewalk, making sure the wheelchair does not roll backward, Figure 3–52.

3. With your body close to the wheelchair, use one single smooth movement to lift the chair by the handles, rolling it up over the curb and pushing it forward, Figure 3–53.

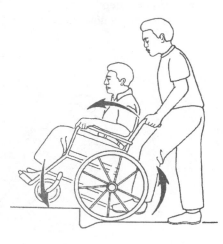

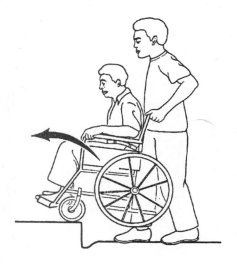

Figure 3–52 Move forward until the front casters pass over the curb and the rear wheels are in contact with the curb. *(Courtesy Everest and Jennings 1983)*

Figure 3–53 Use a lift-roll-push technique to move up onto the curb. *(Courtesy Everest and Jennings 1983)*

4. After the wheelchair is safely on the sidewalk, step up onto the curb.

5. To go down, turn the wheelchair around and pull it to the edge of the curb.

6. Stand below the curb and allow the large wheels to slowly roll down onto the lower level.

7. After the large wheels are on the lower level, tilt the chair to its balance point while lifting the front casters off the curb.

8. When the wheelchair is on the lower level, move backward until you can safely turn the chair around. A second assistant is needed if the curb or step is high.

Procedure: Going Up and Down Stairs

1. Attempt this procedure only if necessary and an elevator is not available. Never use a wheelchair on escalators. You need at least two people who are strong enough to carry the procedure out to its completion. Check the position of the client's extremities and inspect the handgrips for good fit on the chair.

2. To go upstairs, place the wheelchair in backward position, with the rear wheels touching the first step. The strongest assistant is at the rear of the chair, standing on the second step.

3. The assistant in front grasps the chair frame on either side of the client's lower legs, taking care not to grasp a removable part.

4. The rear assistant tilts the wheelchair to its balance point.

5. Working together, all assistants lift and roll the chair up onto the next step, keeping it at the balance point, moving themselves up with the chair.

6. This procedure is continued until the top step is reached.

7. With the chair still at the balance point, the rear assistant rolls the chair back until the assistant(s) in front are off the steps.

8. The rear assistant turns the chair around and gently returns it to the upright position.
9. To go downstairs, the front assistant(s) stands on the third step from the top.
10. The rear assistant tilts the chair to the balance point and rolls it to the edge of the top step. This person is in charge of the procedure.
11. With the front assistant firmly grasping the wheelchair frame, the chair is lowered one step by rolling the large wheels over the edge of the step. All assistants move down one step, Figure 3–54.

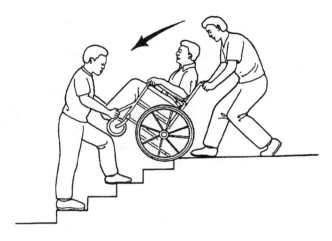

Figure 3–54 Moving a client in a wheelchair down the stairs
(Courtesy Everest and Jennings 1983)

12. Repeat the process until the chair reaches the bottom of the stairs. The rear assistant gently returns the wheelchair to the upright position.

Positioning the Dependent Client in a Wheelchair

The dependent person may slide down in the wheelchair, requiring assistance to regain body alignment. There are several procedures that can be implemented to correct the dependent client's position in the wheelchair.

Procedure 1:
Stand in front of the client and make sure the feet are in alignment and arms are on the armrests. Help the client lean forward and push with the hands and legs as you push against the client's knees.

Procedure 2:
For an alternate method, place a soft towel or small sheet under the client's buttocks and use this as a pull sheet to move the client up in the chair. This requires two people.

Procedure 3:
This method also requires two people. Place the transfer belt around the client's waist. One caregiver stands in back of the wheelchair and grasps the transfer belt with one hand on each side of the client. The other caregiver stands

in front of the client and places his/her hands and arms under the client's knees. On the count of three, this caregiver supports the lower extremities while the other one moves the client back in the chair. This is not recommended for a heavy client.

Procedure 4:

This method also requires two people. Stand in back of the wheelchair and have another caregiver in front of the client. Both caregivers work with knees and hips bent and back straight. Lean forward with your head over the client's shoulder. Instruct the client to fold the arms. Place your arms around the client's trunk. Grasp the client's right wrist with your left hand and grasp the client's left wrist with your right hand. The other caregiver encircles the client's knees with hands and arms. On the count of three, both caregivers lift and move the client up, Figure 3–55.

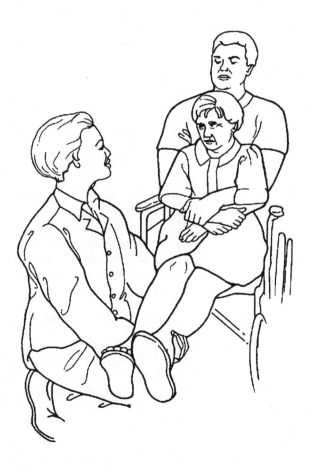

Figure 3–55 Repositioning a client in a wheelchair to maintain body alignment — Procedure #4 *(Courtesy Hegner and Caldwell, Nursing Assistant, 6th ed. [Albany, NY: Delmar Publishers Inc., 1992].)*

Procedure 5:

One person can do this procedure. The client needs to be oriented and able to follow directions. Stand in front of the client. Flex your knees and hips and keep your back straight. Position your feet one on each side of the client's feet. Brace your knees against the client's knees. Have the client lean forward. Lean forward over the client's right shoulder with the client's head under your right arm. Encircle your arms around the client's trunk. The client's arms are folded together, Figure 3–56.

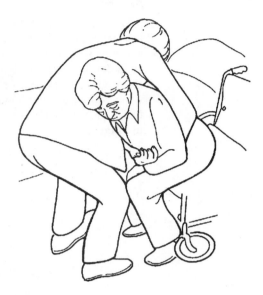

Figure 3–56 Repositioning a client in a wheelchair — Procedure #5.

Rock client forward and on the count of three, when client's weight is over the legs, push against the client's knees to move back in the chair.

If the client can bear weight, it is easier and more beneficial to assist the client to stand and then sit back down, getting the hips to the back of the chair. Wedge cushions placed in the wheelchair will prevent the client from sliding forward.

Wheelchair Activity

Pressure over the ischia is dramatically increased when the client is sitting. Teach the client (and provide assistance if necessary) to periodically relieve the pressure by shifting weight every fifteen minutes. *Be sure wheelchair is locked before beginning any of the following activities involving the client's movement in the chair.*

Procedure: Wheelchair Push-Ups	1. Teach the client to place one hand on each armrest, keeping both elbows bent.
	2. Then have the client lean forward slightly, pushing on the armrests and straightening the elbows while lifting the buttocks off the seat of the wheelchair. Have the client hold this position to the count of five if possible.
Procedure: Leaning	1. Teach the client who cannot do push-ups to place the hands on the armrests or thighs and lean forward slightly and then to each side to relieve pressure on buttocks. (Monitor the client with balance problems to avoid falling out of the chair.)

SUMMARY

Exercise and physical activity are basic human needs. Every client benefits from a program planned for the client's needs and capabilities. Many clients who have the potential for increased functional performance deserve to receive the assistance that is needed to reach their optimal performance. A consistent program of physical activity aids in preventing complications that diminish the quality of life for elderly clients. Improved physical performance brings with it improved self-esteem.

QUESTIONS AND DISCUSSION

1. What nursing interventions can you implement to prevent complications associated with inactivity?
2. Which clients in your care could benefit from an exercise trail?
3. For which of your clients would isometric or isotonic exercises be contraindicated?
4. Which factors would you consider before implementing transfer techniques for specific clients?
5. How would you select an appropriate assistive device and ambulatory gait?
6. Investigate differences in responsibilities for the occupational therapist, physical therapist, and professional nurse for implementing programs of progressive mobilization.

REFERENCES

Alexander, T.T. 1990. *Rehabilitation Nursing Procedures Manual*, 37–120. Rockville, MD: Aspen Publishers, Inc.

Benison, B. and M.O. Hogstel. 1986. Aging and Movement Therapy: Essential Interventions for the Immobile Elderly. *Journal of Gerontological Nursing* 12(12): 8–16.

Cooper, K.H. 1982. *The Aerobics Program for Total Well-Being*. New York: Bantam Books.

Department of Health and Human Services. 1991. *Federal Register*. Health Care Financing Administration.

Dwyer, B.J. and J.M. Bottomley, eds. 1988. Maintaining Strength and Flexibility in Elderly Clients. *Focus on Geriatric Care and Rehabilitation* 1(7): 2–3.

Harrison, W.L. 1988. Exercise for the Older Adult: Guidelines and Safety Precautions. *D.O.N.* (June): 32–36.

Johnson, B.J. 1990. The Hazards of Immobility. Effects on Cardiovascular Function. *American Journal of Nursing* 90(3): 44, 46.

Knight, D.B. and H. Scott. 1990. Contracture and Pressure Necrosis. *Ostomy/Wound Management* 26(January/February): 60–62, 65–67.

Loeper, J. 1985. *Range of Motion Exercises*. Minneapolis: Sister Kenny Institute.

Milde, F.K. 1988. Impaired Physical Mobility. *Journal of Gerontological Nursing* 14(3): 20–24.

National Institutes of Health. 1981. *Exercise and Your Heart*. Washington, DC.

Rankin, D.J. 1989. Intimacy and the Elderly. *Nursing Homes* 38(3): 10–14.

Safety and Handling. 1983. *Wheelchair Prescription Booklet No. 3*. Camarillo, CA: Everest & Jennings, Inc.

Special Committee on Aging, United States Senate. 1990. *Untie the Elderly: Quality Care Without Restraints*. Serial No. 101-H. Washington, DC: U.S. Government Printing Office.

Steinberg, F.U. 1988. In R.D. Sine, S.E. Liss, R.E. Roush, J.D. Holcomb, and G. Wilson, eds. *Basic Rehabilitation Techniques*. Rockville, MD: Aspen Publishers, Inc.

Strumpf, N.E., L.K. Evans, and D. Schwartz. 1990. Restraint-Free Care: From Dream to Reality. *Geriatric Nursing* 11(3): 122–124.

Talbot, D., V. Pearson, and J. Loeper. 1978. *Disuse Syndrome: The Preventable Disability*. Minneapolis: Sister Kenny Institute.

Thompson, L.F. 1990. The Hazards of Immobility. Effects on Respiratory Function. *American Journal of Nursing* 90(3): 47–48.

U.S. Congress. House. Conference Report. *Omnibus Budget Reconciliation Act of 1987*. Washington, DC: U.S. Government Printing Office. 100th Congress, 1st Session, Report 100–495.

Webster, J.A. 1988. Key to Healthy Aging: Exercise. *Journal of Gerontological Nursing* 14(12): 9–15.

Wilson, G.B. 1988. In R.D. Sine, S.E. Liss, R.E. Roush, J.D. Holcomb, and G. Wilson, eds. *Basic Rehabilitation Techniques*. Rockville, MD: Aspen Publishers, Inc.

SUGGESTED READINGS

Brians, L.K., K. Alexander, P. Grota, R.W.H. Chen, and V. Dumas. 1991. The Development of the RISK Tool for Fall Prevention. *Rehabilitation Nursing* 17(2): 67–69.

Coberg, A., D. Lynch, and B. Mavretish. 1991. Harnessing Ideas to Release Restraints. *Geriatric Nursing* 12(3): 133–134.

Cutchins, C.H. 1991. Blueprint for Restraint-Free Care. *American Journal of Nursing* 91(7): 36–42.

Gueldner, S.H. and J. Spradley. 1988. Outdoor Walking Lowers Fatigue. *Journal of Gerontological Nursing* 14(10): 6–12.

Houston, K. and H. Lach. 1991. Restraints: How Do You Score? *Geriatric Nursing* 11(5): 231–232.

Janelli, L.M. 1989. Physical Restraints: How Little We Know. *Nursing Homes* 38(1/2): 10–12.

Johnson, D. 1991. Make Your Own Chairbound Alternatives! *Geriatric Nursing* 12(1): 18–19.

Lewis, C.B. 1989. *Improving Mobility in Older Persons*. Rockville, MD: Aspen Publishers, Inc.

Loeper, J.M., N.A. Flinn, S.J. Irrgang, and M.M. Weightman. 1986. *Therapeutic Positioning and Skin Care*. Minneapolis: Sister Kenny Institute.

McHutchion, E. and J.M. Morse. 1989. Releasing Restraints: A Nursing Dilemma. *Journal of Gerontological Nursing* 15(2): 16–21.

Mion, L.C., S. Gregor, M. Buettner, D. Chwirchak, O. Lee, and W. Paras. 1989. Falls in the Rehabilitation Setting: Incidence and Characteristics. *Journal of Rehabilitation Nursing* 14(1): 17–21.

Neary, M.A., G. Kanski, L. Janelli, Y. Scherer, and N. North. 1991. Restraints as Nurse's Aides See Them. *Geriatric Nursing* 12(4): 191–192.

Rader, J. and M. Donius. 1991. Leveling Off Restraints. *Geriatric Nursing* 12(2): 71–73.

Rubin, M. 1988. The Physiology of Bedrest. *American Journal of Nursing* 88(1): 50–58.

Schilke, J.M. 1991. Slowing the Aging Process with Physical Activity. *Journal of Gerontological Nursing* 17(6): 4–8.

Wiest, M. 1990. The Dilemma of Using Physical Restraints. *Rehabilitation Nursing* 15(5): 267–268.

Woollacott, M.H., ed. 1990. Balance and Falls. *Topics In Geriatric Rehabilitation* 5(2): VII–VIII.

CHAPTER ▮4▮ Maintaining Skin Integrity

OBJECTIVES

- List the causes of pressure-ulcer formation.
- Identify clients at risk for pressure-ulcer formation.
- Describe the components of a preventive protocol for pressure-ulcer prevention.
- List and describe the stages of pressure-ulcer formation.
- Describe the treatment options for repair of pressure ulcers.
- Identify clients at risk for skin cancer.
- Demonstrate the technique of skin inspection for detection of skin cancer.
- Describe the nursing interventions for clients with herpes zoster.
- Identify situations in which other members of the interdisciplinary health care team may contribute to the planning of care for clients with impaired skin integrity.

DESCRIPTION OF THE PROBLEM

Skin care is a major concern for caregivers of the elderly. The aging process brings about changes that cause the skin to become fragile and prone to injury. (See chapter 2, "The Restorative Nursing Process.") Pressure ulcers are the major cause of impaired skin integrity in older adults. Five to ten percent of hospitalized patients suffer skin breakdown; $3.5 billion to $7 billion are spent annually in an attempt to prevent or heal pressure ulcers (Holmes, Macchiano, Jhangiani, Agarwal, and Savino 1987). According to assessment data on 4,951 nursing home residents, nearly 21 percent had pressure ulcers at the time of admission (Mor 1988). The elderly have a fourfold increased risk of death due to associated complications. The cost of nursing time increases up to 50 percent and the cost of treatment is $10,000 to $15,000 per ulcer (Klein, Boarine, Burton, Dobkin, Fowler, Halpin, Martinson, Rhodes, Schindler, and Thompson 1988).

What these figures do not reveal is the traumatic effect of skin breakdown on the client. Pain, immobility, and delayed progress are problems faced by client and caregivers. The cost of nursing time and treatment can be exorbitant. Wound infections, cellulitis, septicemia, and osteomyelitis are complications that result from pressure ulcers. In the elderly, these complications can cause death.

CAUSES OF PRESSURE ULCERS

There are four primary causes of pressure ulcers: pressure, friction, shearing, and moisture. Alteration in nutrition is also a significant factor in skin breakdown.

External pressure, particularly over bony prominences, causes capillary occlusion and prevents the flow of blood to and from tissue cells. The lack of oxygen and nutrients to the cells results in ischemia. Without intervention, cell necrosis occurs. Pressure ulcers develop most often over bony prominences subject to pressure from the bed or chair. Pressure can be induced by restraints, casts, traction devices, splints, orthoses, and tight clothing. Common locations of skin breakdown are the sacrum, trochanter, ischial tuberosity, spinous processes, scapula, lateral malleolus, heels, elbows, and occiput. Areas where two skin surfaces rub together also tend to break down readily.

Pressure greater than 35 mm Hg for one or two hours has been considered sufficient to cause ischemia. Recent studies indicate that higher pressures of 300–350 mm Hg are required to produce ischemia (Iverson-Carpenter 1988).

Shearing occurs when layers of tissue slide on each other. This happens when the head of the bed is raised and the client slides down in bed. The superficial fascia slides, but the sacral skin remains stationary due to the friction of the sheets. The subcutaneous blood vessels are twisted and distorted, preventing blood flow.

When two surfaces move across each other, friction is produced, causing disruption of epithelial cells and accelerating the process of ulceration. This can happen when the client is moved in the bed or chair without a turning sheet. Poor transfer techniques may also produce friction. The continuous presence of moisture from urine, feces, perspiration, or wound drainage results in skin maceration and thus is another causative factor.

Two studies (Iverson-Carpenter 1988) identified decreased body weight as the most effective predictor of skin breakdown. Another study of 232 nursing home patients found that 17 patients with pressure ulcers were classified as severely malnourished based on low serum albumin levels and reduced total lymphocyte count. None of the well-nourished had this problem. A cross-sectional survey of 634 hospitalized adult patients linked hypoalbuminemia due to malnutrition to the development of pressure ulcers (Holmes et al. 1987). Metabolic and cardiovascular diseases, peripheral vascular disease, fractures, fever, infection, stress, old age, edema, general weakness and debilitation, obesity, spasticity, and contractures are additional predisposing factors to impaired skin integrity.

ROUTINE SKIN CARE

1. Bathe the client once or twice weekly and give sponge baths twice daily. This avoids drying the skin. Use patting motions rather than rubbing to prevent tearing the skin.
2. Lubricate skin frequently with moisturizing lotion.
3. Do not use alcohol on the skin because of the drying effect. The use of powder is not recommended. It tends to cake and become abrasive, causing skin breakdown.
4. Give towel and lotion baths to clients in bed. Saturate towels with warm lotion and place over the body, one area at a time, gently patting.
5. Maintain oral fluid hydration and nutritional intake.

6. Advise staff to keep fingernails short and to avoid wearing jewelry.
7. Avoid using tape.
8. Use caution with parenteral injections.
9. Support client's extremities without twisting or grabbing.
10. Inspect skin daily over pressure areas, between the toes, in skin folds and under female breasts.

PRESSURE ULCERS: ASSESSMENT AND PREVENTIVE PROTOCOL

Inspect the client's skin thoroughly within an hour of admission or at the first home visit. Carefully document the size and description of any wounds, bruises, scars, or rashes. Take a photo (with the client's permission) of major skin impairments. This can be used for comparison as healing progresses. Complete a Pressure Ulcer Potential Assessment for all clients upon admission. This will identify those individuals who are at risk for pressure ulcers. Additional preventive measures can then be implemented.*

TABLE 4–1	Pressure Ulcer Potential Assessment*		
Date of Assessment:_____ Nurse: _____ Pressure ulcer present on admission: No _____ Yes _____ Stage _____			
A score of 11 through 20 is moderate risk. A score of 21 through 23 is high risk. Implement all preventive measures.			
	Activity		Total
	—Ambulant without assistance	0	
	—Ambulant with assistance	2	
	—Chairfast	4	
	—Bedfast	6	_____
	Mobility — Range of Motion		
	—Full range of motion	0	
	—Moves with minimal assistance	2	
	—Moves with moderate assistance	4	
	—Immobile	6	_____
	Skin Condition		
	—Hydrated and intact	0	
	—Rashes or abrasions	2	
	—Decreased turgor, dry	4	
	—Edema, erythema, pressure ulcers	6	_____
	Predisposing Disease Process		
	—No involvement	0	
	—Chronic, stable	1	
	—Acute or chronic, unstable	2	
	—Terminal	3	_____

Continues

---

* Adapted from Fowler, Evonne. 1985. Skin Care of Older Adults. *Journal of Gerontological Nursing* 2(November): 44.

Level of Consciousness —Alert —Slow verbal response —Responds to verbal or painful stimuli —Absence of response to stimuli	0 1 2 3	_____
Nutritional Status —Good (Eats 75% or more of required intake) —Fair (Eats less than 75% of required intake) —Poor (Minimal intake, consistent weight loss) —Unable/refuses to eat/drink, emaciated	0 1 2 3	_____
Incontinence—Bladder —None —Occasional (less than 2/24 hours) —Usually (more than 2/24 hours) —Total (no control) **Incontinence—Bowel** —None —Occasional (formed stool) —Usually (with semiformed stool) —Total (no control, loose stool)	0 1 2 3 0 1 2 3	_____ _____

Implement the preventive protocol for clients who receive a score indicating at risk status for pressure sore formation.

TABLE 4–2	Protocol for Clients at Risk for Pressure Ulcers
OBJECTIVE	INTERVENTIONS
Relieve pressure	❑ Establish positioning schedule. ❑ Place pressure-relieving mattresses, cushions on bed, chair. ❑ Teach client wheelchair exercises (See chapter 3). ❑ Stand and/or ambulate resident in chair frequently. ❑ Use wheelchair for transporting only. ❑ Allow resident to sit on bedpan, commode, or toilet for only brief periods. ❑ Check areas of pressure under casts, braces, splints, slings, prostheses.
Relieve friction and shearing	❑ Use turning sheet for positioning in bed and chair. ❑ Keep head of bed lower than thirty degrees unless contraindicated. ❑ Use supportive devices to prevent sliding in chairs. ❑ Use appropriate transfer techniques. ❑ Do not use powder on skin. ❑ Place bed cradle under top covers.
Prevent moisture/maceration	❑ Implement scheduled toileting or bladder retraining program. ❑ Use absorbent incontinent briefs or pads. ❑ Check incontinent clients frequently. Wash and rinse thoroughly. Apply moisture barrier. ❑ Avoid use of plastic/rubber sheets, protectors.
Prevent spasticity and contractures	❑ Avoid quick, rough movements. ❑ Do range-of-motion exercises at least twice daily.

Continues

	❏ Administer oral antispasmodics if ordered.
Maintain hydration/nutritional status	❏ Assess nutritional status. ❏ Investigate causes of anorexia. ❏ Correct underlying nutritional deficits. ❏ Encourage additional fluids unless contraindicated. ❏ Give high protein supplement if necessary. ❏ Monitor weight weekly.
	Continue with routine skin care. Do skin checks with each position change.

STAGES AND CLASSIFICATION OF PRESSURE ULCERS

Treatment of pressure ulcers is determined by the stage of the ulcer. Staging is a controversial issue and there is no one universally accepted method. The four-stage system described here is used in many health care settings.

In stage I, the skin is intact, warm, pink, red, or mottled. The skin blanches on touch and the redness does not disappear within fifteen minutes of pressure relief. The client with normal sensation will complain of pain in the area. While the skin is not yet broken in stage I, the underlying damage to tissue and blood vessels is already extensive. The ischemia caused by pressure results in edema and dilatation of the blood vessels. This causes the tissue layers between the skin layers and underlying bone to become thickened and distorted, Figure 4–1.

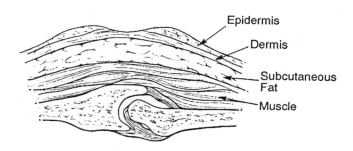

Figure 4–1   Stage 1 pressure ulcer

Stage II is a partial-thickness ulcer. There is a blister, crack, or superficial break in the epidermis. The surrounding skin is red or dusky. A partial-thickness ulcer is confined to the epidermal and dermal layers, Figure 4–2. The ulcer is painful because the nerve endings in the dermal layer are exposed.

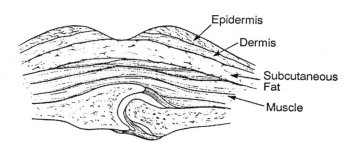

Figure 4–2   Stage 2 pressure ulcer

In stage III, the ulcer has progressed to a full-thickness skin ulcer. There is deep tissue involvement and exposure of subcutaneous tissue, Figure 4–3. Deep full-thickness wounds extend to the fascia. Exudate is usually present that may or may not be purulent. The ulcer margin may be red and indurated. Stage III pressure ulcers have the potential for becoming necrotic with formation of slough or eschar. Sinus tracts or undermining can occur. There is an increased risk of developing pressure ulcer-associated complications.

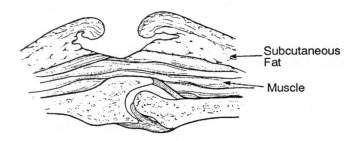

Figure 4–3   Stage 3 pressure ulcer

In stage IV, deep fascia is penetrated, exposing muscle and bone, Figure 4–4. Necrotic tissue and eschar are usually present with infection and drainage. The risk for complications is very high.

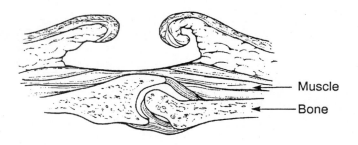

Figure 4–4   Stage 4 pressure ulcer

This staging system communicates only the depth of the ulcer. Referring to a pressure ulcer by stage does not necessarily indicate whether there is necrotic material or exudate present or whether the wound is granulating. Without any information about the actual wound status, it is difficult to select a treatment regime. A system has been developed by Marion Laboratories called the Three Color Concept. Wounds are classified by color (Moriarty 1988).

During the yellow stage, the tissue is soft and necrotic. Color of the wound ranges from ivory to yellow. Purulent drainage is usually present, indicating infection. Eschar, pus, fibrous material, and other cellular debris may be present in the black stage. In the red stage, ulcers range in color from pale pink to beefy red, and are revascularized, free of necrotic tissue, and ready to heal.

TREATMENT AND REPAIR OF PRESSURE ULCERS

Prompt healing of pressure ulcers is a priority issue in the client's plan of care. In the elderly client with health problems, a pressure ulcer is likely to develop into a chronic wound. It will never be fully healed, leaving the client continually at risk for associated complications. An enterostomal therapist should be consulted for unusual cases of skin impairment.

There are two body mechanisms for repair of tissue damage: regeneration and scar formation. In regeneration, the destroyed tissue is replaced with the same type of healthy tissue. The epidermis and most of the structures of the dermis can regenerate. Thus, partial-thickness wounds will heal by regeneration. There is no loss of function and little or no scar formation (Doughty 1990).

Scar tissue replaces destroyed tissue in the wound during the process of scar formation. Tissues unable to regenerate heal by scar formation. The subcutaneous, fascia, and muscle tissues of full-thickness wounds heal by this process. Scar tissue is much weaker than normal tissue. The area is thereafter more prone to breakdown (Doughty 1990).

Routine Nursing Interventions

Any treatment will be ineffective if the underlying causes for the pressure ulcer are not corrected. Continue with all preventive measures described in Table 4–1. A pressure ulcer cannot heal without adequate tissue perfusion.

The first concern is to keep the client off the pressure ulcer. Pressure-relieving interventions are described in Table 4–1.

Dehydration causes a decrease in blood volume and an increase in blood viscosity. This impedes tissue perfusion. Increase fluid intake to 2500–3000 ml unless it is contraindicated. Devise a schedule that will provide the client with a specific amount of fluids every waking hour.

Consult with the dietician for a nutritional assessment. (See chapter 5.) Wounds need adequate protein stores in order to heal. Adults need 45–55 grams of protein daily or 0.6 grams per kilogram of body weight. It is estimated that a draining pressure ulcer loses 30 grams of protein daily. This means clients with draining pressure ulcers would need to double their protein intake.

Continue with routine skin care and the preventive protocol. Use a cleansing solution on the ulcer that promotes healing. Normal saline is physiologically neutral and is nonirritating to healthy tissue. Lactated Ringer's solution contains electrolytes and is conducive to tissue growth. Use a gentle, flushing technique for cleansing. Vigorous irrigation or scrubbing may impede epithelialization. Whirlpool baths or irrigation with syringe and needle may be needed for infected or necrotic wounds.

Cleansing solutions used in the past have been found to be detrimental to the healing process. Hydrogen peroxide, povidone-iodine, acetic acid, and Dakin's solution are often irritating to the healthy skin surrounding the wound. New capillaries in the granulation tissue are disturbed and they are often toxic to fibroblasts. Epithelialization may be impeded and collagen synthesis impaired. Hydrogen peroxide can cause subcutaneous gas, leading to embolisms. Povidone-iodine has been noted in some cases to absorb through skin into the circulation, causing iodine uptake. This affects renal function (*Nursing 91*).

All pressure ulcers are contaminated but not all are infected. Monitor clients with pressure ulcers for clinical signs of infection: elevated temperature; elevated white blood cell count; copious, purulent, foul smelling drainage; erythema and induration of the wound (Van Rijswijk and Cuzzell 1991). Remember that older adults may not present with elevated temperature or elevated white blood cell count as readily as a younger person. Evidence of adjacent cellulitis, osteomyelitis, bacteremia, and sepsis requires the use of systemic antibiotics. Obtain an order for a culture and sensitivity so the physician can order the appropriate antibiotic medication. To collect the specimen, cleanse around the wound with normal saline to remove skin organisms that can contaminate the culture. Rotate the swab while wiping it along the wound edges. Avoid wiping over eschar. Send the specimen to the laboratory immediately (*Nursing 91*). The effectiveness of topical antibiotics is controversial.

Debridement

Tissue repair cannot begin if the wound is covered with eschar. Evaluate the wound for vascular status before debridement is initiated. Dry ischemic wounds may not have sufficient blood flow to support wound healing. After removal of the eschar, the open wound will likely become infected. If left dry, the necrotic tissue may come loose by itself, causing less tissue loss. There are four debridement procedures: surgical, mechanical, chemical, and autolytic.

Surgical debridement may be done with or without grafting. The procedure may include local excision, removal of bony prominences, split- or full-thickness grafting, transposition of muscle into ulcerated areas, and creation of rotational skin flaps (Keyes and Tenta 1987).

Mechanical debridement is accomplished with the application of wet-to-damp dressings. (Wet-to-dry dressings disrupt new granulation tissue when removed. Remove before they are dry.) This procedure may be beneficial only in ulcers where limited debridement is needed and there is minimal drainage. The use of normal saline and lactated Ringer's solution for the dressings will support cell formation. Soak 4" x 4" dressings in solution, wring out excess moisture, and apply to wound. Change the dressing every three to four hours. Apply a dry secondary dressing to absorb excess drainage. Use wet-to-damp dressings only until epithelialization begins. If dressings with wide mesh are used, the granulation tissue may extend between the mesh fibers and be damaged when the dressing is removed.

Chemical debridement requires the use of enzymatic agents. The necrotic wound debris is chemically digested and liquified. These agents may not be successful in penetrating thick eschar. Sutilains, streptokinase, collagenase, and fibrinolysin are examples of enzymatic agents. Follow the manufacturer's instructions explicitly. Many chemical debriding agents are inactivated by certain irrigation fluids and by soap and other products with hexachlorophene. Some experts recommend the use of chemical debridement only to supplement surgical debridement (*Nursing 91*).

Autolytic debridement requires the use of occlusive/semiocclusive dressings to create a moist environment. The body's white blood cells liquify the eschar and necrotic debris.

Topical Therapy

There are a variety of dressings available for the treatment of pressure ulcers. The effectiveness of any dressing is dependent on the faithful implementation of the procedures described earlier. Principles for healing require a moist environment, wound insulation, and protection from trauma and infection. Other factors in selecting a therapy include the need for debridement, the amount and type of drainage, and the presence of dead space. Selection of topical therapy should also take into consideration the stage of the pressure ulcer, the cost-effectiveness of the treatment, and reimbursement approval. Allow the therapy a reasonable length of time to bring about improvement of the wound before changing protocols.

Transparent dressings are also described as thin-film, semipermeable, or semiocclusive. They can be used on shallow abrasions, skin tears, and partial-thickness and shallow, full-thickness wounds with minimal exudate (*Nursing 91*). The dressings allow for exchange of oxygen and moisture vapor, but do not allow passage of fluid or bacteria. This decreases the incidence of secondary infection. Exudate forms from white blood cells and serum, bathing the wound, and providing a moist environment. The dressing is left in place up to seven days unless there are signs of maceration, infection, or leakage. The wound can be easily visualized through the transparent dressing. The hydrophobic surface of the dressings prevents contamination of the wound with stool and urine. The client can bathe or shower without disrupting the dressing (Doughty 1990).

Transparent dressings also have limitations. Because they are nonabsorptive, leakage occurs if they are used on wounds with heavy fluid accumulation. The dressings may not adhere when applied to moist areas. Removal of the dressing requires skill to avoid tearing the adjacent skin. Remove the dressing from the outer edges toward the center. Hold the skin firmly while gently peeling the dressing back.

Transparent pouch dressings are used in the same manner as regular transparent dressings. Pouch dressings have the capacity to contain larger amounts of drainage. The pouch receives the excess fluid, which then evaporates through the pouch film. To summarize the characteristics of transparent dressings: they debride by autolysis, protect from trauma and infection, insulate, and maintain a moist wound base.

Hydrocolloid collusive wafers contain hydroactive and absorptive particles. These interact with wound exudate to form a gel that promotes healing. The dressings can be used for partial-thickness wounds and shallow, full-thickness wounds (*Nursing 91*). Hydrocolloids provide moderate absorption while maintaining a moist wound surface. Necrotic tissue is liquified by autolysis. The outer layer is hydrophobic, preventing contamination and allowing the client to bathe without disturbing the dressing. The pores of the dressing are too small for bacteria to enter, thus decreasing the risk of secondary infection (Doughty 1990).

Hydrocolloid dressings are easy to apply, even to areas like the coccyx. However, they may tend to wrinkle, soften, and may become dislodged when applied to uneven surfaces. The wrinkles can cause pressure on the wound surface. Remove the dressing and apply a new one. Tape all sides of the dressing and check such areas frequently. Change hydrocolloid dressings when they leak or have an odor. They generally require removal every twenty-four to seventy-two hours (Fowler, Cuzzell, and Papen 1991). Removal of the dressing may leave a residue on the skin. Wash with soap and water to remove, but avoid scrubbing which would damage the skin. If the residue is not completely removed, leave it and cover with the new dressing. The residue will eventually wear off. These dressings are not appropriate for all pressure ulcers. They should not be used on wounds that are infected, have deep tracts, or have large amounts of drainage. Hydrocolloids are also contraindicated for wounds at risk for anaerobic bacterial infection. To summarize characteristics of hydrocolloid dressings: they debride by autolysis, are absorptive, insulate, protect from infection and trauma, and maintain a moist wound base.

Gel dressings are available in liquid gel, sheet, and granular forms. They are appropriate for partial-thickness wounds and to liquify necrotic tissue (*Nursing 91*). Sheet forms are occlusive if the plastic backing is left on one side and semiocclusive when both plastic backings are removed. For other forms, an additional occlusive dressing is necessary to protect the ulcer from bacteria and contaminants such as urine and stool. Gels are moist, soothing, moderately absorptive, and nonadhesive. They maintain a moist wound surface unless allowed to dry out. Liquid gels require frequent reapplication to avoid dehydration (Doughty 1990). To summarize characteristics of gels: they debride by autolysis, are absorptive, fill dead space, insulate, and protect from infection and trauma.

Polyurethane foam dressings are semipermeable wafers that contain hydroactive particles. They are used for partial-thickness and shallow, full-thickness wounds with minimal exudate (*Nursing 91*). The surface is hydrophobic. The dressings do not adhere to the wound or surrounding skin, so removal is atraumatic. To summarize the characteristics of polyurethane foam dressings: they are absorptive, protect from trauma and infection, insulate, and maintain moisture.

Dextranomers — absorption flakes, beads, and granules — are used only on draining wounds. They are designed to reduce edema and absorb exudate, odor, and bacteria. Depending on the brand, they may be applied dry, in a paste, or mixed to form a solution. The product is placed on the wound surface and covered with dressings. These products can be used on deep, draining wounds but are contraindicated in the presence of sinus tracts or bone involvement. The treatment is carried out one to four times a day. The wound must be thoroughly cleansed before reapplication, with all traces of previous applications removed. To summarize dextranomers: the procedure requires more frequent reapplication than many other treatments; the granules may be difficult to remove from deep wounds; they absorb large amounts of drainage.

Calcium alginate wound dressings are manufactured from seaweed. The sodium alginate in brown seaweed is converted into a nonwoven calcium alginate dressing. They are available as fibrous squares and as a long, loose packing. These dressings are used for exudating wounds. When the dressing comes in contact with the wound, it forms a gel. They are contraindicated for dry wounds or those needing debridement. Before application of the dressing, the wound needs to be irrigated with normal saline. The surrounding skin is dried and the dressing is applied to the moist wound surface. A secondary dressing is required to secure the calcium alginate dressing. Gauze or semipermeable film dressings can be used as the secondary dressing. The volume of exudate determines the frequency of dressing change. For heavily draining wounds, one or two changes may be needed daily. Before redressing, irrigate the wound with normal saline to remove remaining gel without damaging the healing tissue (Barnett and Odugbesan 1988). To summarize the characteristics of calcium alginate dressings: they absorb exudate, insulate, protect from trauma, and maintain a moist wound base. The dressing has no inherent antimicrobial properties.

PRESSURE-ULCER DOCUMENTATION

Document the treatment of pressure ulcers and the progression of healing accurately and consistently. There must be objective data to evaluate the wound status.

1. Use posterior and anterior body forms to indicate location of skin wound. Pictures may be taken throughout the healing process.
2. Type of wound: pressure ulcer, skin tear, stasis ulcer
3. Classification of wound using the accepted system of the facility or agency: the four stage method or color concept method
4. Size of wound: length, width, and depth using the standard for the facility, either inches or centimeters
5. The appearance of the wound and surrounding tissue: color, presence of inflammation or tunneling
6. Presence of drainage: description, type, odor, and amount
7. Presence of necrosis, eschar, thrombosis
8. Treatment used; solution used for cleaning or irrigation, type of topical medications, and type of dressing.
9. Implementation of preventive interventions

PREVENTION AND TREATMENT OF SKIN TEARS

10. Summary of client/family teaching

Skin tears are another major cause of skin impairment in older adults. The fragile, tissue paper-like skin can separate with little provocation. The lack of elasticity contributes to the problem. Skin tears frequently occur when the client moves unexpectedly as a caregiver is holding an extremity during a bath or other procedure. Prompt treatment will avoid further skin damage and the onset of infection.

1. Gently cleanse with sterile normal saline.
2. Smooth the undamaged skin flap and cover with a polyurethane film dressing.
3. Damaged skin flaps may need debridement.

(SEE ROUTINE SKIN CARE FOR PREVENTION OF SKIN TEARS.)

OTHER SKIN IMPAIRMENTS

Skin Cancer

Skin cancers account for 40 percent of all cancers. One out of every seven persons will develop skin cancer during his/her lifetime. About 90 percent of these are thought to be due to sun exposure (Lawler 1991). Individuals whose occupations and recreational activities expose them to the sun have an increased risk of developing skin cancer. Caucasians with red or blond hair, blue or green eyes, fair skin that burns or freckles easily, and a family history of skin cancer are also at risk (Maguire 1991).

Prevention of Skin Cancer.

The majority of skin cancers may be preventable. The American Cancer Society, Skin Cancer Foundation, and the American Academy of Dermatology recommend the following precautions.

1. Avoid sun exposure between 10:00 A.M. and 3:00 P.M. This is when ultraviolet rays are most intense.
2. Wear a hat and tightly woven protective clothing that covers the arms and legs. Wear sunglasses when exposed to the sun.
3. Apply a sunscreen with an SPF (Sun Protection Factor) of 15 or more before sun exposure. An SPF of 15 means that if it is properly applied, the user can stay in the sun fifteen times longer before burning than without a sunscreen. The recommended application is about 5½ teaspoons applied fifteen to thirty minutes before exposure to maximize effectiveness (Lawler 1991).
4. Avoid tanning parlors.
5. Photosensitivity may be a side effect of certain medications and cosmetics. Check with the physician or pharmacist if these products are being used.

Detection of Skin Cancers.

Skin cancers are easy to detect. It is recommended that skin self-examination be performed once a month after a shower or bath (Lawler 1991). The procedure may be difficult for elderly individuals with impaired vision and diminished joint flexibility. The nursing assistants in long-term care should be taught to thoroughly inspect the client's skin during the bathing procedure. In the home setting, family members or the home-health aide may do this.

Procedure: Skin Self-Examination

1. Make sure the room is well-lighted, and that nearby there are a full-length mirror, a hand-held mirror, a hand-held blow **dryer**, and two chairs or stools, Figure 4–5. Undress completely.

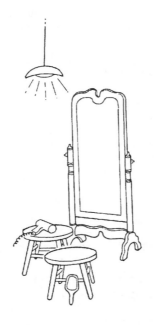

Figure 4–5   Step 1 *(Adapted, courtesy American Cancer Society, Inc.)*

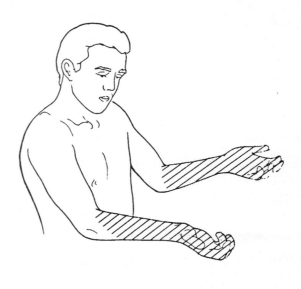

Figure 4–6   Step 2 *(Adapted, courtesy American Cancer Society, Inc.)*

2. Hold your hands with the palms face up, Figure 4–6. Look at your palms, fingers, spaces between the fingers, and forearms. Then turn your hands over and examine the backs of your hands, fingers, spaces between the fingers, fingernails, and forearms.
3. Now position yourself in front of the full-length mirror. Hold up your arms, bent at the elbows, with your palms facing you, Figure 4–7. In the mirror, look at the backs of your forearms and elbows.
4. Again using the full-length mirror, observe the entire front of your body, Figure 4–8. In turn, look at your face, neck, and arms. Turn your palms to face the mirror and look at your upper arms. Then look at your chest and abdomen, pubic area, thighs, and lower legs.
5. Still standing in front of the mirror, lift your arms over your head with the palms facing each other. Turn so that your right side is facing the mirror, Figure 4–9. Look at the entire side of your body — your hands and arms, underarms, sides of your trunk, thighs, and lower legs. Then turn, and repeat the process with your left side.
6. With your back toward the full-length mirror, look at your buttocks and the backs of your thighs and lower legs, Figure 4–10.
7. Now pick up the hand-held mirror. With your back still to the full-length mirror, examine the back of your neck, your back, and buttocks, Figure 4–11. Also examine the backs of your arms in this way. Some areas are hard to see, so you may find it helpful to ask your spouse or a friend to assist you.
8. Use the hand-held mirror and the full-length mirror to look at your scalp, Figure 4–12. Because the scalp is difficult to examine, also use a hand-held

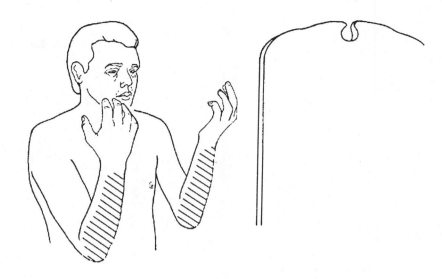

Figure 4–7 Step 3 *(Adapted, courtesy American Cancer Society, Inc.)*

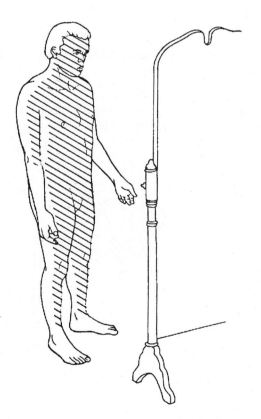

Figure 4–8 Step 4 *(Adapted, courtesy American Cancer Society, Inc.)*

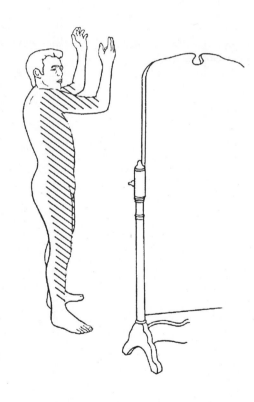

Figure 4–9 Step 5 *(Adapted, courtesy American Cancer Society, Inc.)*

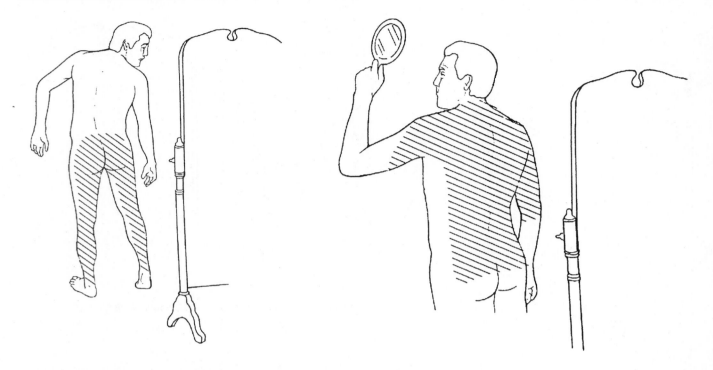

Figure 4–10 Step 6 *(Adapted, courtesy American Cancer Society, Inc.)*

Figure 4–11 Step 7 *(Adapted, courtesy American Cancer Society, Inc.)*

blow dryer turned to a cool setting to lift the hair from the scalp. You may wish to ask your spouse or a friend to assist you with this step.

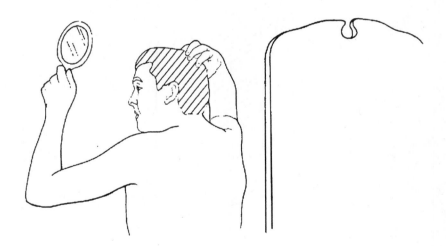

Figure 4–12 Step 8 *(Adapted, courtesy American Cancer Society, Inc.)*

9. Sit down and prop up one leg on a chair or stool in front of you, Figure 4–13. Using the hand-held mirror, examine the inside of the propped-up leg,

beginning at the groin area and moving the mirror down the leg to your foot. Repeat the procedure for your other leg.

10. Still sitting, cross one leg over the other. Use the hand-held mirror to examine the top of your foot, the toes, toenails, and spaces between the toes, Figure 4–14. Then look at the sole or bottom of your foot. Repeat the procedure for the other foot.

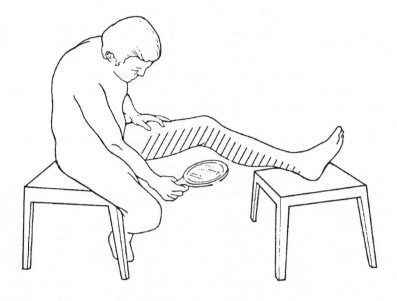

Figure 4–13 Step 9 *(Adapted, courtesy American Cancer Society, Inc.)*

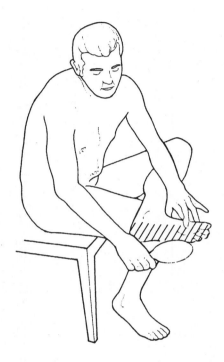

Figure 4–14 Step 10 *(Adapted, courtesy American Cancer Society, Inc.)*

Types of Skin Cancer.

There are three major types of skin cancer: basal cell carcinoma, squamous cell carcinoma, and malignant melanoma.

Two-thirds of skin cancers are diagnosed as basal cell carcinoma. This type occurs most frequently in middle-aged and elderly individuals. A lesion usually develops on sun-exposed areas of the body, with 80 percent found on the head and neck (Lawler 1991). The lesion appears as a red, scaly patch or as a nodule with an umbilicated, ulcerated center. Ulceration, pruritus, and bleeding are common. Ninety to 95 percent of basal cell carcinomas are cured when treated with surgery or radiation. These cancers are not usually life-threatening and metastasis is rare (Maguire 1991).

Squamous cell carcinomas usually form on sun-damaged skin or from preexisting skin lesions. Seventy-five percent of these skin cancers occur on the head. The appearance of the lesions varies. They may be slightly elevated, oval or circular, scaly, and keratotic. Others appear as a fungating mass. Seventy-five to 80 percent of squamous cell carcinomas are cured with surgery or radiation. Metastasis is rare; but lesions that invade the deep dermal layer may metastasize to the proximal lymph glands and to the lungs, bone, and brain (Maguire 1991).

Malignant melanoma can develop on any epithelial surface but is found most often on the skin. The incidence of melanoma has increased more than one-thousand times in the last fifty years. Melanoma develops in moles or nevi on the skin and is found primarily on the head and trunk of males and the extremities of females (Lawler 1991). In people of African heritage, melanoma tends to occur in less pigmented areas such as the palms of the hands and the soles of the feet.

Melanoma is detected by a change in color that may be dark brown, black, or red, white, and blue. The surface of the lesion is characterized by scaliness, erosion, ulceration, oozing, bleeding, and crusting. The size may enlarge suddenly or continuously and the shape develops an irregular margin. There may be itching, tenderness, or pain present (Friedman, Rigel, and Kopf 1990). Wide-excision surgery is the primary mode of treatment. Of all skin cancers, melanoma has the greatest potential for metastasis. The lymph nodes, skin, lung, brain, liver, and bones are common sites of metastasis. However, lesions less than 0.76 mm thick are almost 100 percent curable. With metastases, fewer than 20 percent live ten years or more (Maguire 1991).

Herpes Zoster

Herpes zoster (shingles) occurs when the dormant varicella (chicken pox) virus is reactivated in the body. After an infection of chicken pox during childhood, the virus becomes dormant within the spinal or cranial dorsal root ganglia. The reactivation may be triggered by a compromised immunologic state, chronic debilitation, acute illness, local trauma, stress, or the presence of lymphomas. After reactivation, the virus travels along the sensory nerve to the skin area innervated by that ganglia (Cuzzell 1990). Older adults are more likely to suffer from herpes zoster because of their diminishing immunologic response.

Severe pain, itching, and burning may precede the eruption of the rash by four or five days. The pain is often severe, unrelenting, and exhausting. The rash is unilateral, following the pathway of a nerve, and is usually localized to the thoracic and cervical regions. The rash begins with erythematous plaques and progresses to vesicles filled with clear fluid that becomes purulent. The rash continues to appear for five to seven days. The lesions break open with seeping and crusting. Healing occurs within ten to fourteen days with frequent residual scarring. In some cases, postherpetic pain can persist for months or years after the lesions have disappeared. The incidence of this neuralgia increases with the age of the client. Left untreated, herpes zoster can spread to systemic involvement of the lungs, liver, or central nervous system. Treatment is directed toward relief of pain, alleviation of itching, and prevention of infection. Analgesics are often ineffective in controlling pain. Alternative methods for pain relief, such as biofeedback, transcutaneous nerve stimulation (TENS), and antidepressants, may need to be investigated. Astringent compresses soften and loosen the crusts. Topical antimicrobial agents may be indicated if lesions are ulcerative or gangrenous to help prevent infection. Change the dressings every eight to twelve hours, cleansing the area with sterile saline before reapplication. The physician may order an antiviral medication. In older adults, oral prednisone given early in the course of the disease decreases the risk of postherpetic neuralgia (Thompson, McFarland, Hirsch, Tucker, and Bowers 1989). For localized infections, the Centers for Disease Control recommends the use of gloves for touching the lesion secretions until the lesions are crusted. The client should be placed in a private room if the client's personal hygiene is poor. In disseminated cases or for immunocompromised clients, a private room is always necessary. The use of masks, gowns, and gloves is recommended (Garner and Simmons 1984).

SUMMARY

Skin care of elderly clients is a priority for the nursing staff. The changes resulting from aging predispose the client to skin breakdown and subsequent infection.

The incidence of skin cancer is high among the general population. The risk for skin cancer increases with age. The nurse can assist in the prevention and early detection of skin cancers through teaching and skin inspection.

QUESTIONS AND DISCUSSION

1. How many of the clients in your care are at risk for the formation of a pressure ulcer?
2. What nursing interventions can you implement with your clients to prevent pressure ulcers?
3. Which treatment options are available in your facility or agency?
4. What are the advantages and disadvantages of each treatment option?
5. Which of your clients are at risk for skin cancer?
6. Can you develop a teaching program for prevention and detection of skin cancer?

REFERENCES

Barnett, A.H. and O. Odugbesan. 1988. Intensive Therapy and Clinical Monitoring. *Medical Tribune UK Ltd.* (May–June).

Coburn, L. 1990. Preventing Pressure Ulcers. *Nursing 90.* 20(12): 60–62, 63.

Cuzzell, J.Z. 1990. Derm Detective: Clues: Pain, Burning and Itching. *American Journal of Nursing* 90(7): 15–16.

Doughty, D. 1990. The Process of Wound Healing: A Nursing Perspective. *Progressions* 2(1): 3–5, 8–12.

Fowler, E., J.Z. Cuzzell, and J.C. Papen. 1991. Healing With Hydrocolloid. *American Journal of Nursing* 91(2): 63–64.

Friedman, R.J., D.S. Rigel, and A.W. Kopf. 1990. *Early Detection Of Malignant Melanoma: The Role of the Physician Examination and Self-Examination of the Skin.* Atlanta: American Cancer Society, Inc.

Garner and Simmons. 1984. *CDC Guidelines for Isolation Precautions in Hospitals.* Atlanta: Centers for Disease Control, U.S. Department of Health and Human Services.

Holmes, R., K. Macchiano, S.S. Jhangiani, N.R. Agarwal, and J.A. Savino. 1987. Nutrition Know-How: Combatting Pressure Sores — Nutritionally. *American Journal of Nursing* 87(10): 1301–3.

Iverson-Carpenter, M.S. 1988. Impaired Skin Integrity. *Journal of Gerontological Nursing* 14(3): 25–29.

Keyes, G.R. and L.T. Tenta. 1987. *The Pressure Sore Manual.* Springfield, IL Department of Public Aid.

Klein, L., J. Boarine, C. Burton, K. Dobkin, E. Fowler, J. Halpin, J.D. Martinson, W.M. Rhodes, S. Schindler, and G. Thompson. 1988. *Pressure Ulcers in the Nursing Home Patient: A Practical Nursing Reference.* Sugarland, TX: Dow Hickam, Inc.

Lawler, P.E. 1991. The Prevention of Skin Cancer: A Nursing Challenge. *Oncology Nurse Exchange* 13(2): 1–2.

Maguire, A.M. 1991. Skin Cancers. In S.B. Baird, M.G. Donehower, V.L. Stalsbroten, and T.B. Ades, eds. *A Cancer Source Book for Nurses.* 259–69. Atlanta: American Cancer Society, Inc.

Mor, V. 1988. One of Five Persons Admitted to Nursing Homes Have Decubitus Ulcers. *The Brown University Long-Term Care Letter* 1(2): 1–2.

Moriarty, M. 1988. How Color Can Clarify Wound Care. *RN* 51(9): 49–54.

Thompson, J.M., G.K. McFarland, J.E. Hirsch, S.M. Tucker, and A.C. Bowers. 1989. *Mosby's Manual of Clinical Nursing.* 2d ed. St. Louis: C.V. Mosby Co.

Van Rijswijk, L. and J.Z. Cuzzell. 1991. Managing Full-Thickness Wounds. *American Journal of Nursing* 91(6): 18, 22.

SUGGESTED READINGS

Wound Care Update 91. *Nursing 91* 21(4): 47–50.

Cuzzell, J.Z. 1990. Trial and Error Yields to Knowledge. *American Journal of Nursing* 90(10): 53–54, 58–60.

Dimant, J. and M.E. Francis. 1988. Pressure Sore Prevention and Management. *Journal of Gerontological Nursing* 14(8): 18–25.

French, E. and K. Ledwell-Sifner. 1991. A Method for Consistent Documentation of Pressure Sores. *Rehabilitation Nursing* 16(4): 204–7.

Jahnigen, D. 1988. Pressure Sores: Etiology and Management. *Clinical Report on Aging* 2(4): 14–15.

Jester, J. and V. Weaver. 1990. A Report of Clinical Investigation of Various Tissue Support Surfaces. *Ostomy/Wound Management* 26(January–February): 39–45.

Knight, D.B. and H. Scott. 1990. Contracture and Pressure Necrosis. *Ostomy/Wound Management* 26(January–February): 60–62, 65.

Krasner, D. 1990. *Chronic Wound Care: A Clinical Source Book for Healthcare Professionals*. King of Prussia, PA: Health Management Publications, Inc.

Payne, R.L. and M.L. Martin. 1990. Epidemiology and Management of Skin Tears in Older Adults. *Ostomy/Wound Management* 26(January–February): 26–37.

Tenpas, D.M. 1990. Multidisciplinary Team Approach to Skin Care. *Ostomy/Wound Management* 26(January–February): 50–52, 56–58.

CHAPTER ■5■ Alterations in Nutrition

OBJECTIVES

❑ Identify the components of a nutritional assessment.
❑ List the factors that may influence food choices.
❑ Describe the possible causes and nursing interventions for inadequate food ingestion.
❑ Identify the signs of impaired swallowing.
❑ Describe how to feed a client with impaired swallowing.
❑ List the signs and symptoms of dehydration.
❑ Describe interventions to prevent dehydration.
❑ Implement the nursing care related to enteral feedings.
❑ Identify responsibilities of other interdisciplinary health care team members for maintaining adequate nutrition in elderly clients.

NUTRITION AND THE ELDERLY

Food sustains and is a source of pleasure, often serving as the focal point for social gatherings and business affairs. Cultural heritage, religious rites, ethnic practices, and family traditions are linked with food, its preparation, serving, and consumption. For the disabled older adult, eating can be a complicated matter. The 1988 Surgeon General's Report on Nutrition and Health indicates that three million of the country's elderly residing in the community require assistance with basic activities related to food consumption, such as shopping, meal preparation, or eating. Three-fourths of the elderly receiving home care require therapeutic diets. Government programs have been in place for many years in an attempt to improve and maintain the nutritional status of the elderly. The Administration on Aging established the Nutrition Program for the Elderly in 1973 to expand food and nutrition services to include communities and homes, as well as hospitals. The Congregate Meals program serves two million people and the Home-Delivered Meals program serves one-half million people. The Food Stamp Program, under the auspices of the United States Department of Agriculture, serves qualified people of all ages, including two million older adults (United States Government 1988).

The physiological, psychological, sociological, and economic changes of aging often compromise the nutritional status of older adults. These changes can interrupt or interfere with any stage of the nutritional processes of ingestion, digestion, and absorption. Chronic disease processes and medications can also interfere with the body's absorption and utilization of nutrients.

There is a lack of available data on nutritional requirements and recommended intakes for older adults. Present standards for adults over age fifty are for the most part identical to those for ages twenty-three to fifty. These standards fail to consider the great heterogeneity of adults whose ages may differ by as much as fifty years. The dietary needs of healthy, active, older adults do not differ greatly from those for younger people. However, many older adults are neither healthy nor active. Current recommended dietary allowances (RDA) can be used in the absence of more specific guidelines, but the caloric requirement for individuals over age seventy-five is reduced to 75–80 percent of that of young adults. Dietary guidelines recommend two to four servings daily of fruit, three to five servings of vegetables, two to three servings of dairy products, two to three servings of meat, and six to eleven servings of grains. No more than 30 percent of the daily calories should come from fat (Hallfrisch 1991). The elderly require a balanced daily intake of vitamins, minerals, water, carbohydrates, fat, and slightly increased amounts of protein. For the disabled client, one of the basic and most challenging nursing responsibilities is assisting the client to maintain adequate nutritional status.

NUTRITIONAL ASSESSMENT

Nutritional care and evaluation are an interdisciplinary responsibility, requiring the services of the nutritionist or dietician. Consultation with the pharmacist for information regarding the impact of specific drugs on food utilization may be necessary. The speech pathologist can make a swallowing evaluation and suggest interventions for swallowing disorders. Exercises and activities to facilitate self-feeding are prescribed by the occupational therapist. Because the condition of the mouth greatly influences eating habits and abilities, the dentist and dental hygienist are also important members of the team. Assessment of nutritional status upon admission to the health care system detects existing deficiencies and provides opportunity for early intervention. Complications related to altered nutrition can be avoided and recuperative abilities enhanced. There are several components to a complete nutritional assessment, including anthropometric, hematologic, and biochemical measurements; a review of socioeconomic status; and evaluation of functional or physical impairments. The procedure can be adapted to serve the individual needs of each client.

Observation of Physical Appearance

The cells of the skin, hair, and gastrointestinal tracts are replaced most rapidly. Signs of altered nutritional status will be reflected in these areas first. Many of the signs are nonspecific and by themselves do not provide conclusive answers.

TABLE 5–1	Signs of Possible Undernutrition
Hair	Sparse, dull, dry, thin, straight, easily plucked; uneven color
Face	Loss of color, scaling around nostrils; dark areas on cheeks, under eyes; parotid glands enlarged; facial edema
Eyes	Dull; membranes dry, pale, or inflamed; inflamed ring around cornea; xanthelasma around eyes; triangular, gray spots on conjunctivae; corners of eyelids inflamed, fissured
Lips	Red, swollen; fissures at corner of mouth
Tongue	Swollen, smooth; scarlet or purple color; sores or abnormal papillae
Gums	Spongy, bleeding
Teeth	Cavities; discolored; teeth missing or erupting abnormally
Neck	Thyroid gland swollen
Skin	Lack of subcutaneous fat; dry, flaky, hyperpigmentation; tight, drawn, cutaneous flushing, petechiae
Nails	Brittle, ridged, spoon-shaped
Musculoskeletal	Muscles weak, wasted; legs out of alignment, joints swollen, nodules on ribs
Nervous system	Irritability, disorientation; complaints of tingling of hands, feet; loss of proprioception; diminished ankle, knee reflexes
Cardiovascular	Rapid, irregular heart rate, enlarged heart; hypertension; enlarged spleen

(Cataldo and Whitney 1986)

Anthropometric Measurements

Anthropometric measurements are physical measurements that reflect the individual's growth and development. They are not difficult to take, but practice and skill are necessary to obtain accurate, useable results. The reader is referred to a text on nutrition for further information on norms for these measurements.

The use of anthropometric measurements for evaluating body composition in the elderly is controversial because of the changes of body fat distribution during aging. The information derived from the measurements is useful when considered with all other aspects of the assessment.

The triceps skin fold (TSF) measurement is obtained with skin fold calipers and estimates the amount of subcutaneous body fat. This information is useful in predicting risk for pressure sores. The measurement is taken with the client lying on the right side. The trunk should be straight, with knees flexed and left arm resting along the trunk. First locate the point midway between the tip of the acromion and the olecranon. Pinch a fold of skin and subcutaneous fat about one centimeter above the midpoint and apply the calipers over the fatfold at the midpoint, Figure 5–1. Read the measurement to the nearest 1.0 mm (Chumlea, Roche, and Mukherjee 1987).

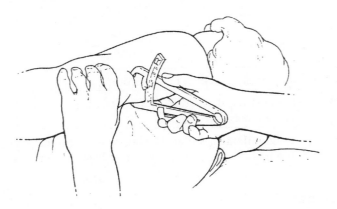

Figure 5–1 Triceps skin fold measurement *(Adapted, with permission, courtesy Ross Laboratories, Columbus, OH 43216)*

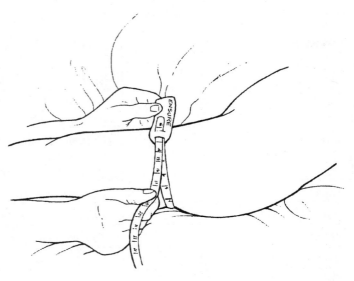

Figure 5–2 Midarm circumference *(Adapted, with permission, courtesy Ross Laboratories, Columbus, OH 43216)*

The midarm circumference (MAC) is an index of the arm's total area. Using the nondominant arm, have the client lie in the supine position. Flex the client's elbow to ninety degrees with the hand across the stomach. Measure from the acromion to the olecranon and divide the measurement by two. Mark this spot and, with the client's arm hanging loosely at the side, measure the arm at midpoint to obtain the midarm circumference (Chumlea, et al. 1987), Figure 5–2.

Midarm muscle circumference correlates with total body muscle mass and reflects the caloric adequacy of the client's previous diet. The midarm muscle circumference (MAMC) is calculated:

$$MAMC = MAC - (3.14 \times TSF)$$

(Hargrave 1979).

Height and Weight

Height and weight measurements also provide useful assessment data. It is sometimes difficult to obtain an accurate height measurement on an elderly client. If the client is unable to stand or has structural deformities such as kyphosis, the measurement for knee height can be used to approximate height. A triangle, Figure 5–3, and caliper, Figure 5–4, are required for the measurement (Chumlea, et al. 1987).

To measure knee height, have the client lie in the supine position with left knee and ankle each bent at a ninety-degree angle. Place the fixed blade of the caliper under the heel of the left foot. Place the movable blade on top of client's thigh, at least two inches behind the kneecap. From the side of the calf, make sure the shaft of the caliper passes over the anklebone and just behind the head of the fibula. Hold the shaft of the caliper parallel to the shaft of the lower leg. Apply pressure to compress tissue, and take the measurement. Record measurement to nearest 0.1 cm. Repeated measurements should agree within 0.5 cm. Use knee height with other data or anthropometric measurements to compute stature or weight. Compare computed measurement with previous measurements (actual

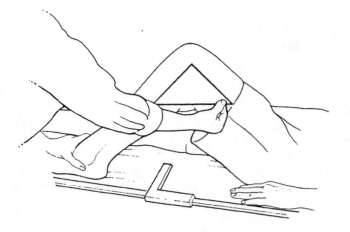

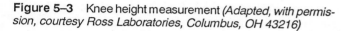

Figure 5–3 Knee height measurement *(Adapted, with permission, courtesy Ross Laboratories, Columbus, OH 43216)*

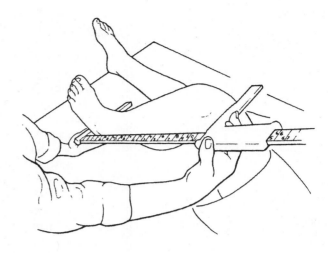

Figure 5–4 Knee height measurement *(Adapted, with permission, courtesy Ross Laboratories, Columbus, OH 43216)*

or computed) and with reference tables or graphs to determine change and to aid with interpretation of measurements.

Take and record the client's actual body weight, usual body weight, and ideal body weight. If the individual's usual weight has varied significantly from the ideal for several years, the use of height and weight tables to assess present weight status is meaningless. Compare the actual body weight with usual body weight to determine the client's present status. A 5-percent weight loss in one month is considered significant and greater than 5 percent is severe. A 7.5-percent loss over a three-month period is significant and greater than 7.5 percent is severe. Over a six-month period, 10-percent weight loss is significant and anything greater is considered a severe weight loss. This formula determines the percentage of loss:

$$\% \text{ of body weight loss} = \frac{\text{usual weight} - \text{actual weight}}{\text{usual weight}} \times 100$$

When evaluating weight loss, determine if the client is on a weight-loss diet or if the daily caloric intake is less in the facility than the client is used to eating. Determine whether the client was edematous when initially weighed and with treatment has lost weight (Health Care Financing Administration 1991).

To estimate weight change for the client with an amputation, an entire lower extremity equals 18.5 percent of total body weight and an entire upper extremity equals 6.5 percent of total body weight.

Laboratory Data

Note: Laboratory values may vary depending on the testing methods used by the laboratory. Refer to the normal values of the testing laboratory.

Hematocrit is a measurement of the percentage of red blood cells by volume in whole blood. The measurement depends on the number and the size of red blood cells. During periods of critical illness, the measurement may be high as a result of increased concentrations of blood glucose and sodium, which cause swelling of the red blood cells. Reference values for men: 40 percent to 54 percent; reference values for women: 37 percent to 47 percent. Hemoglobin is a protein in red blood cells. Low levels of hemoglobin are an indication of anemia. Dehydration can result in high levels. Reference values for men: 14–18 g/dl; reference values for women: 12–16 g/dl (Loeb 1991).

Serum transferrin is an iron-carrying protein in the blood. The concentration of the protein increases if iron stores are diminished and it increases with protein deficiency. Transferrin does not carry all the iron it can.

The total iron binding capacity (TIBC) assesses the transferrin level in terms of the amount that would be carried if the transferrin was saturated with iron. The percentage of saturation is determined by dividing serum iron levels by the TIBC. Clients with iron deficiency anemia have an increase in iron binding capacity, a low transferrin saturation value, and decreased serum iron level. Normal values for iron: 60–190 µg/dl; normal values for TIBC: 250–420 µg/dl (Pagana and Pagana 1986).

Unlike carbohydrates and fats, proteins are not stored by the body. Proteins are continuously broken down into amino acids in the intestinal mucosa. Serum proteins are a reserve source of nutrition for body tissues. Albumin and globulins make up the total proteins in serum. The total protein test is a chemical determination of albumin plus globulin. Advanced malnutrition or protein deprivation results in decreased levels. Severe drops in albumin lead to edema, and decreased levels of gamma globulin weaken the body's resistance to infection. When protein depletion occurs, the lymphocytes appear to decrease in number, making this a useful measurement of nutritional status. Normal values for total protein: 6–8 g/dl; normal values for albumin: 3.2–4.5 g/dl; normal values for globulin: 2.3–3.4 g/dl (Pagana and Pagana 1986).

Urea, the end product of protein metabolism, is formed in the liver from ammonia and excreted in the urine. This is the primary method of eliminating nitrogen from the body. The blood-urea-nitrogen (BUN) levels reflect protein intake and renal excretory capacity. Normal values: 8–20 mg/dl (Loeb 1991). Decreased blood-urea-nitrogen levels (BUN) may be another indication of malnutrition.

In antigen skin testing, antigens to which most people are immune are injected under the skin. After forty-eight hours, a raised, hardened area will be observed in a well-nourished person. The body of a malnourished person will not be able to develop a response due to the depressed immune system.

Some elderly clients may have abnormal laboratory values due to certain disease processes. Abnormal values should be considered in conjunction with the client's clinical condition.

Quality and Quantity of Food Intake

Refer to the admission assessment for preliminary information. (See chapter 2, "The Restorative Nursing Process.") When questioning the client concerning food intake, categorize intake into the four basic food groups to evaluate possible deficiencies or record percentages of intake, such as 75 percent or 50 percent of food eaten by end of meal. Resume this documentation during periods of unusual nutritional demands, e.g., when there are infections or pressure ulcers. Instruct the client at home to enter food intake in a food diary.

Many factors influence individual food choices. Review the initial assessment for clues to a need for more detailed information concerning the quality and quantity of food eaten. The client may lack financial resources, cooking facilities, or transportation for marketing. Functional limitations may interfere with the ability to prepare food. Consider religious practices and ethnic traditions. Psychosocial factors such as depression and grieving affect appetite. Obtain information concerning the client's allergies and whether or not the client has been following a therapeutic dietary regime. The client's responses may indicate a need for nutritional instruction.

Evaluation of nutritional status can be determined by the data derived thus far. An analysis of the information may result in a nursing diagnosis of alterations in nutrition.

ALTERATIONS IN NUTRITION, LESS THAN BODY REQUIREMENTS

Current federal regulations for long-term-care facilities set these criteria for indicating malnutrition/dehydration: malnutrition can result from any factor that interferes with ingestion, digestion, or absorption. The processes of digestion and absorption may be disrupted by diseases, drugs, surgical procedures, or treatment regimes. Nursing intervention alone will not resolve these problems. Problems with ingestion on the other hand, can frequently be alleviated with the appropriate approach, and may require consultation with other members of the interdisciplinary team.

Causes and Interventions for Inadequate Ingestion

Food must be eaten before it can be digested and absorbed for use by body cells. Several variables influence this process. A review of the interdisciplinary assessment may reveal the presence of problems interfering with ingestion.

Appetite or the desire to eat arises from interpretation of sensory stimuli, an intact neural mechanism in the hypothalamus, and an awareness of feelings of hunger. Sensory deficits appear to be a natural consequence of aging. Diminished olfactory, gustatory, and visual senses affect the enjoyment of food. This can cause the client to become anorexic. The use of salt-free herbs and spices heightens the flavor of food without adding sodium content. Garlic powder, basil, anise seed, oregano, lemon, savory, sage, thyme, and marjoram can be used alone or in combination during cooking or added at the table. Planning meals with a variety of textures, colors, and flavors also enhances appetite. Describe the meal for the visually impaired client so he/she can mentally visualize it. (See chapter 20.)

Appetite is also influenced by the mealtime environment. Unpleasant odors, noises, and visual stimuli dampen the desire to eat, even for a hungry person. It is not uncommon in nursing homes to have problems arise from unpredictable behavior or distasteful habits of clients. Staff members need to act on these in a timely and effective manner to avoid dampening the occasion for the others.

Cloth table covers, centerpieces, and colorful dishes are more pleasing to the eye than are plastic and disposable materials. Wall coverings, drapes, and wall hangings contribute to a festive atmosphere. Lighting should be adequate and free from glare. Round tables for six or eight are more conducive to socialization than long tables. Assigned, consistent seating with compatible tablemates reduces anxiety associated with frequent changes.

Because impaired hearing is so common among the elderly, food servers need to be aware of the problems created by background noise (including music) that can interfere with mealtime conversations. Turn off TV sets and create a calm atmosphere with limited traffic flow. Serving in an efficient and unhurried manner facilitates eating pleasure.

The cognitively impaired client may be unaware of hunger or be unable to attend to the task of eating as a result of memory loss, disorientation, or short attention span. The client with psychosocial symptoms such as depression, anxiety, agitation, and paranoia may be too preoccupied to eat or may lack the motivation to eat without assistance. These problems are also discussed in the disease-specific chapters of this book.

Food intake is also dependent upon the individual's ability to get the food from plate to mouth. Perceptual deficits and physical impairments can restrict this ability. The client with apraxia, even in the absence of physical limitations, is unable to use eating utensils. The utensil and its use may be recognized, but the client cannot pick up the utensil and use it to put food in the mouth. The presence of apraxia may be readily noted by observing the client at mealtime.

Agnosia is the inability to recognize common objects such as food or eating utensils. The client with agnosia may not recognize food or utensils as relating to food and eating. The client may use the utensils inappropriately, e.g., trying to comb hair with a spoon. Agnosia may also be readily noted through observation.

Clients with central nervous system damage frequently exhibit perseveration, which is a continued repetitive movement. These clients may constantly stir the food, tap the spoon on the plate, or make chewing motions long after the food is ready to swallow.

Spatial perceptual deficits make it difficult to relate where one's body is in space and in relationship to other objects. This can result in overreaching and spilling or underreaching and dropping items.

Persons with these perceptual deficits may benefit from gentle verbal cues or the use of hand-over-hand techniques by the caregiver. Perceptual deficits are discussed further with the case studies in section III. Evaluation and recommendations by the occupational therapist may be required for persons with perceptual deficits.

The client with decreased range of motion or contractures in the neck and joints of the upper extremities may be unable to flex the neck and get the hand to the mouth. The most essential joint movements for self-feeding are flexion of the neck, flexion and extension of the elbow, supination and pronation of the forearm, flexion and extension of the fingers, and opposition of the thumb. The client with limited strength and endurance may be too weak to eat. Incoordination and tremors of the upper extremities result in spilling and the inability to handle food and utensils. The client may be unable to grasp the eating utensils or may have a problem with grasp-release. The use of adaptive eating aids can overcome some of the difficulties associated with perceptual and physical impairments. Assistance is usually needed by these clients at mealtime.

Clients who require close supervision or help with eating because of physical impairments are usually served meals in a common area apart from the other residents. This enables staff to monitor and provide the necessary assistance. Seating arrangements should allow easy access to clients for feeding or for emergency interventions. Special semicircular tables facilitate feeding, with clients sitting on the outside of a semicircular table and the caregiver on the inside. Assist the dependent client to the bathroom or check for incontinence before each meal. Give all the clients the opportunity to wash their hands even if they are fed. Check to see that hearing aids, eye glasses, and dentures are in place. Position clients appropriately. Clients with physical impairments can often feed themselves if the food is prepared first. Teach caregivers to check the tray, open and pour beverages, and remove covers and paper wrappings. Open condiments, butter the bread, and cut the meat. Check food temperatures and tell the client what is on the tray. Visually impaired clients need special assistance. (See chapter 20.) Provide adaptive aids if the care plan so indicates. After setting up the tray, check frequently to see if additional help is needed. Offer choices and have food substitutes available at mealtime. Clients unable to feed themselves require time. When the caregiver is comfortably seated, the tendency to rush is decreased. If the caregiver is seated, it avoids the need for the client to look up, thereby hyperextending the neck and increasing the risk of swallowing problems. Give the client choices in the sequence of eating. If this is not possible, alternate foods and alternate solids and liquids.

Restorative programs for self-feeding may be appropriate for clients with perceptual, cognitive, or physical impairments. The functional assessment provides data about which steps of self-feeding the client is unable to complete. Consultation with the occupational therapist may be necessary for clients with perceptual deficits before initiating a program. Start with small goals, such as lifting a glass to the mouth. Bringing the glass to the mouth and drinking from it may be as far as the client will progress. Use simple, direct verbal cues, such as "Here is your glass. Now take a drink of milk." Hand-over-hand assistance is provided by placing the utensil or glass in the client's hand, placing your hand over the client's, and guiding the object to the client's mouth. Continue to set more complex goals as long as the client advances and does not become frustrated. Adaptive eating aids are available to help overcome many of the obstacles that interfere with hand-to-mouth actions. Restorative programs for self-feeding are further addressed in the chapters on disease processes.

Poor positioning impedes the eating process, even for the individual who has adequate eating skills. This may be a result of unilateral neglect, loss of proprioception, lack of attention from nursing staff at mealtime, or seating the client in an inappropriate chair. Transfer clients to regular chairs if possible. The table surface should be high enough to allow easy visual and physical access to utensils. The client should not have to reach more than twelve inches for the food. Assist the client to assume good body alignment with the neck slightly flexed, the shoulders up and back, hips and knees flexed at a ninety-degree angle, and feet flat on the floor. The design of some wheelchairs makes it impossible to get the chair close enough to the table for problem-free eating. If clients must remain in these chairs for meals, consider lowering the chair or raising the table, whichever is most appropriate. Wheelchair brackets are available to lower the seat by two inches. These are economical and easy to attach.

In addition to appetite and the ability to get food to the mouth, the process of ingestion and the beginning of digestion require the ability to bite, chew, and manipulate food in the oral cavity for movement into the pharynx. The condition of the mouth may be overlooked in the effort to determine reasons for poor nutritional status. Age-related changes of the oral cavity, together with self-care deficits in personal hygiene, predispose the elderly to problems that cause loss of appetite, difficult chewing, and pain from oral lesions.

Plaque is constantly forming on the teeth along the gum line. When plaque and sugar combine, acid is formed that literally eats a hole in the tooth. Inadequate brushing and flossing lead to gingivitis which, untreated, progresses to periodontal disease. Resorption of bone and shrinkage of the gingiva occur exposing the root of the tooth. Without dental attention, nutritional deficiencies will follow due to impaired chewing and oral pain associated with eating. Dentures can also develop plaque, causing changes in the dentures, irritating the gums (Illinois Department of Public Health 1984).

Problems associated with biting and chewing may be avoided with a structured, consistent program of oral care. Supply clients with soft toothbrushes, toothpaste, and dental floss. For independent clients, check to see that mouth care is completed regularly and thoroughly. Instruct caregivers in correct brushing techniques for dependent clients. Brush teeth or dentures at least twice a day with commercial cleansers or baking soda. To clean dentures, ask the client to remove them. If the client cannot do this, the caregiver places a finger above the edge and uses a rocking motion to break the suction. Denture stains are removed with an ultrasonic cleaning unit or by soaking overnight in a solution of one teaspoon household bleach in eight ounces of cool water. (*Do not place any partial or full denture containing metal in this solution. The metal will corrode.*) Provide two brushes for denture wearers, one for dentures and one for the mouth. If the client is not going to wear the dentures after cleaning, store them in cool water or cleansing solutions to prevent warping (Illinois Department of Public Health 1984). The oral cavity of the edentulous client also needs attention. Use a soft brush with a small amount of paste or diluted mouthwash. Use lemon-glycerin swabs cautiously. Glycerin is drying to mouth tissues and the acidity of the lemon juice may erode tooth enamel. Toothettes® are not as effective as brushes for removal of tooth debris, but may be appropriate for clients with sensitive, fragile mouths. Label denture cups and brushes, cleaning them daily and changing frequently. Identify dentures upon admission to the health care facility. Standards require a permanent marking system in each facility. Laws in some states require the marking of dentures as they are fabricated.

Conduct an oral screening as a part of every client's ongoing health assessment. Inspect and palpate all areas of the mouth — lips, throat, tongue, cheeks, floor, roof, teeth or dental ridges, and gums. Document and report white areas, red areas or patches, ulcers, masses, swelling, pigmentations, decayed teeth, and swollen or bleeding gums. Make arrangements for a dentist or dental hygienist to see clients regularly and make referrals as necessary. Neglect of oral hygiene and dental care will quickly impair appetite and interfere with eating.

After chewing and preparing food for ingestion, the bolus must be swallowed. For some clients, this step may be the cause of inadequate nutrition.

Oral dryness (xerostomia) may be noted in clients who are receiving drug therapy (anticholinergics, antidepressants, antipsychotics). Radiation and chemotherapy contribute to oral dryness. Other health problems, such as multiple sclerosis and rheumatoid arthritis, are sometimes associated with dry mouth. This condition can lead to infections, dental caries, discomfort, and malnutrition. Synthetic salivas may be beneficial in alleviating dryness and preventing associated complications. (See chapter 10 for further information.)

Impaired swallowing (dysphagia) is defined as a state in which the individual has difficulty transferring food from the oral cavity to the stomach. Visual and olfactory stimulation, combined with appetite, activate the swallowing center in the brain stem. The first phase of swallowing is completed when food is chewed and formed into a bolus. This movement requires teeth for chewing and grinding, adequate secretions from the salivary glands, and movements of the lips, tongue, and cheeks. In the second phase, the bolus is propelled toward the pharynx, which is open to receive it. The swallowing reflex is triggered as the food bolus is transferred through the pharynx into the esophagus during the third phase. To be successful, this muscular movement must be complex, precise, and rapid so respirations are only briefly interrupted. The opening to the airway must be protected to prevent aspiration. In the fourth phase, peristalsis moves the food through the esophagus into the stomach. The fifth, seventh, ninth, tenth, eleventh, and twelfth cranial nerves control the primary muscle groups involved in the normal swallowing process. Pathologic swallowing disorders can result from tumors, infections, impactions, diverticula, laryngectomy, hiatal hernia, tracheostomy tube, strictures, vascular abnormalities, or cervical spine displacement. Almost any disease of the central nervous system or peripheral nerves can produce a neurogenic swallowing disorder as a result of muscular weakness, incoordination, or paralysis.

Clients with impaired swallowing frequently complain of "food getting stuck" while eating. Other symptoms include the presence of food in the oral cavity and evidence of aspiration, coughing, choking, nasal dripping, gurgly voice, and drooling. Consult the speech pathologist for the diagnosis, cause, severity, and treatment of the condition. Video recorded fluoroscopy is often used to make a diagnosis.

When impaired swallowing is suspected, check these criteria before feeding the client.

❑ Client is adequately alert and responsive.

❑ Client displays control of oral muscle movement noted by absence of drooling.
❑ Client can produce an audible cough.
❑ Client can voluntarily swallow.
❑ Check the gag reflex by gently stroking the right and left pharyngeal walls with a tongue blade.

(DiIorio and Price 1990)

Techniques for Clients with Impaired Swallowing

❑ Allow the client to rest before eating. Fatigue increases the risk of aspiration.
❑ Place client in an upright position at a sixty- to ninety-degree angle before, during, and for one hour after eating, whether in bed or chair.
❑ Maintain the head in midline with the neck slightly flexed during swallowing. Keep the head in alignment. Use pillows for propping if necessary so the client is comfortable.
❑ Sit facing the client and avoid any impression of haste. Minimize distractions from the surrounding environment, keep conversation minimal, and do not ask questions requiring an answer until a few seconds after swallowing is completed. All of the client's attention has to focus on eating.
❑ One step at a time, ask the client to feel the spoon on the lips and then the tongue.
❑ Use a regular metal teaspoon for feeding, giving only one-half teaspoonful of food at a time.
❑ Allow the client to see and smell the food, giving verbal descriptions if necessary.
❑ Place the food on the intact side of the mouth. Teach the voluntary swallow by instructing the client to hold the food in the mouth while thinking about swallowing, and then to swallow twice (Price and DiIorio 1990). Look for the rise of the larynx to indicate that swallowing is completed. Check for a clear mouth before proceeding.

Begin with foods that require very little manipulation. Concentration can then be directed toward swallowing rather than chewing. Pureed foods are often difficult to swallow because more control is required to manipulate them through the oral cavity. Semisolid foods of medium consistency — such as mashed potatoes, casseroles, scrambled eggs, custards, and puddings — usually work well. Liquids are also difficult to control. Because water is colorless, tasteless, and odorless, it may present problems in the beginning. This is because of the minimal sensory stimulation associated with water — the client may be unaware of the water in the mouth. Avoid milk and milk products because they stimulate the production of saliva. When giving fluids, begin with a full glass so the client does not have to tilt the head back which increases the risk of aspiration. Do not automatically pour the liquid into the client's mouth. If small sips cannot be taken, place a small amount (5 ml) on the floor of the mouth behind the lower front teeth. A straw requires adequate sucking ability. A straw may be difficult to use and distracting to the client. Short straws with wider diameters are easier to manage. Hold the straw so the client does not have to "chase" it around the glass. A commercial thickener added to liquids does not change the taste and makes the liquid easier to manage.

As progress is made, the client can attempt biting, chewing, and the manipulation of food with more texture within the mouth. Avoid ground meats or other foods that do not readily form a bolus. Fresh white bread tends to become like glue if the person has trouble manipulating the tongue. When the client begins eating solid foods, place the food in the mouth on the lower molars. Instruct the client to concentrate on chewing. When chewing is completed, have the client then concentrate on swallowing. Use a gloved finger or instruct the client to remove food that is pocketed in the cheek on the weak side of the mouth.

Clients with impaired swallowing should be fed only by qualified persons who have been instructed in the use of appropriate feeding techniques, the procedure for obstructed airway (Heimlich maneuver), and cardiopulmonary resuscitation (CPR). A registered nurse, suction equipment, and oxygen must be present.

ENTERAL NUTRITIONAL SUPPORT

Clients unable to maintain nutritional status by traditional means may require feeding through an enteral tube. Feedings may be administered by any of these routes: nasogastric, nasoduodenal, nasojejunal, esophagostomy, gastrostomy, and jejunostomy. *The guidelines presented here are general in nature and may vary somewhat depending on the route of administration and individual facility policy.*

TABLE 5–2	Nursing Care of Clients Receiving Enteral Feedings
	❑ Use a small-bore, flexible feeding tube if possible. However, a small-bore tube may enter the bronchus during insertion of a nasogastric tube without causing respiratory distress or coughing.
	❑ Attach a nasogastric tube securely to the nose and face and gastrostomy tube to the abdominal wall. Place client in a thirty- to forty-five-degree position during feeding and for one hour afterward. Maintain this position at all times for continuous feedings.
	❑ Check tube placement before each feeding and at least once a day with continuous feedings. Initial or questionable placement should be checked with an X ray. Placement can also be confirmed by checking the aspirated gastric contents for pH. An acidic pH (1.0 to 4.0) should be an indication that the tube is in the stomach. An alkaline pH may indicate small bowel or lung placement.
	❑ Check the gastric residual before each intermittent feeding and once every four hours for continuous feedings. Aspirate gastric contents, measure, and return to client's stomach. If more than 100 ml was removed, wait for one-half to one hour and recheck. If there is still more than 100 ml, notify the physician. A large amount of residual increases the risk of aspiration.
	❑ Flush tubing before and after intermittent feedings with 20–50 ml warm water. Flush every four hours during continuous feedings. This keeps the tube patent, prevents fluid from adhering to the inside of the tube, and maintains water intake. The tube may rupture due to pressure created by using a small syringe. Using a 50-ml syringe will prevent tube rupture.
	❑ Administer feedings at room temperature. Do not allow a container to hang for longer than four hours. (Closed-system commercially prepared feedings may hang up to 24 hours.)
	❑ Administer continuous feedings slowly at first — at a rate of 25–30 ml per hour — and use half-strength concentrations. If there are no complications within twenty-four hours, gradually increase the rate. After the rate has reached the desired level, gradually increase the concentration until it is full strength.

Continues

❑ Check intermittent feedings every half hour and prn. Check continuous feedings every hour and prn.

❑ Change containers and tubing every twelve to twenty-four hours.

❑ Record intake and output every eight hours and total every twenty-four hours. Calculate this intake separately from other sources.

❑ Initially monitor blood glucose, electrolytes, and blood urea nitrogen frequently until the values are stabilized.

❑ Check vital signs every four hours initially, then every eight hours.

❑ Observe for signs of aspiration, nausea, vomiting, diarrhea, and fluid and electrolyte imbalance.

❑ Provide meticulous mouth care every two hours. Check and clean insertion sites at least every eight hours.

❑ Clients receiving enteral feedings need activity. For the immobile person, give passive range-of-motion exercises at least twice daily. Clients can be assisted to sit in a chair and to ambulate periodically throughout the day.

❑ Provide psychosocial support. The client is denied the experience of visualizing, smelling, tasting, chewing, and swallowing food.

❑ To administer medications, use a liquid form if possible. Crush tablets finely and dissolve in warm water. Do not crush enteric-coated or timed-release tablets or capsules. Gelatin capsules can be opened and the powder dissolved in warm water. Flush tubing with 20–30 ml warm water before and after administering medication. Do not mix medications together. If more than one must be given at the same time, rinse the tube with 5 ml warm water between medications. If medication should not be given with food, schedule it between intermittent feedings. If the client is receiving continuous feedings, check with the pharmacist and physician. If medication is best absorbed from the stomach, check with the pharmacist on the advisability of administering these medications through duodenal or jejunal tubes.

(Bockus 1991, Walsh and Banks 1990)

There are many liquid formulas available for both oral supplementary feedings and for enteral feedings. The choice of formula is determined by the needs of the client and is ordered by the physician.

ALTERATIONS IN NUTRITION, MORE THAN BODY REQUIREMENTS

A number of older adults are considered overweight (10 percent over ideal body weight) or obese (20 percent or more over ideal body weight). This situation may reflect a combination of sedentary activity patterns, decreased metabolic needs, and lack of basic nutritional knowledge. An overweight or obese individual may still be deficient in essential nutrients and manifest clinical signs of malnutrition that need to be corrected.

The success of a weight-loss plan often depends on the factors that motivate the client to eat. After admission to a long-term-care facility, the planning, preparation, and distribution of food by staff are often enough to assure compliance with the dietary regime. The client does not have to make food selections and a nutritious, balanced diet is assured. This is particularly true if the problem is lack of knowledge, misinformation, or poor eating habits.

Counseling and educating the client on the reasons for weight loss are important. Find out what foods the client is especially fond of and consult with the dietician for including these in the client's food plan if at all possible. Dining room seating can be arranged so that clients with similar restrictions sit together. The compulsive eater, on the other hand, may continue with previous habits by taking the leftovers of fellow diners or asking family members to bring in favorite foods. It is unrealistic to expect a quick change in eating habits. In some cases, these habits have been established for more than half a century. No more than a two-pound weight loss per week should be expected. Weighing too frequently can be discouraging to the client since weight can fluctuate daily.

The client at home may benefit from joining a weight loss group in the community. The established, reputable programs are based on meeting required daily allowances and developing healthy eating habits. Liquid diets have received considerable attention recently and are controversial as to their safety and effectiveness. For the elderly client, these diets are probably inappropriate or should be undertaken only with strict medical supervision and management. It is important to help the client plan an exercise program in conjunction with the nutritional regime. (See chapter 3.) Some clients with caloric restrictions may also have other dietary concerns.

THERAPEUTIC DIETARY MANAGEMENT

Food restrictions are common among older adults living with a chronic disease. Education of the client increases compliance with the dietary regime. However, bombarding the client with information is overwhelming, confusing, and discouraging. A lifetime of eating habits are entwined with values, traditions, and beliefs that are not readily altered. Emphasize the positive, offering as many choices as possible. Unless severe complications are a threat, it may be possible to relax the restrictions somewhat for occasional special events. Discussing the benefits to be derived from compliance may increase the client's motivation. Educate the client's family too so they can give the client encouragement and support.

DEHYDRATION AND THE ELDERLY

The elderly are at risk for fluid-volume deficit related to diminished capacity of the kidneys to conserve needed fluids. Thirst is not experienced as readily in an elderly client as it is in a younger person. In addition, elderly persons often restrict their fluid intake voluntarily out of fear of incontinence. Immobility, disorientation, and functional impairments are additional predisposing factors for the onset of dehydration. A high-fiber diet without sufficient fluid intake can be dangerous. Monitor the client and maintain fluid intake to prevent dehydration.

Assessment for Dehydration

Observe:
- oral mucous membranes for dryness
- for weight loss
- laboratory data: electrolytes, BUN, hematocrit, hemoglobin, creatinine
- for signs of fainting and orthostatic hypotension (These may be indicators of dehydration.)
- for signs of acidosis: increases in pulse and respiration, decreased blood pressure
- mental status for increased disorientation
- skin turgor (This may not be accurate in the elderly due to the normal loss of elasticity.)
- urinary output: note color and specific gravity
- loss of additional fluids through body excretions and drainage

Prevention of Dehydration

Prevent dehydration by providing:
- ❏ fluid intake at 1500–2000 ml, unless contraindicated
- ❏ fresh water within reach of the client in a utensil the client can handle
- ❏ ice, if desired and not contraindicated
- ❏ additional fluids with medications and snacks
- ❏ for fluids lost through body excretions and drainage
- ❏ for regular toileting to allay client's fear of incontinence

Continue with nutritional monitoring and evaluation throughout the client's term of care. In the long-term-care facility, establish procedures for noting and recording food intake. The onset of an infection, fever, pressure ulcer, edema, or any condition causing loss of body fluids alters food requirements and should be reported and acted on immediately. Weigh clients monthly or more often if indicated. During care plan conferences, communicate to other departments any food restrictions placed on individual clients. Discharge planning for homebound clients should include an evaluation of the ways and means by which the client will meet nutritional needs after discharge.

Teach the person at home or the caregiver to keep a diary for recording food intake and weight. For the person at home, shopping and food preparation are often the biggest obstacles to adequate nourishment. Community resources, such as the Home-Delivered Meal Program, may need to be utilized. The Congregate Meals Program provides healthful meals in a social setting in the community. Many older adults find this a welcome change from eating alone. Both of these programs will consider individual medical restrictions. In many communities, there is access to free public transportation to food sites.

Check the client's living quarters periodically for stored food. Alterations in the senses of smell and vision can prevent the client from detecting food spoilage.

SUMMARY

Food may be one of the few pleasures remaining to the frail, older adult. Meals may be the best times of the day. The act of eating is more than the ingestion of food to meet physical requirements. It reaches across all human need levels, fulfilling a variety of needs for each person. Clients should have opportunities for socializing during meals with other clients. Families should have opportunities to join their loved ones for meals for special occasions and at other times of their choice.

QUESTIONS AND DISCUSSION

1. Which components of the nutritional assessment are regularly completed on the clients in your facility or agency?
2. Which factors influence the food choices of your clients?
3. Assess a client to determine the reasons for a loss of appetite.
4. Assess a client for the presence of perceptual deficits that may be interfering with the client's ability to eat.
5. Teach a nursing assistant to feed a dependent client.
6. What precautions are necessary when feeding a client with impaired swallowing?
7. Devise a care plan for a client with a permanent enteral feeding tube.
8. For what situations would you consult with other members of the interdisciplinary health care team?

REFERENCES

Bockus, S. 1991. Troubleshooting Your Tube Feedings. *American Journal of Nursing* 91(5): 24–28.

Cataldo, D.B. and E.N. Whitney. 1986. *Nutrition and Diet Therapy: Principles and Practice*. St. Paul: West Publishing Company.

Chumlea, W.C., A.F. Roche, and D. Mukherjee. 1987. *Nutritional Assessment of the Elderly through Anthropometry*. Columbus, OH: Ross Laboratories.

DiIorio, C. and M.E. Price. 1990. Swallowing: An Assessment Guide. *American Journal of Nursing* 90(7): 38–41.

Hallfrisch, J. 1991. Dietary Needs of Older People. *Nutrition & the M.D.* 17(7): 1–3.

Hargrave, M. 1979. *Nutritional Care of the Physically Disabled*. Minneapolis: Sister Kenny Institute.

Health Care Financing Administration. 1991. *Survey Procedures: Interpretive Guidelines*. U.S. Government.

Illinois Department of Public Health. 1984. *A Guide for Oral Hygiene Care in Extended Care Facilities*. Springfield, IL: Illinois Department of Public Health.

Loeb, S., ed. 1991. *Diagnostic Test Implications*. Springhouse, PA: Springhouse Corporation.

Pagana, K.D. and T.J. Pagana. 1986. *Pocket Guide to Laboratory and Diagnostic Tests*. St. Louis: The C.V. Mosby Company.

Price, M.E. and C. DiIorio. 1990. Swallowing: A Practice Guide. *American Journal of Nursing* 90(7): 42–46.

United States Government. 1988. *Surgeon General's Report on Nutrition and Health*. Washington, DC: Department of Health and Human Services.

Walsh, S.M. and L.A. Banks. 1990. How to Insert a Small-Bore Feeding Tube Safely. *Nursing 90* 20(3): 55–59.

SUGGESTED READINGS

Buelow, J.M. and D. Jamieson. 1990. Potential for Altered Nutritional Status in the Stroke Patient. *Rehabilitation Nursing* 15(5): 260–63.

Camp, D. and N. Otten. 1990. How to Insert and Remove Nasogastric Tubes Quickly and Easily. *Nursing 90* 20(9): 59–64.

Collinsworth, R. and K. Boyle. 1989. Nutritional Assessment of the Elderly. *Journal of Gerontological Nursing* 15(12): 17–21.

Deal, T. and D. Anderson. 1989. Dental Care: Problems and Suggested Solutions. *Nursing Homes* 38(1): 17–20.

DeLetter, M.C. 1991. Nutritional Implications for Chronic Airflow Limitation Patients. *Journal of Gerontological Nursing* 17(5): 21–26.

Donohue, P.A. 1990. When It's Hard to Swallow: Feeding Techniques for Dysphagia Management. *Journal of Gerontological Nursing* 16(4): 6–9.

Emmick-Herring, B. and P. Wood. 1990. A Team Approach to Neurologically Based Swallowing Disorders. *Rehabilitation Nursing* 15(3): 126–32.

Hogstel, M.O. and N.B. Robinson. 1989. Feeding the Frail Elderly. *Journal of Gerontological Nursing* 15(3): 16–20.

Kolodny, V. and A.M. Malek. 1991. Improving Feeding Skills. *Journal of Gerontological Nursing* 17(6): 20–24.

Pettigrew, D. 1989. Investing in Mouth Care. *Geriatric Nursing* 10(1): 22–24.

CHAPTER ■ 6 ■ Alterations in Bowel Elimination

OBJECTIVES

- ❑ Distinguish between rectal, colonic, and perceived constipation.
- ❑ Identify the components of bowel assessment.
- ❑ List the objectives of a bowel-management program.
- ❑ Describe the elements of a bowel-management program.
- ❑ Identify situations that may require consultation with other members of the interdisciplinary health care team.

DESCRIPTION OF THE PROBLEM

Although many older adults have bowel problems, there is no real evidence that age in itself results in a change in bowel habits. The limited studies available indicate that age has no significant effect on intestinal motility in the absence of a history of constipation or laxative use (Castle 1988). Sensations for the urge to defecate may be diminished due to decreased nerve sensation in the colon (Eliopoulos 1987). Normal defecation is dependent on food intake. It takes sixteen to twenty-four hours for ingested food to be digested and eliminated. Muscular contractions and peristalsis propel the feces into the rectum. The internal sphincter relaxes and the external sphincter contracts to allow defecation. Both sympathetic and parasympathetic innervation are necessary for defecation to occur (Resnick 1985). This process is affected by many factors, such as the nature of the food, absorptive capacity of the colon, intestinal motility, muscular exercise, and emotional state of the individual.

Constipation is a common problem among older persons. Rectal constipation is characterized by stool retention and delayed elimination. This type of constipation results from environmental factors, impaired mobility, impaired communication, self-care deficits, weak pelvic floor muscles, or emotional disturbances (McShane and McLane 1988). The individual with colonic constipation experiences delay in the passage of food residue, also resulting in the elimination of dry, hard stools. Abdominal distention and pain, lack of appetite, complaints of rectal pressure, and headache are frequently noted. Palpation of the left lower quadrant will show tenderness. The temperature and white blood cell count may be elevated (Sine 1988). Constipation can result from malnutrition, sensory-motor deficits, chronic disease processes, ileus, and decreased peristalsis. Perceived constipation is the nursing diagnosis for those situations in which the client overuses laxatives, suppositories, or enemas daily to move the bowels (Gordon 1991).

Incontinence is another problem related to alterations in bowel elimination, characterized by an involuntary passage of stool. This may be a result of an underlying disorder of the lower digestive tract, depression, neurogenic disease, or fecal impaction.

ASSESSMENT

Distinguishing between recent onset and chronic constipation is necessary before establishing a program of bowel management. In the absence of other causes, constipation or other changes in bowel habits may be a sign of colon carcinoma. Several factors can contribute to chronic constipation. Identification of these factors through careful assessment is a prerequisite to successful alleviation of the problem. A review of the initial assessment (see chapter 2) will provide information concerning bowel habits in regard to frequency and consistency of stools, incontinence, associated pain or discomfort, and the use of laxatives, enemas, or suppositories. Eating and drinking patterns and exercise habits have significant impact on bowel regularity. Consider the client's ability to get to an accessible bathroom. Many medications have a constipating effect, including nonsteroidal anti-inflammatory drugs, anticholinergic agents, minerals (iron and calcium), opiates, antihistamines, psychotropics, and some antihypertensives. Review the medical diagnoses and the presence of depression or other psychosocial disorders.

Question the client concerning elimination routine. The disruption of this routine as a result of a change in environment is often the chief cause of constipation. Evacuation at a specific time of day, eating certain foods, toileting after drinking a hot beverage upon arising, or reading while on the toilet may be well-established habits that were previously effective.

Inspect the abdomen, auscultate for bowel sounds, percuss the abdomen, and then palpate. A rectal examination may reveal the presence of hemorrhoids or fissures that can interfere with bowel elimination. The presence of an impaction can also be determined.

NURSING MANAGEMENT

The objectives for a bowel-management program are to establish regular evacuation of the colon and to prevent constipation, impaction, involuntary stool, and diarrhea. Successfully reaching these objectives can facilitate other restorative measures and improve the client's self-respect and dignity. Client problems with bowel elimination may require consultation with other members of the interdisciplinary health care team. Successful bowel-training programs are dependent upon some degree of trunk stability and mobility. The physical therapist may suggest measures to increase mobility before initiating the program. Food intake has an influence on bowel regularity. The dietician may be consulted for suggestions for increasing fiber in the client's diet. Information and recommendations from the pharmacist may be useful in evaluating the effect of the client's medications on a bowel-management regime. Use a flow sheet to document the time and place of evacuation, the consistency and amount of stool, and whether or not a suppository or enema was given. Implementing the program often requires a change in the lifetime habits of the client. This may be easier in the institutional setting where it is possible to reinforce the teaching as needed and to monitor the client's progress.

Nutritional Recommendations

Food and fluid intake are major factors in the alleviation of chronic constipation. Dietary fiber adds bulk and stimulates peristalsis. Because food travels through the intestines in less time, there is less water absorbed by the large intestine and the stool remains soft and bulky. Whole grain cereals and breads, fresh fruits, and raw vegetables are good sources of fiber. Fine bread crumbs can be added to other foods such as oatmeal or puddings for clients who have trouble chewing and swallowing. At least ten grams of dietary fiber per day are recommended. This can be obtained from four slices of whole wheat bread, 1.1 ounce of bran, or 2.9 ounces of shredded wheat. Other good sources of fiber are kidney beans, pinto beans, raspberries, boysenberries, corn on the cob, and spinach (Shoaf 1991). Fiber should be added to the diet gradually to avoid gas formation, bloating, cramping, and diarrhea.

Fiber requires adequate fluid intake in order to do its job in the intestines. A total of 2500 to 3000 ml per day with large amounts of water included in this amount is recommended. Older clients often resist drinking fluids because of fear of bladder incontinence. Coffee and tea may be irritating to the bladder and may also have a diuretic effect which tends to decrease the body fluids needed to lubricate and soften the stool (Resnick 1985). Lactase deficiency is common with aging. Lactose is fermented in the intestines, causing bloating and gas formation. Individuals with lactase deficiency should avoid ingesting milk or milk products. The physician may order a calcium supplement in these cases.

Exercise

Physical activity helps stimulate intestinal motility. Exercise is therefore an essential component of the bowel management program. Walking for twenty or thirty minutes a day is good exercise for those who can ambulate. Wheelchair exercises and even movement in bed are helpful in maintaining regularity. Abdominal- and perineal-muscle-strengthening exercises increase the ease of defecation.

Scheduling

To establish regularity and avoid bowel incontinence, it is necessary to adhere to a schedule determined by the client's previous habits. For most individuals, this is usually about thirty minutes after a meal when the gastrocolic reflex reaches peak effect. Assist the client to the toilet or commode within a half hour after eating, allowing ten to twenty minutes for defecation. If a bedpan must be used, raise the head of the bed high enough to allow gravity to assist in the movement of feces down the colon. Physical comfort, privacy, and consistency are necessary for success.

Evacuation Aids

Suppositories are not a permanent part of the bowel management plan, but their use can assist in establishing a normal, regular bowel pattern (Davis, Nagelhout, Hoban, and Barnard 1986). Insert the suppository about one hour before the meal that precedes toileting. Gradually decrease the use of the suppositories until the client can defecate without them. This may take six to eight weeks. Laxatives and enemas are used only as emergency measures and are not considered part of a bowel-management program.

TABLE 6–1	Summary of Evacuation Aids	
DESCRIPTION	ACTIONS	ADVERSE EFFECTS
Stimulants/irritant laxatives Senna, cascara, danthron, castor oil, glycerine suppositories, bisacodyl, phenolphthalein	❑ Increase peristalsis, acting mainly on transverse and descending colon ❑ Inhibit absorption of water	❑ May cause abdominal cramping ❑ Excessive use causes diarrhea, fluid and electrolyte imbalances, or cardiac and respiratory distress. ❑ Prolonged use leads to disappearance of nerve cells in colon, resulting in loss of peristalsis.
Saline or osmotic laxatives Magnesium sulfate, magnesium citrate, magnesium hydroxide, sodium phosphate	❑ Water is attracted osmotically into lumen of large intestine to increase bulk and promote peristalsis.	❑ Large doses can cause diarrhea, leading to dehydration and fluid and electrolyte imbalance. ❑ Saline laxatives may be hazardous for clients on sodium restriction or with congestive heart failure.
Lubricants Mineral oil	❑ Coats and softens fecal mass	❑ Mineral oil can be aspirated into the lungs. Any left in pharynx at bedtime can seep into bronchioles, eventually causing fibrosis. ❑ May be absorbed and localized into various areas of digestive system, especially if given with docusate sodium
Bulk laxatives Psyllium seed, psyllium hydrocolloid, psyllium hydrophilic mucilloid, methylcellulose, karaya gum	❑ Bulky gel is formed in intestines, stimulating peristalsis ❑ One to 3 doses/day are usually needed to promote regular defecation. ❑ Must be taken with sufficient water	❑ Dehydration and intestinal disorders may occur if taken over prolonged periods. ❑ Some bulk laxatives contain up to 50 percent dextrose and may be contraindicated for persons with diabetes. ❑ May combine with and decrease absorption and activity of salicylates and digitalis drugs

Continues

Stool softeners Docusate calcium, docusate sodium	❑ Helps water penetrate and soften hard, dry stools, easing passage of stools through colon ❑ Only effective if adequate fluids are taken	❑ Docusate sodium reduces digestive capacity of gastric juices on dietary proteins — volume of stomach secretions is decreased, producing inhibitory effect on pepsin.
Cleansing enemas Soapsuds, tap water, saline	❑ Introduction of fluid into rectum, stimulates peristalsis	❑ Too much stool may be removed, leaving a long interval before the next defecation; or too much moisture may be absorbed from stool remaining in colon, causing further constipation. An enema cycle is established. ❑ Blood pressure may rise during enema administration and evacuation

Digital stimulation may be needed if suppositories are ineffective or for clients with a spinal cord injury or neurological disorder. Insert a lubricated, gloved finger into the client's rectum about 1–2 cm and gently rotate the finger for thirty to sixty seconds. This procedure relaxes the anal sphincter and promotes elimination (Quinless 1988).

RECTAL IMPACTION

The leakage of loose stool around a rectal impaction may be misinterpreted and wrongly treated as diarrhea. A rectal examination will reveal the presence of hard stool if the impaction is low. Administer an oil retention enema and if there are no results, follow it with a tap water enema. Removing stool digitally is considered a last resort to be used when rectal impaction is present and all other efforts to initiate elimination have failed. Measure the client's pulse before and periodically throughout the procedure. Vagal stimulation can slow the heart rate and induce arrhythmias, especially in the person with chronic cardiovascular disease. Nursing assistants should not be responsible for this procedure. An impaction high in the bowel will not be detected by rectal examination. Further medical investigation and diagnostic tests may be needed to establish a reason and to plan treatment for probable impaction.

DIARRHEA

Another alteration in bowel elimination of the elderly includes diarrhea, which is defined as the frequent passage of liquid or unformed stool and flatus. If impaction has been ruled out and diarrhea persists, further assessment is required. Take the client's temperature, pulse, and respirations to determine if physical illness is present. Discontinue the administration of any evacuation aids. Evaluate food and fluid intake and assess the medication regime. Drugs are frequently the cause of digestive disturbances in elderly clients. Consult with the physician if this is the case.

Diarrhea resulting from a bacterial infection can spread rapidly in a long-term-care facility. If a client persists with loose stools, consult with the physician and request a stool specimen for laboratory culture. The consistent use of universal precautions for all clients reduces the risk of spreading the infection. Meticulous attention is required to prevent skin breakdown in the perineal area as a result of the diarrhea. In the majority of cases, alterations in bowel elimination are functional, with no actual organic change in the bowel (Ellickson 1988).

SUMMARY

Many older clients can resolve their problems related to bowel function by participating in a bowel-management program. Education of both the client and the staff helps ensure the success of a program. Constipation and bowel incontinence can be prevented by improving intake of dietary fiber and fluids, exercising regularly, and adhering to a routine that is successful for the client. Like all other aspects of restorative care, alleviation of one problem tends to prevent others from occurring and thus improves the quality of life for elderly clients.

QUESTIONS AND DISCUSSION

1. Why is it necessary to distinguish between rectal, colonic, and perceived constipation?
2. What questions would you ask the client when you are assessing bowel function?
3. What dietary recommendations would you give to the client with rectal constipation?
4. Discuss client problems that would benefit from consultation with other members of the interdisciplinary health care team.

REFERENCES

Castle, S.C. 1988. Constipation and Aging. *Clinical Report on Aging* 2(6): 8–10.

Davis, A., M.J. Nagelhout, M. Hoban, and B. Barnard. 1986. Bowel Management. *Journal of Gerontological Nursing* 12(5): 13–17.

Eliopoulos, C. 1987. *A Guide to the Nursing of the Aging.* Baltimore: Williams and Wilkins.

Ellickson, E.B. 1988. Bowel Management Plan for the Homebound Elderly. *Journal of Gerontological Nursing* 14(1): 16–19.

Gordon, M. 1991. *Manual of Nursing Diagnosis 1991–1992.* St. Louis: Mosby-Year Book, Inc.

McShane, R.E. and A.M. McLane. 1988. Constipation: Impact of Etiological Factors. *Journal of Gerontological Nursing* 14(4): 16–19.

Quinless, F.W. 1988. Nurse's Guide to Successful Bowel Training. *Nursing 88* 18(11): 32n.

Resnick, B. 1985. Constipation, Common but Preventable. *Geriatric Nursing* 6(4): 213–15.

Shoaf, L.R. 1991. Fluid and Fiber Needs and Drug Implications. *Nursing Homes* 40(2): 16–20.

Sine, R.D. 1988. Identification and Management of Bowel Problems. In R.D. Sine, W.E. Liss, R.E. Roush, J.D. Holcomb, and G. Wilson, eds. *Basic Rehabilitation Techniques*, 58–62. Rockville, MD: Aspen Publishers, Inc.

SUGGESTED READINGS

Yakabowich, M. 1990. Prescribe with Care: The Role of Laxatives in the Treatment of Constipation. *Journal of Gerontological Nursing* 16(7): 4–11.

CHAPTER 7 Alterations in Bladder Elimination

OBJECTIVES

- Describe the expected changes of aging that predispose the elderly client to incontinence.
- Define the six types of incontinence.
- Identify the components of a nursing assessment for bladder incontinence.
- Select the management techniques that would be most appropriate for urge, reflex, and stress incontinence.
- Identify the criteria for determining the probability of success for bladder retraining and habit training.
- List several nursing interventions to prevent urinary tract infections.
- Identify members of the interdisciplinary health care team who could provide assistance in the management of clients with alterations in urinary elimination.

DESCRIPTION OF THE PROBLEM

Urinary incontinence, defined as the involuntary loss of urine from the bladder (Gordon 1991), is a common problem among older adults. This is not a normal process of aging, although the expected alterations that affect the genitourinary system predispose to its occurrence. Several age-related changes affect the process of urine formation and elimination. (See chapter 2, "The Restorative Nursing Process.") Bladder capacity is less, causing increased frequency of urination and nocturia in both men and women. The bladder and perineal muscles weaken, resulting in increased difficulty in emptying the bladder, and retention of urine. Males with enlarged prostates may experience dribbling. Incidence of stress incontinence increases in women (Christ and Hohloch 1988). The incidence of urinary incontinence may be underreported as many elderly clients view it as an unpleasant but expected consequence of aging. Estimates indicate that incontinence ranges from 7 percent in men to 18 percent in women (Thomas and Morse 1991).

The Consensus Development Conference on Urinary Incontinence in Adults (1988) presented questions on this topic to nurses, physicians, and researchers. Sponsored by the National Institutes of Health, testimony and research findings were presented to a panel of experts who developed a consensus answer for each question. The conclusions reached by the conference will provide direction for improvement in the care and treatment of people with incontinence. The panel found that health care professionals and clients often consider incontinence normal in old age and fail to investigate the problem. Although most cases of urinary incontinence can be alleviated, controlled, or cured, more than one-half of those with incontinence have had no evaluation or treatment. This may be partially due to the fact that the subject is neglected in medical and nursing education programs. Incontinence costs Americans more than $10 billion each year, creating a significant impact on the financial resources of older adults (National Institutes of Health 1988).

Incontinence is second only to dementia as a feared consequence of aging. These two problems are the major reasons for nursing home placement. Loss of bladder and/or bowel control is demoralizing and humiliating, leading to social isolation, diminished feelings of self-worth, progressive functional decline, and depression.

Persons who are incontinent can often lead normal lives if the problem is controlled. Institutionalization of the client may be delayed or avoided and the quality of life for individuals in any setting is greatly enhanced. Identification of the problem is necessary before interventions can be established. Studies show that only 10–30 percent of primary care physicians and nurses are aware of incontinence in ambulatory clients. Only 15 percent of incontinent residents in nursing homes are identified as having a problem (Pannill 1987). Health care professionals need to obtain information from the client during the initial assessment. Asking simple, open-ended questions in a sensitive, nonjudgmental manner will establish the presence of incontinence. Further assessment can provide data on associated symptoms and may indicate a need for urological evaluation. The individual who is continent but finds it necessary to go to the bathroom frequently also requires intervention. Nine voidings per day and two or less during the night are considered the norm (Wells 1990).

CAUSES AND TYPES OF INCONTINENCE

Urinary continence requires a competent bladder and sphincter mechanism, such that maximum urethral pressure always exceeds intravesical pressure. Normal voiding occurs when urinary bladder contractions are coordinated with sphincter relaxation. Incontinence can occur whenever this process is disrupted by disease or anatomic or physiologic factors. Persons with normal bladder and urethral functions may become incontinent in the presence of systemic illness or genitourinary disease such as urinary tract infection.

The North American Nursing Diagnosis Association (1990) lists five types of incontinence: functional, reflex, stress, total, and urge (Gordon 1991). Functional and urge are the most common forms of incontinence in elderly clients, although an individual may experience more than one type.

Functional Incontinence

In functional incontinence, bladder emptying is unpredictable and complete. The involuntary passage of urine is related to impairment of cognitive, physical, or psychological functioning or to environmental barriers (Newman, Lynch, Smith, and Cell 1991). Cognitive impairments may be due to dementias or other neurological disorders that result in disorientation, memory deficits, or the inability to recognize and use the toilet/commode. Impaired communication may be another cause of functional incontinence.

Physical reasons for functional incontinence are related to impaired mobility or loss of manual dexterity, which prevents the individual from getting to the bathroom, transferring to the toilet, or manipulating the clothing. Diminished vision and placement in a strange environment can make it difficult for the client to find the bathroom. An unusually large output from diuretics, diabetes, or an increased intake are contributing factors. Psychological impairments may be due to loss of motivation, depression, anger, frustration, or perceived rewards associated with incontinence. Environmental etiologies include inaccessible toilets or unavailable caregivers.

Symptoms associated with functional incontinence are dependent on the etiology. Observation over a period of time may reveal a change in behavior or facial expression indicating a need to void. However, clients with dementia are eventually unaware of the link between the toilet and voiding (Warkentin 1992) and do not generally exhibit any signs of the need to void. Physically impaired clients frequently become frustrated and angry at a situation over which they feel they have no control.

Urge Incontinence

Urge incontinence is defined as the involuntary passage of urine occurring immediately after the sensation of bladder fullness is perceived (Gordon 1991). Frequency and nocturia are common. Bladder irritation (resulting from infections, tumors, or stones), the use of caffeine or alcohol, an enlarged prostate, and atrophic vaginitis, are contributing factors to urge incontinence (Swearingen 1992).

Reflex Incontinence

Reflex incontinence is due to a neurogenic bladder and is found in clients with central nervous system or spinal cord injury. It occurs because the transmission of signals from the reflex arc to the cerebral cortex is impaired (Swearingen 1992). Uninhibited bladder contractions cause loss of urine in the absence of symptoms of urgency. Voiding is under reflex control, occurring when the bladder fills, often establishing a predictable pattern. There is diminished or even no awareness of bladder fullness and the urge to void.

Stress Incontinence

Increased abdominal pressure raised above urethral resistance causes stress incontinence associated with coughing, laughing, or straining. Leakage occurs because of weakness of the urethral sphincter or weakened pelvic floor musculature (Newman et al. 1991). The urethrovesicular angle is altered, resulting in more pressure on the sphincters. This can occur because of urethral or vaginal prolapse, cystocele, rectocele, atrophic vaginitis, obesity, chronic overdistention, or multiple pregnancies. The problem may arise in males after transurethral prostatectomy as a result of damage to the proximal urethra (Newman et al. 1991). Characteristics include dribbling, frequency, and urgency.

Total Incontinence

Total incontinence is defined as the unpredictable, involuntary, continuous loss of urine. There may be a lack of awareness of bladder filling or of incontinence occurring (Gordon 1991). This classification is used when other types of incontinence have been ruled out or after treatment has failed.

Retention or Overflow Incontinence

This is generally referred to as urinary retention, characterized by a chronic inability to void, resulting in bladder distention with small frequent voidings or dribbling (Newman et al. 1991). There are many possible etiologies, including neurogenic disorders, congenital anomalies, enlarged prostate in the male, drug therapy, removal of indwelling catheter, impaired communication, environmental barriers, fecal impactions, loss of muscle tone, or depression.

NURSING ASSESSMENT OF INCONTINENCE

An assessment of bladder function may take several days to complete. Review the physical assessment and history with special attention to those factors that contribute to incontinence. Assess the client's ability to get to the bathroom by walking or per wheelchair, to transfer on and off the toilet, and to manipulate clothing. Note communication skills, mental status, and psychosocial status. Evaluate the environment for distance to the bathroom and accessibility of appropriate toileting facilities.

Identify any medical diagnoses or previous surgeries related to bladder dysfunction and review the client's drug regime. Review laboratory tests for the presence of urinary tract infection or changes in renal function. The physician may order additional diagnostic urology tests based on the assessment, the client's signs and symptoms, and the results of previous blood tests and urinalyses. Several classes of drugs can affect bladder function.

- ❑ Diuretics cause more urine to be produced, causing urgency leading to incontinence.
- ❑ Anticholinergics may diminish urgency, but retention of urine can occur because of increased strength of the bladder outlet or because the bladder is relaxed (depending on the particular medication).
- ❑ Psychotropic and pain medications may diminish awareness of the urge sensation, resulting in urinating before getting to the toilet. Constipation may be another side effect, leading to fecal impaction which can predispose to incontinence.
- ❑ Antihypertensives relax the smooth muscle of the bladder neck, increasing the risk for involuntary bladder emptying.

(Newman et al. 1991, Wendland and Ouslander 1986, Jeter 1992).

Both evaluation and treatment must be completed on an individual basis, considering cognitive, functional, and psychosocial status as well as residence of the client. Document the pattern of incontinence for several days to determine the frequency, amount, and circumstances of voiding. The use of a checklist simplifies this procedure. The usefulness of the information obtained is dependent on the accuracy of the individuals completing the document.

TABLE 7–1	Assessment for Bowel and Bladder Management

To be completed by a registered nurse and reviewed every 90 days or as frequently as needed based on outcome and response.

Resident _____ Adm. No. _____ Date _____

Diagnoses _____ Birth date _____

Bladder Function

History of infection or other urinary problems _____

Urinalysis: Date _____ Protein _____ Glucose _____ Ketones _____

RBC _____ WBC _____ Bacteria _____ Crystals _____ Sp.Gr. _____

Culture: Date _____ Result _____ Treatment _____

BUN _____ Ser.Creatinine _____ Tot.Pro. _____ FBS _____

To be completed after two-week assessment period

Frequency of voiding _____ Average amount _____

Is client aware of need to void? _____ Urgency? _____

Dribbling? _____ Incontinence preceded by laughing, sneezing _____

Medications affecting bladder function/continence

_____, _____

_____, _____

Mental status

Short-term memory _____ Orientation _____

Able to express self _____ Able to follow directions _____

Reaction to incontinence _____

Hydration Baseline

Daily average fluid intake: Days _____ Eve. _____ Night _____

Mobility/Self-care skills

Ambulatory/self _____ Cane _____ Walker _____

Requires assist of 1 or 2 _____ Weight bearing _____

Propels self by w/c _____ Transfers self _____

Requires assistance _____

Can manage clothing _____ Cleans self after toileting _____

Washes hands _____

Bowel Function

Bowel history: Impaction _____ Constipation _____ Incont. _____

Present pattern: Frequency _____ Time _____ Consistency _____

Recent changes: Color _____ Bleeding _____ Pain _____

Laxatives/elim. aids _____

Methods to initiate defecation _____

Medications affecting bowel function

_____, _____, _____

Continues

Evaluation for management program

Plan _____

Rationale _____

_____

Nurse _____

GENERAL PRINCIPLES OF TREATMENT

MANAGEMENT TECHNIQUES

The treatment of incontinence is based on assessment findings and is directed to preserving renal health by preventing overdistention of the bladder and urinary tract infection. The goal is to avoid incontinence, thereby reducing anxiety, fear, anger, and embarrassment and restoring self-respect and dignity.

Incontinence can be managed in several ways. Behavioral techniques are used frequently. Most drugs used in the treatment of incontinence have not been studied in well-designed clinical trials. However, some cases of stress and urge incontinence respond well to pharmacologic treatment. Surgery is successful in selected situations. A number of products are available for the palliative management of incontinence if all other treatments are ineffective or inappropriate. The use of indwelling catheters is to be avoided unless all methods are inappropriate or ineffective.

Behavioral Techniques

These methods are noninvasive and usually free of side effects. Success is dependent on the motivation and cognitive awareness of the client and the commitment of the caregivers.

Kegel Exercises.

The exercises developed by Dr. Arnold H. Kegel in 1940 have been described in different ways by many authors. This technique is used for management of stress incontinence for clients with intact cognitive function. The goal is to strengthen the pelvic floor musculature and the squeezing action that holds back the flow of urine, thereby preventing incontinence. Tell the client to try to stop the flow of urine while voiding, hold for a few seconds, and then restart the flow. Then instruct the client to contract the anus (as if holding back a bowel movement) without tensing the muscles of the legs, buttocks, or abdomen. These two activities are repeated ten to twenty times, four times a day (Swearingen 1992). The program takes six to twelve weeks and has been reported to benefit 30–90 percent of the women starting the program. Continued exercise is required for continued benefit.

Training Programs.

Greengold and Ouslander (1986) define three bladder-training procedures: scheduled toileting, habit training, and bladder retraining. These programs are designed for postcatheter management, but the first two have been used successfully for other clients as well.

Scheduled toileting involves a fixed schedule of toileting — usually every two hours. Techniques are used to facilitate voiding and emptying the bladder completely. This program is used frequently in nursing homes and is successful in reducing the number of incontinent episodes. Strong commitment is required of the caregivers to ensure adherence to the schedule. Persons with functional incontinence, including those who have severe cognitive deficits, benefit from a program of scheduled toileting (Warkentin 1992). Caregivers in the community can be taught to implement this program, relieving the client's frustration and embarrassment. Clients who are functionally incontinent because of impaired mobility should be assessed to determine the feasibility of improving their mobility status, thus increasing their ability to get to the toilet.

Habit training involves the toileting of clients according to their individual patterns of voiding. Reinforcement techniques can be used with this program. Several days may be needed previous to implementation to establish a schedule for the client. The flexibility necessary for this program requires commitment and time on the part of the staff. In the client's home, this program may be just as feasible as scheduled toileting once the pattern is established (Greengold and Ouslander 1986).

Bladder retraining restores a normal pattern of voiding and continence. Candidates for this program must be mentally and physically capable of independent toileting and have the motivation to cooperate with the caregivers. After the assessment, a schedule is established with progressive shortening or lengthening of toileting intervals. Adjunctive measures may include techniques for triggering and bladder emptying, attention to the time and amount of fluid intake, and intermittent catheterization, if necessary (Greengold and Ouslander 1986).

Prompted voiding requires the staff to prompt the client to toilet at regularly scheduled intervals and give social reinforcement for appropriate toileting behavior. This approach was implemented by Kaltreider and associates in a thirteen-week study carried out in a nursing home with sixty-five women. Each participant was checked every hour from 7:00 a.m. to 9:00 p.m. to determine wet/dry status. The clients were prompted to go to the toilet, given assistance if necessary, and praised for successful toileting. Those who were dry on the scheduled check were provided with social reinforcement. The most successful candidates were found to be those who were the most cognitively alert and those with the most severe incontinence (Kaltreider, Hu, Igou, Yu, and Craighead 1990).

Biofeedback.

Biofeedback teaches the client how to improve voluntary control over urine storage. Visual or auditory instrumentation is used to help the client learn correct responses. Manometric biofeedback is one of the newest forms of therapy used to treat clients with stress and urge incontinence. The bladder is filled with sterile water, and bladder pressure is monitored. A rectal probe measures the pressure of the external sphincter muscle and increases in abdominal pressure. Clients receive instant visual feedback on a monitor and learn how to coordinate and control the bladder and muscles. Three to five sessions of one hour each are spaced over a two-week interval. In addition, clients are taught to alter behavioral responses that contribute to incontinence. At this time, there is a lack of data on the long-term follow-up effectiveness of biofeedback (Schmidt and Russ 1989).

Surgical Techniques

Surgical procedures have been employed to correct stress incontinence in women. These operations elevate or suspend the urethra and provide support during activities that create stress or straining. The difference in the two procedures is the approach and the location of the sutures used for the urethral suspension.

The Marshal-Marchetti-Krantz or Burch procedure is used for clients with stress incontinence not responsive to conservative treatment. An abdominal incision is made and the abdominal muscles are separated to approach the urethra from above. The tissue next to the urethra is elevated with sutures to the pubic bone or adjacent ligaments (Staskin 1988).

The Stamey, Pereyra, and Raz techniques involve a vaginal incision to approach the urethra from below. Sutures are passed through the space behind the pubic bone with a specialized needle. The sutures are then secured over the abdominal muscles after making a small abdominal skin incision (Staskin 1988).

Benign prostate hyperplasia is a common occurrence among men as they age. Urge incontinence results from prostatic enlargement and is caused by involuntary bladder-muscle contractions. If the prostate completely obstructs the urethra, retention of urine occurs, with overflow incontinence. For these cases, a transurethral resection of the prostate (TURP) usually provides complete relief from the voiding difficulties.

The bladder pacemaker is a surgically implanted electrical device that stimulates the nerves responsible for urination. Entry is made through the back with an electrode attached to one component of a nerve root and an electrode connected to a receiver implanted under the skin of the lower abdomen. The receiver is activated on demand by the client with a remote-control hand-held unit. This procedure attempts to restore the client's ability to retain urine and maintain control over sphincter muscles in persons with central nervous system involvement resulting from spinal cord injury, stroke, multiple sclerosis, Parkinson's disease, and diabetes. Thorough assessment and urodynamic evaluation are required before the procedure is attempted. After implantation, the client is monitored for two or three days to evaluate the success of the pacemaker (Tanagho 1986).

The artificial urinary sphincter (AUS) is an hydraulic system of silicone rubber implanted to allow the client to void at appropriate times. A cuff is placed around the urethra, a pump is implanted in the scrotum or labia, and a reservoir is placed in the lower abdomen. To empty the bladder, the pump is squeezed to transfer fluid from the cuff to the reservoir, allowing the urethra to open. The fluid remains in the reservoir for three to five minutes, gradually moving back to the cuff by gravity to reestablish continence. The surgery takes one to two hours, with a hospital stay of three to seven days. To ensure healing, the pump is not activated for two or three months after surgery (Hammond 1984).

The Transurethral Teflon Injection is completed in twenty or thirty minutes with local anesthesia. It is considered experimental by the Food and Drug Administration. Teflon is injected into the damaged sphincter muscle, causing a bulge into the urine channel. The procedure provides enough resistance to avoid leakage but permits urination (Hoff 1985).

THE MANAGEMENT OF UNCONTROLLABLE OR INCURABLE INCONTINENCE

Not all cases of incontinence in the elderly can be controlled or cured. In those situations, avoidance of soiling is the focus of management. A drip collector may be an appropriate device for men who experience only a small amount of urine leakage. These cuplike devices enclose the penis or penis and scrotum and are held in place by a belt or pins. When applied correctly, the collector is not seen under the clothing.

External condom catheters are efficient devices if used properly. Strict attention must be given to cleanliness and correct application. Teach the client or caregiver to gently wash, rinse, and dry the penis thoroughly before application. Use a nondrying soap or incontinent wash. A plasticizing film (available in home health stores), applied to the skin before applying the catheter, protects the penile skin from urine and the irritation of frequent removal and reapplication. The newer forms of condom catheters do not rely on adhesives. Instead, there is a retention ring within the catheter that is inflated with air for a secure fit. External catheters are also available for women.

The period of wearing is gradually extended according to the tolerance of the client. The device is cleaned and reapplied every twenty-four hours. Meticulous hygiene and inspection of the perineal area are required. The manufacturer's instructions should be followed for application and care.

A compression clamp may be appropriate for the male client who experiences constant dribbling. The device is available only by prescription and the client must have the ability to apply and remove the device without assistance. The intervals of clamping are timed to avoid overfilling of the bladder and damaging pressure to the penis. If the clamp is not used correctly, skin problems, tissue trauma, and overstretching of the bladder can occur (Duffy 1989).

Clean intermittent catheterization (CIC), done by the client, is recommended by many specialists as the procedure of choice for incontinence that cannot be controlled by other methods. Sterile technique is not necessary when self-catheterization is done in the home. Studies have documented that this technique reduces the incidence of urinary tract infections, reflux, renal and bladder stones, and hydroureteronephrosis. In addition, the client experiences greater feelings of independence and is not impaired by the constant presence of an indwelling catheter. Advocates of CIC feel that no individual is too old to do the procedure as long as manual dexterity is present. Teach the client which body parts are involved, preparation, and insertion of the catheter. Stress the importance of draining the bladder every three to four hours during the day whether at home or elsewhere and as needed during the night. This procedure may not be effective or appropriate for persons with total sphincter incompetence, urethral stricture, or for severe uninhibited bladder contractions (Kaplan).

Indwelling catheters are the treatment of choice only if a behavioral program to improve bladder function has been attempted and failed, intermittent catheterization is not practical, or the use of absorbent products is inappropriate. There are a number of complications associated with the long-term use of indwelling catheters, including bacteremia, acute and chronic pyelonephritis, urethral abscesses, bladder and renal stones, renal failure, and death (Greengold and Ouslander 1986). Clinical conditions indicating the need for an indwelling catheter include cases of urinary retention with persistent overflow incontinence, symptomatic infections and/or renal dysfunction, skin wounds or pressure sores that are contaminated by urine, and the care of terminally ill or severely impaired clients for whom changes of clothing and linen are uncomfortable or disruptive.

TABLE 7–2	Guidelines for Catheter Care
	❑ Catheterization procedures should be carried out only by persons with knowledge of the procedure and of sterile techniques.
	❑ Wash hands thoroughly before and after any manipulation of the catheter site or apparatus.
	❑ Use universal precautions when there is the possibility of contact with urine.
	❑ Use as small a catheter as possible with as small a bulb as possible. This minimizes urethral trauma. A #16 catheter with 5-ml bulb is usually adequate. Leaking around the catheter does not justify the use of a larger catheter.
	❑ Properly secure the catheter after insertion to prevent movement and urethral traction. For males, tape catheter to the abdomen when the client is lying down. When the male client is up, tape the catheter laterally to the upper anterior thigh. For female clients, tape catheter to the inner thigh.

Continues

❑ Maintain a sterile, closed drainage system. Bladder irrigation or changing to a leg bag are the only exceptions.

❑ Leg bags are worn only when the client is in the chair or ambulating (never in bed). A new sterile bag should be used each time. If this is not practical, carefully disinfect the bag between uses.

❑ Disinfect catheter/tubing junction before disconnecting.

❑ Date tubing and drainage bags and change regularly, according to facility policy.

❑ Empty drainage bags at least once every eight hours. Use a separate collecting container for each client. The spigot should not touch the container.

There is a large number of absorbent products available to help minimize the problems encountered by people with incontinence. When selecting a product for one client or several, consider absorbency, bulk, noise level (before, during, or after use), comfort, availability, cost, ease of changing, disposability, special fitting, deodorizing features, and compactness. Pad and pants systems include an absorbent pad held in place by underpants. After use, the pads are changed and the pants remain in place. These systems may not be effective when lying down, so alternative protection must be used at night or for nonambulatory clients. Absorbent briefs are designed for major bladder- and/or bowel-control programs. Clients using the pad and pants system during the day may change to the briefs for at-home and nighttime protection. The use of these products is contributing to the environmental problems of waste disposal. Reusable diapers are available and need to be considered in view of these critical problems.

AVOIDING URINARY TRACT INFECTIONS AND IRRITATIONS

The structural and functional changes of the genitourinary system that occur with aging predispose the elderly to urinary tract infections. Incidence is greater in women than men, because of a shorter urethra and the proximity of the urethra to the vagina and anus. Bacteriuria in older women is frequently associated with fecal incontinence (Warren 1992). Asymptomatic bacteriuria is common in older women, but most experts feel that therapy is not warranted (Warren 1992). Stringent personal hygiene practices will decrease the risk of infection and prevent skin breakdown in the incontinent client.

After each incontinent episode, cleanse the skin with a wash made for this purpose. Most soaps are alkaline and tend to irritate the skin. Vanishing creams made for incontinence keep the skin moisturized. Avoid the use of alcohol or thick ointments that are difficult to remove. Substitute cornstarch for talcum powder; the latter can be abrasive to the skin. The use of a barrier film provides additional protection against skin breakdown. A fungal rash may occur if the client is taking antibiotics. This will only heal with an antifungal cream or powder that requires a prescription.

Avoid the use of too many diapers and underpads between the person and the bed since these trap moisture and heat. Cotton underwear is more absorbent and less irritating than synthetic underwear, especially under slacks. Eliminate the use of fabric softeners when laundering underwear.

Advise female clients to avoid douching (unless ordered by the physician), vaginal deodorants, and tampons. Bath oils, bubble bath, bath salts, and colored toilet paper may also increase irritation of the genital area. In the presence of functional limitations, female clients may have difficulty in cleansing after toileting. Provide instructions on correct techniques to avoid contaminating the urethral area.

For sexually active clients, incontinence need not interfere. Instruct clients to completely empty the bladder and wash the genital area thoroughly both before and after sexual intercourse. The presence of an indwelling catheter need not preclude sexual activity. Males can fold the catheter up along the penis and place a condom over the penis, holding the catheter in place. Females can tape the catheter so that it remains out of the way of the vaginal orifice. Care must be taken in both instances to avoid any pull on the catheter and subsequent irritation to the urethra.

Encourage and assist clients to maintain high oral intake of fluids. Drinking juices with a high acidic content, such as cranberry juice, may decrease the risk of infection and reduce odors. Drinking large amounts of alcoholic beverages and those with caffeine can cause bladder irritation.

Personal hygiene measures and sufficient fluid intake are usually effective in preventing unpleasant odors associated with incontinence. For stubborn cases, chlorophyll deodorant tablets (chlorophyllin copper complex) are available without prescription for internal use. Taking 100–200 mg daily will eliminate odors in two to ten days (Jeter 1989).

There is no excuse for the environment to be permeated with the smell of stale urine in the long-term-care facility or in the home. Rigorous housekeeping practices and nursing measures eliminate the formation of odors.

EMOTIONAL STRESS RELATED TO INCONTINENCE

Incontinence is one of the most demeaning problems faced by disabled adults. Feelings of anxiety and diminished self-esteem result in social isolation, depriving the individual of opportunities for personal growth and enjoyment. The attitudes of family members and facility caregivers have a tremendous impact on the client's ability to deal with the problem. With the assistance of caregivers, the client can continue to participate in meaningful activities without fear of having an accident.

SUMMARY

Tremendous strides have been made in the last decade by researchers and clinicians in their attempts to increase the quality of life for persons dealing with incontinence. Nursing homes are implementing programs to alleviate incontinence, thus avoiding the use of indwelling catheters. In some states, Medicaid reimbursements are wisely based on retraining and maintenance programs rather than on the number of catheters in the facility. This progress is only a beginning.

Education of physicians, nurses, and the public is needed to eliminate the myth of incontinence as normal aging. Problems are not resolved unless the problems are recognized and acted upon. Quality of life for the elderly need not be diminished by incontinence.

QUESTIONS AND DISCUSSION

1. Complete an assessment for a bowel- and bladder-management program on one or more of your incontinent clients.
2. From the data you have collected, can you determine the types of incontinence that your clients are exhibiting?
3. Which management programs do you think would be most effective?
4. Which members of the interdisciplinary team could be utilized in the management of incontinent clients?

REFERENCES

Centers for Disease Control. 1981. Guidelines for Prevention of Catheter-Associated Urinary Tract Infections. *Guidelines: Nosocomial Infections*.

Christ, M.A. and F.J. Hohloch. 1988. *Gerontologic Nursing*. Springhouse, PA: Springhouse Publishing Company.

Duffy, L.M. 1989. When All Else Fails, Men Can Use a Compression Clamp. *The HIP Report* 7(1): 2.

Gordon, M. 1991. *Manual of Nursing Diagnosis 1991–1992*. St. Louis: Mosby-Year Book, Inc.

Greengold, B.A. and J.G. Ouslander. 1986. Bladder Retraining. *Journal of Gerontological Nursing* 12(6): 31–35.

Hammond, G.W. 1984. The Artificial Urinary Sphincter. *HIP* 2(1).

Hoff, S. 1985. Transurethral Teflon Injection for Urinary Incontinence. *HIP* 3(4).

Jeter, K.F. 1989. A New Look at Odor Control. *The HIP Report* 7(3): 1.

———. 1992. Medications: How They Affect Your Bladder. *The HIP Report* 10(1): 1.

Kaltreider, D.L., T. Hu, J.F. Igou, L.C. Yu, and W.E. Craighead. 1990. Can Reminders Curb Incontinence? *Geriatric Nursing* 11(1): 17–19.

Kaplan, W. Clean Intermittent Catheterization. *The Informer*. The Simon Foundation.

National Institutes of Health. 1988. Urinary Continence in Adults. *Consensus Development Conference Statement*.

Newman, D.K., K. Lynch, D.A. Smith, and P. Cell. 1991. Restoring Urinary Continence. *American Journal of Nursing* 91(1): 28–34.

Pannill, F.C. 1987. Urinary Incontinence. *Clinical Report on Aging* 1(3): 6–9, 11–12.

Schmidt, D. and K.L. Russ. 1989. Manometric Biofeedback for Stress and Urge Incontinence. *The Informer* (Fall Issue).

Staskin, D.R. 1988. Operations for the Treatment of Genuine Stress Incontinence in Female Patients. *The Informer*. The Simon Foundation.

Swearingen, P.L., ed. 1992. *Pocket Guide to Medical-Surgical Nursing*. St. Louis: Mosby-Year Book, Inc.

Tanagho, E.A. 1986. Bladder Pacemaker. *HIP* 4(1).

Thomas, A.M. and J.M. Morse. 1991. Managing Urinary Incontinence with Self-Care Practices. *Journal of Gerontological Nursing* 17(6): 9–14.

Warren, J.W. 1992. Asymptomatic Bacteriuria in Aged Women. *Geriatric Focus on Infectious Diseases* 2(1): 12–13, 16.

Warkentin, R. 1992. Implementation of a Urinary Continence Program. *Journal of Gerontological Nursing* 18(1): 31–36.

Wells, T. 1990. Conquering Incontinence. *Geriatric Nursing* 11(3): 133–35.

SUGGESTED READINGS

Keller, P.A., S.P. Sinkovic, and S.J. Miles. 1990. Skin Dryness: A Major Factor in Reducing Incontinence Dermatitis. *Ostomy/Wound Management* 30(September–October): 60–64.

Moore, K.N. 1991. Intermittent Catheterization: Sterile or Clean? *Rehabilitation Nursing* 16(1): 15–18.

Oldham, K.F. and J.G. Ouslander. 1987. *Rehabilitating for Continence in Long-Term Care*. Pasadena: Beverly Foundation.

Perry, J.D. 1990. The Role of Home Trainers in Kegel's Exercise Program for the Treatment of Incontinence. *Ostomy/Wound Management* 30(September–October): 46–48, 50–51, 53–57.

Scheve, A., B. Engel, K. McCormick, and E. Leahy. 1991. Exercise in Continence. *Geriatric Nursing* 12(3): 124.

Wendland, C.J. and J.G. Ouslander. 1986. *A Rehabilitative Approach to Urinary Incontinence in Long-Term Care*. Pasadena: The Beverly Foundation.

Wroblewski, J. 1990. Terodiline: A New Compound for the Treatment of Urge Incontinence. *Ostomy/Wound Management* 30(September–October): 22–26, 28–29.

SECTION **III**

Interdisciplinary Team Management of Older Adults with Chronic Disease Processes

INTRODUCTION

The third section of this book includes case studies of clients with specific health problems. A description of the problem provides the reader with general information about the disease process in regard to pathophysiology, clinical manifestations, diagnosis, and prevalence of the disease. The presentation of the case study is followed with a list of strengths that are utilized in planning the client's care. The interdisciplinary assessment includes findings from nursing and from other disciplines that would be involved in the client's care. In some situations, a problem may be relevant only to nursing, in which case there is no assessment data from other disciplines. Problems are described in the nursing diagnosis format. Interventions are suggested for each identified problem. Because the focus of this book is restorative nursing, directions for nursing interventions are specific. The success of restorative nursing is dependent on a successful interdisciplinary health care team approach. When it is appropriate to the problem, suggestions are given for collaboration with other disciplines. Nurses providing long-term care frequently find themselves in situations where professionals from other disciplines are only available on a consulting basis. The nursing interventions are suggested with this in mind. The health problems that are presented were selected because of the frequency with which they occur in the elderly population.

8 A Restorative Approach to Caring for the Client with Impaired Thought Processes

OBJECTIVES

❑ Describe the stages and correlating symptoms of Alzheimer's disease.
❑ Distinguish between depression, dementia, and delirium.
❑ List the criteria for establishing a medical diagnosis of dementia.
❑ Establish nursing interventions that will maintain the client's skills and abilities as long as possible, prevent complications, avoid catastrophic reactions, and preserve the client's dignity.
❑ Provide support for clients' families.
❑ Identify the role of the interdisciplinary health care team in the management of the client with a dementia.

DESCRIPTION OF THE PROBLEM

Impaired thought processes are defined as a discrepancy between manifested cognitive operations and expected cognitive operations for chronological age (Gordon 1991). The problem can arise from several etiologies, including dementia. There are several forms of dementia classified as organic mental disorders. All types of dementia are characterized by impaired cognitive function, impaired memory and judgment, and behavioral disturbances (Hogstel 1990).

Multi-infarct dementia is one type of dementia caused by cerebral vascular disease. It is characterized by an uneven presentation of deficits, with some functions being affected while others are not. The symptoms may vary from one day to the next because of the fluctuation in blood flow to the brain cells (American Psychiatric Association 1987). Pick's disease and Creutzfeldt-Jakob disease are other forms of dementia. Pick's disease is similar to Alzheimer's disease. The onset usually occurs after age seventy and affects more women than it does men. The numbers of neurons in the frontal and temporal lobes decrease (Hogstel 1990). Creutzfeldt-Jakob disease is caused by a type of virus called a *prion*. Prions are "unconventional" viruses identified as causative factors for a number of chronic, progressive brain diseases. Creutzfeldt-Jakob disease is the most common of these, but has a frequency of only one case per one million population. Onset occurs between the fifth and sixth decade and it affects men and women equally. The characteristics of the disease are similar to other dementias. The disease progresses rapidly, with death occurring within nine to twelve months after onset (Garbarino and Katz 1992).

Alzheimer's disease is the most common dementia, affecting over four million people in this country. It is progressive, irreversible, with insidious onset, and has no regard for race, color, sex, socioeconomic status, intellectual level, or occupation. Age of onset varies, but the disease is more common after age sixty-five (Alzheimer's Association 1990). It affects the cells of the cerebral cortex, affecting the functions of language, memory, calculation, learned movements, sensory recognition, and motor function. Microscopic lesions in the brain reveal neuritic plaques primarily in the frontal cortex and hippocampus. Neurofibrillary tangles are found in the hippocampus and temporal lobes (Chipps, Clanin, and Campbell 1992).

Diagnosis

Medical diagnoses for all dementias are established by ruling out other conditions with similar symptoms. A history, complete physical examination, blood studies, neurological and psychiatric testing, magnetic resonance imaging, electroencephalogram, and brain scan are suggested.

The Short Portable Mental Status Questionnaire (SPMSQ), the Mini-Mental Status Examination, the FROMAJE test, Cognitive Capacity Screening, and Philadelphia Geriatric Center Mental Status Questionnaire are examples of assessment tools that may be used to evaluate mental status. Several factors can alter the validity of the findings. Medications, impaired verbal communication, sensory deficits, and cultural and ethnic differences may affect the outcome. Testing should be avoided during stressful situations and in noisy, public places. Most tools consist of questions that evaluate some or all of the areas listed in Table 8–1.

TABLE 8–1	Mental Status Examinations
	❑ Orientation —date, day, month, year —name of this place, town, state, country —age, birth date, telephone number, address ❑ Memory —distant (years ago) —recent (several hours ago) —immediate (a few minutes ago) ❑ Knowledge of current events ❑ Reasoning ability ❑ Judgment ❑ Arithmetic ❑ Language

There are many reversible and treatable processes that can mimic the symptoms seen in a dementing illness. Symptoms of depression and delirium in older clients may be overlooked with the assumption that these are the result of a dementia. Clients may also have depression or delirium superimposed upon the dementia. In no case should the signs of dementia be considered normal aging.

TABLE 8–2	Distinguishing Dementia, Depression, Delirium
DEMENTIA	❑ Gradual onset, irreversible, chronic, progressive, long duration ❑ Sensorium clear ❑ Short attention span ❑ Consistent impairments ❑ Client struggles to remain independent, plays down shortcomings, confabulates to fill in answers, does not admit to memory loss (in early stages). ❑ Mood fluctuates ❑ May have thoughts of suicide in early stages
DELIRIUM	❑ Acute onset; may be reversed or alleviated with prompt, appropriate treatment; short duration; fluctuating course ❑ Sensorium clouded ❑ Perceptual disturbances ❑ Associated with trauma, infections, cardiovascular disease, alcohol intoxication or withdrawal, side effects from medications, metabolic disturbances

Continues

DEPRESSION	❑ Variable onset, reversible with treatment, long or short duration
	❑ Feelings of hopelessness, worthlessness, helplessness
	❑ Difficulty concentrating, thinking
	❑ Short-term memory intact
	❑ Oriented
	❑ Inconsistent impairments
	❑ Marked dependency
	❑ Changes in appetite, sleep patterns
	❑ Depressed mood and physical symptoms of depression
	❑ May have recurring thoughts of death, suicide

(Hogstel 1990).

If there is no evidence of other organic or functional cause, the following features must be present to establish dementia.
❑ Impairment of short-term and long-term memory
❑ Impairment in abstract thinking and/or impaired judgment and/or aphasia, apraxia, agnosia, "constructional difficulty" (inability to copy designs or arrange blocks in designs)
❑ The above disturbances interfere with work, usual social activities, or relationships.
❑ Personality change

(American Psychiatric Association 1987)

Alzheimer's disease can be positively diagnosed only by microscopic examination of the brain by biopsy or autopsy.

Symptoms of Dementia

The person with Alzheimer's disease progresses through several stages of mental and physical deterioration which may occur rapidly or may proceed slowly over a number of years. The first stage lasts from one to three years. One of the first symptoms is short-term-memory loss. It is important to differentiate the loss associated with Alzheimer's disease from age-associated benign memory impairment. The person with Alzheimer's forgets whole experiences rather than just parts of an experience and will rarely remember later, even with prompting. This memory loss results in an inability to process new information, making learning difficult at first and impossible in later stages.

Long-term memory remains intact for a surprisingly long time, but all memories are eventually lost. During the first stage, the person can function with reminders and instructions but is absentminded, has decreased concentration abilities, and becomes careless in appearance and actions. Changes in affect are noted, with either an increase in emotional reactions or a flattening of response. Vocabulary diminishes and the client will use word substitutes to fill in conversational gaps. Mistakes in judgment often have to do with social behavior or handling of money, causing distress to the family. New experiences are avoided as the individual realizes an inability to cope with unfamiliar situations. Time and spatial disorientation usually occur at the end of the first stage. With a supportive family, the client generally remains at home through this stage of the disease (Hogstel 1990).

The second stage lasts from two to ten years, with progression of existing symptoms. Appetite remains good and may be insatiable, without the client gaining weight. The client has great difficulty making decisions or plans. Arithmetic skills and writing skills are lost (agraphia). The ability to read words may remain intact but comprehension is diminished (alexia). Wandering begins during the second stage. The client may walk aimlessly for hours, unaware of environmental hazards. Wandering, lack of judgment, impulsiveness, and disorientation create a dangerous situation. The client may go outside in freezing weather without a coat, oblivious to the cold, or walk into the middle of traffic on a busy street. Pacing may also be present and is associated with anxiety, differentiating it from wandering. By the end of this stage, the client has lost impulse control and has symptoms of delusions, anger, and fear. Many families continue to care for the client at home through most of the second stage. Physically, the client is usually healthy and strong unless there are other underlying disease processes. If attentive caregivers assist with grooming and hygiene, the client may not appear ill to other people. Spouses often become so adept at shielding and compensating for the client that other family members may not even realize the extent of the illness (Hogstel 1990).

Communication becomes more difficult, with a gradual inability to verbalize meaningfully. The client eventually becomes aphasic. Hyperorality is noted by the constant mouth and tongue movements. Sundowning is a change in behavior that occurs late in the day or during the night (Gwyther 1985). It is characterized by increased confusion, agitation, and wandering. This causes severe problems for family members as they realize they are now "on duty" twenty-four hours a day. Catastrophic reactions occur because the individual cannot cope with situations that are too stimulating or overwhelming. These reactions are not necessarily dramatic or violent but can last for hours and are unsettling to the client and caregivers (Gwyther 1985). Hallucinations and delusions are common, often causing behavioral reactions. The client eventually loses the function of sensory recognition, which is an inability to recognize common objects (agnosia). As the brain cells responsible for learned movements deteriorate, the client is unable to use common objects (apraxia) appropriately. Perseveration phenomena may be observed as the individual repeats certain activities over and over, such as rocking or moving a body part. Eventually, the client does not recognize loved ones or self. Incontinence may begin during the end of the second stage. Many clients are admitted to nursing homes by the end of the second stage. Most families, no matter how supportive, simply do not have the emotional or physical resources to provide care twenty-four hours a day, seven days a week. By this time, they are exhausted and unable to cope with the constant demands.

The third stage lasts eight to twelve years. During this final stage, the client requires total care. Hyperorality is noted with constant lip licking, chewing, and sucking motions. There is complete loss of self, as the person is but a shell of the person that used to be. There is no verbal response, although the client may perseverate phrases and syllables. Apathy replaces previous episodes of catastrophic behavior, but irritability may occur if the client is uncomfortable or inundated by environmental stimuli. Seizures may occur in the later stages of Alzheimer's disease. The family also needs care and comfort as they witness the continuing deterioration and experience the loss of the person they love. Respite care for the family is important throughout the duration of the client's illness (Hogstel 1990).

Nursing Care for Dementia

Nursing care is directed to structuring a calm, safe environment, providing physical and intellectual stimulation in accordance with the client's capabilities, and preserving the dignity of a human being. Throughout the illness, the restorative aspect of nursing care is aimed at maintaining intact skills and abilities as long as possible and preventing complications. Once the client loses a skill, it is lost forever and cannot be restored. Compassion, patience, creativity, and a sense of humor are prerequisites for employees who can provide a consistent, structured, but flexible routine in a peaceful environment. It is important that caregivers understand how the use of self influences the behavior of the person with Alzheimer's or other dementias. The wrong approach and inappropriate interactions can precipitate agitation and catastrophic reactions.

TABLE 8–3	Guidelines for Caregivers of Clients with a Dementia

- ❑ In the early stages, the client realizes he/she is slipping and is helpless to do anything about it. This can precipitate depression and anger.
- ❑ The client is usually very skillful during the first stage at covering up deficits in an attempt to remain "normal."
- ❑ The client has the same needs as anyone else: physical needs, a need for safety, and for love, belonging, and esteem. Assess these needs when attempting to uncover the cause of unusual behaviors. Avoid focusing so closely on the dementia that other health problems are neglected.
- ❑ Once the client loses a skill, it is lost forever. Value the client's present skills by concentrating on remaining strengths.
- ❑ Be sensitive to the client's body language and to your own. Be aware of your own comfort level when providing care, because the client will identify it and respond accordingly.
- ❑ When planning care, consider whether an identified problem is the client's or whether it is a staff problem. If it is not detrimental to the client or other clients, maybe it is not a problem.
- ❑ Assist the client to perform at optimum level, but do not expect too much.
- ❑ Catastrophic reactions are frequently precipitated by the environment or the caregivers. Prevent these reactions by adapting the environment and caregivers to the client. Simplify the environment and eliminate sources of distraction and noise. Television may be particularly disturbing since the client cannot separate the program from reality. Use soothing, peaceful, unpatterned colors for decor. Mirrors may be upsetting. Avoid overwhelming the client with too much stimuli.
- ❑ Personalize the client's room with familiar pictures, afghans, nontoxic plants, and memorabilia.
- ❑ Because of the short attention span, distraction is a very effective technique.
- ❑ Redirect the client's energies. If his/her hands interfere with accomplishing personal care, give him/her a washcloth or something safe to hold.
- ❑ If a client is upset and refuses to allow care to be given, let it go and try later. Do not allow staff to enter into power struggles with the client. Never argue or attempt to "reason" with the client. Avoid giving lengthy, complicated explanations.
- ❑ Avoid putting the client on the spot by asking questions he/she may not be able to answer.

Continues

❑ Use physical and chemical restraints only if the life of the client or other clients is in danger and only if all alternatives have failed.

❑ Consistency is the key to success: caregivers, routine, environment.

❑ Provide the client with reassurance, affection, and dignity.

CASE STUDY

Mrs. Sylvia Lewis, seventy-four years old, was admitted to the nursing home by her husband and daughter. She was diagnosed six years ago after a complete examination at an Alzheimer's diagnostic center. Mr. and Mrs. Lewis own a local business and have always been active in several community organizations and charities. The disease progressed slowly the first two years after diagnosis. Mrs. Lewis managed fairly well at home even though she was alone during the day while her husband operated the business. Before leaving the house, Mr. Lewis prepared breakfast and assisted his wife with bathing and dressing. At noon each day, he returned home to prepare lunch and attend to any other needs of Mrs. Lewis. Six months ago, Mr. Lewis noted a rapid decline in his wife's condition. Not being able to leave her alone anymore, he arranged for adult day care while he was working. He sold the business shortly thereafter to devote his time to caring for his wife at home. In the last six weeks, Mrs. Lewis had been up several times during the night wandering around the house. She made telephone calls, turned on the stove, and left water running in the sink. The daughter came on weekends to help with her mother's care, but Mr. Lewis is exhausted and unable to continue providing the care and attention that his wife needs. Although they would rather keep Mrs. Lewis at home, he and the daughter agree this is the best solution.

Strengths

❑ Physically healthy and ambulatory
❑ Remains dry if toileted regularly
❑ Healthy appetite; no problems chewing or swallowing
❑ Completes basic activities of daily living with verbal cues and hand-over-hand assistance
❑ Has supportive husband and daughter

Interdisciplinary Assessment

Nursing.

Mrs. Lewis often thinks she is at the office where she and her husband operate their business. She paces around the nursing unit, approaching staff and visitors, asking them if they know where her husband is and what time he is coming to work. Reminders of where she is and when her husband will arrive appear to calm her, but within a few minutes, she is asking the same questions. Mrs. Lewis frequently misplaces her glasses and purse. This causes her to become upset when she cannot find them.

Activities.

Mrs. Lewis is unable to participate in group activities because of a limited attention span. She becomes agitated when staff attempt to involve her in the activity.

Social Services.

A mental status examination revealed a loss of short-term memory. Long-term memory is relatively intact. Mrs. Lewis is disoriented as to time and place.

Nursing Diagnosis

Alterations in thought processes related to progressive dementia and characterized by disorientation to time and place, loss of short-term memory, inability to concentrate, and periods of agitation.

Nursing Interventions

❑ Distract Mrs. Lewis with other activities when she repeatedly asks the same questions. Boredom is sometimes the cause of restlessness in persons who were formerly busy and productive. If she is able to comprehend, write a note that indicates the time her husband will arrive. When she thinks she is at the office, ask her to tell you about the business and the work she did. This reaffirms her worthiness, allowing her to feel comfortable with her memories. Providing Mrs. Lewis with familiar "office supplies" (paper, envelopes, cards) may increase her comfort.

❑ Provide Mrs. Lewis with clues: "Good morning Mrs. Lewis, my name is Donna and I will help you today"; "It's a sunny, warm, June day today." Do not ask questions that may put her on the spot ("Do you know what day this is?") and do not correct her unless she asks for reaffirmation of information. For example, if she says "It's Monday," do not say "No, it's Tuesday." If she asks whether it's Monday or Tuesday, give the correct response.

❑ Place a sign on her door if she no longer recognizes her name. Arrange to have a staff member assist her when she needs to go to other parts of the building.

❑ Help Mrs. Lewis keep track of her possessions by putting items back in the same place all the time. Avoid changing her room. Identify everything with her name so staff will know who owns the item if it is misplaced.

Collaboration: Interdisciplinary Team

❑ Consult with the occupational therapist for appropriate activities that will meet the changing needs of Mrs. Lewis. The following suggestions may be implemented by activities, social services, or nursing.

❑ Reminiscing is healthful and satisfying. Have the family bring in snapshots and photos. Use these as a way of stimulating conversations and memories about people and events important to her. Other familiar objects can also be used for this purpose. Discussions centered on holiday traditions, child raising, and historical events are just a few examples. Staff must be sensitive to the emotions of the client during reminiscing. Unpleasant or unhappy long-term memories may be triggered, causing agitation or catastrophic reactions.

❑ Painting and drawing allow for self-expression. Provide large sheets of paper and washable, edible fingerpaints, watercolors, or large crayons.

❑ Modeling with nontoxic clay gives opportunity for hand, wrist, and finger exercise as well as self-expression. These activities are also effective for sensory stimulation by bringing attention to colors and the feeling of the paint or clay.

❑ Raised gardens can be a source of enjoyment when clients plant seeds, monitor the progress of growth, pull weeds, and water the plants. Colors, smells, and textures can be utilized for sensory stimulation.

❑ Ask staff or visitors to bring in friendly pets to visit. Such visits require close supervision of clients and animals. These visits are very gratifying and the most confused person will respond to a gentle kitten or puppy on the lap.

❑ Music is enjoyable for listening or as an accompaniment for exercise or dancing.

❑ Dolls and stuffed animals may give pleasure.

❑ If Mrs. Lewis participated in religious activities and worship before admission, she will continue to enjoy these at the nursing home.

Activities must be geared to the cognitive level of the client. Expressions of enjoyment are the criteria for the success of the activity. Regardless of intellectual level, the client is not a child but an adult who has lived several years, with a vast collection of experiences and memories.

Outcome

Mrs. Lewis will

❑ Remain calm and avoid experiencing agitation and anxiety as a result of the disorientation and memory loss.

(The issue here is not whether she is oriented but whether she can cope with her environment.)

TABLE 8–4	Thoughts on Reality Orientation
	❑ Individuals with irreversible dementia live in the past. To force them into reality may not be where they would choose to be. ❑ Reality may be established for clients in the very early stages, with large numbered clocks and calendars throughout the facility. ❑ Reality can be confirmed with social conversation: "I noticed the tulips were in bloom today as I walked from the parking lot into the nursing home." ❑ Reality is reinforced when we answer the client's questions concerning what day it is, when lunch will be served, what activities are scheduled, and what time visitors will arrive. ❑ It is not kind to drill a client on the day, the month, or the year. The client may answer after a reminder, but will probably forget as soon as you leave the room. Does it matter? ❑ If the client waits contentedly every evening for her husband to come and is oblivious to the fact that he does not come, it is not appropriate to remind her that he died six years ago. Do not reinforce false beliefs, but be kind. Ask her to tell you about her husband and their life together. She may gradually work up to the present time and present reality. ❑ For the aged person, who has lost a spouse, children, health, and home, how important is the present? If the client has to "get home to care for the children," please allow the client to live in that satisfying, happier time. ❑ If we are concerned with behaviors, it is caring, rather than constant reminders of reality, that creates improvement. Learn to go with the moment. Connect with clients by accepting them as they are and communicating with them on their level. Sing, recite poems with them, laugh with them.

Interdisciplinary Assessment

Nursing and All Departments.

Mrs. Lewis is unaware of unsafe environmental conditions when she wanders. Her wandering may take her off the nursing unit, making it difficult for nursing staff to keep track of her. She also wanders away during activities. Staff from all departments have observed Mrs. Lewis in other parts of the building.

Nursing Diagnosis

High risk for injury related to wandering behavior, impaired judgment concerning ingestion of inedible items and use of common objects, loss of impulse control, and the inability to recognize sensory cues indicating danger.

Nursing Interventions

❑ Maintain a safe environment in which Mrs. Lewis can safely wander. Check frequently for the presence of her identification bracelet. Keep an up-to-date snapshot in her medical records.
❑ Keep her bed in the lowest position and make sure the brakes are set, or have the wheels removed. Evaluate the need for side rails. Raised side rails are sometimes a greater risk for falls.
❑ Have someone walk with her when possible. Her husband and daughter may be willing to do this when they visit. Security systems are expensive to install but are worth considering because of the benefits to clients and staff.
❑ Do safety checks on Mrs. Lewis every thirty minutes.

Collaboration: Interdisciplinary Team

❑ Alert all staff to her behavior. Discreetly post her snapshot at the reception desk so the receptionists know who she is and can help keep track of her whereabouts.

(Some of the following interventions are not necessary in nursing homes but may be valuable for families of clients at home.)
❑ Lock up sharp and pointed tools and household items as well as anything that is potentially poisonous, such as medicines, alcohol, and cleansing chemicals. Keep poisonous houseplants out of reach.
❑ Heavy, fragile, or valuable objects are best removed from the environment. Arrange the furniture so the client does not bump into it. Remove area rugs and pad sharp corners of tables and chests. Place electrical appliances out of reach. Devices are available that prevent turning on stove burners and that cover electrical outlets. Cover hot radiators and place shields over thermostats. Place electrical cords and telephone wires out of the client's reach.
❑ Install hand rails, rubber mats, and a slip-proof chair in the tub or shower. Regulate water temperature to avoid burns.
❑ Place gates on staircases and slide locks on outside doors.
❑ Persons with dementia may become frightened during fire drills. Provide assurance and support at these times.

Medications may be used in an attempt to prevent the wandering, thus reducing the risk for injury. However, the use of antipsychotic drugs imposes other risks.

TABLE 8–5	The Use of Psychotropic Medications
	❑ Resort to the use of chemical restraints only if all other interventions are ineffective and: —client displays psychotic or agitated behavior that presents danger to client or others or —delusions, hallucinations cause client severe distress ❑ Remember that these symptoms may be caused by a medical problem other than dementia. Evaluate the client carefully. ❑ Psychotropic drugs themselves may aggravate behavior. ❑ Combinations of drugs may contribute to confusion. ❑ Clients on multiple drugs have increased risk for adverse interactional effects. ❑ It is preferable to use one rather than a combination of drugs. Initiate treatment with ¼–⅓ the usual dose. If necessary, increase dosage gradually. ❑ Monitor closely for extrapyramidal effects of medication: —apathy, akinesia (slow, shuffling movements), drooling, dysphagia, muscular rigidity, tremors, restlessness, involuntary eye movements —tardive dyskinesia: protrusion of tongue, puffing of cheeks, chewing, involuntary trunk and extremity movements —diminishing functional abilities for ADLs. ❑ Supervise client's activities. ❑ Monitor: B/P, bowel activity, appetite, fluid intake, pulmonary function. ❑ Review client's condition regularly to determine if continued use of medication is justified. ❑ Refrain from the use of psychotropic drugs unless the benefits outweigh the risks. Consult with the pharmacist if all other interventions are ineffective for: situations associated with psychotic or agitated behavior that presents danger to the client or others, and delusions or hallucinations that cause the client unrelenting distress.

Outcome

Mrs. Lewis will
❑ Remain free of injury while retaining as much independence and freedom as possible.

Interdisciplinary Assessment

Nursing.

Mrs. Lewis is physically capable of completing tasks related to activities of daily living but needs reminders and assistance. She does not recognize (agnosia) or know how to use the items commonly used for these tasks (apraxia).

Nursing Diagnosis

Self-care deficits (total) related to memory loss, apraxia, and agnosia.

Nursing Interventions

❑ Utilize Mrs. Lewis's remaining ability to complete activities of daily living with verbal cues and hand-over-hand assistance. Instruct staff to avoid the temptation to do these tasks for her. They also need to watch for signs of frustration and irritation and intervene when it is appropriate.

❑ Make preparations for the task at hand and then tell Mrs. Lewis "I'm going to help you with your bath now" (or brush your teeth, etc.). Gently take her hand and walk her to the bathroom. If she resists, wait a while and try the task again later. Delay the procedure if she is already agitated.

❑ Hand her the correct item with a short, simple instruction, one step at a time: "Here is your toothbrush, please brush your teeth." Demonstrate with the appropriate motions if necessary.

❑ If Mrs. Lewis perseverates with a task, e.g., washing her face over and over, gently take her hand, praise her efforts, and direct her hand to another part of her body.

❑ Consider tub baths rather than showers as they are frequently less threatening and can also be more relaxing. Maintain privacy, covering Mrs. Lewis with a towel if necessary. Check the room temperature of the bathroom before bringing Mrs. Lewis in. Do not leave her alone in the tub.

❑ Ask the family to bring in clothing that is easy to manipulate so Mrs. Lewis can maintain self-dressing skills as long as possible. Jogging suits, velcro closures, and front opening dresses are appropriate. As she is dressing, hand her one piece at a time.

❑ If antidepressants or antianxiety medications are prescribed, dry mouth may be a side effect, increasing the risk of decay and periodontal disease. Phenytoin (Dilantin® which may be prescribed for seizures) can cause swelling and overgrowth of gum tissue if meticulous oral care is not maintained.

❑ Arrange for Mrs. Lewis to go to the hairdresser regularly. If she loses the ability to sit still long enough to complete this task, seek the family's permission for a short, attractive, "wash and wear" style.

❑ Assist Mrs. Lewis to maintain an attractive, well-groomed appearance. Provide her with a mirror and compliment her on her appearance. Help her apply makeup and nail polish if this is her usual routine.

Collaboration: Interdisciplinary Team

❑ Arrange for the dentist or dental hygienist to examine Mrs. Lewis's mouth regularly to evaluate changes in the oral cavity due to medications.

Outcome

Mrs. Lewis will
❑ Complete the activities of daily living with minimal assistance. (As her

disease progresses, the amount of assistance needed will increase, until she requires total care.)

Interdisciplinary Assessment

Nursing.

Mrs. Lewis usually experiences incontinence while she is searching for the bathroom. Assessment data reveal no other problems associated with urinary tract complications.

Nursing Diagnosis

Functional incontinence related to memory loss and disorientation.

Nursing Interventions

❏ Place Mrs. Lewis on a toileting schedule. Each time you take her to the bathroom, tell her where you are going and point out landmarks or signs that identify the toilet. After a few times, she may be able to find her way alone with just a reminder.
❏ Provide clothing that is easy to manipulate.
❏ Avoid the use of indwelling catheters since this will predispose her to additional problems. As Mrs. Lewis's ambulatory skills deteriorate, toileting will become more of a problem. Adult incontinent pads are a better choice when she reaches this stage. She will then be at risk for skin impairment and will need to be placed on a pressure-ulcer prevention program.

Outcome

Mrs. Lewis will
❏ Remain continent
❏ Remain free of skin impairments related to incontinence

Interdisciplinary Assessment

Nursing.

Mrs. Lewis generally enjoys eating and completes her meals if she receives assistance and reminders. If left alone, she forgets to eat or plays with her food and utensils. At this time, she has no problems with chewing or swallowing.

Dietary.

Mrs. Lewis is at her usual body weight.

Nursing Diagnosis

High risk for alterations in nutrition, less than body requirements, related to decreased attention span, agnosia, and apraxia.

Nursing Interventions _____

❑ Toilet Mrs. Lewis before each meal.

❑ Position her so she is close to the table with her feet flat on the floor.

❑ Prepare food before placing it in front of her — cut her meat and vegetables, open beverage cartons, pour her coffee.

❑ Limit the need for selection by giving her one course at a time and only the utensil needed to eat that course. Remove condiments and other nonessentials from the tray or table.

❑ Avoid using plastic or paper dishes and utensils for safety reasons. Use Dycem® or a wet washcloth under the dishes to prevent slipping. A plate guard keeps food on the plate. Fill cups and glasses only partially full.

❑ Patterned dishes are confusing. Mrs. Lewis may try to pick the pattern off the dish.

❑ Check food temperatures, especially if the food was warmed in a microwave oven.

❑ Because of the apraxia and agnosia, Mrs. Lewis will need help. Place a glass or utensil in her hand and give brief, simple instructions, using hand-over-hand techniques if necessary. If she has trouble getting started with the mechanics of eating, moisten her lips and give her a small amount of liquid to swallow. She may be more successful drinking from the glass than using a straw.

❑ Maintain a position of slight head flexion for eating to facilitate swallowing. Watch for signs of aspiration.

❑ Perseveration may be noted by continuous chewing after the food is ready to be swallowed. If this is a problem, gently touch her cheek or lips with your finger and instruct her to swallow.

❑ Eliminate environmental distractions, such as noise. Turn off televisions or radios. Move Mrs. Lewis if there are noisy residents in the eating area. Allow Mrs. Lewis plenty of time to finish her meal.

❑ Mrs. Lewis will eventually need to be fed. A thickener may be needed to prevent liquids from drooling out of her mouth. If hyperorality occurs, coordinate the insertion of the spoon with the movements of her tongue. Avoid serving pureed foods as long as possible. Nutritional value is diluted if the foods are pureed with water. Mixing pureed foods together or syringe feeding are two practices that should be avoided.

❑ Nasogastric or gastrostomy feedings may need to be considered in the terminal stage of dementia. The decision to insert a feeding tube must be based on any advance directives that Mrs. Lewis may have made while she was still mentally competent. In the absence of directives, her husband may be required to serve as surrogate for Mrs. Lewis in making these decisions, depending on the laws of their state.

❑ Monitor Mrs. Lewis's fluid intake. Dehydration is common among clients who forget to drink or who do not experience thirst.

❑ Record her weight monthly, more often if her appetite diminishes.

Collaboration: Interdisciplinary Team _____

❑ As Mrs. Lewis's eating skills deteriorate, ask the dietary department to prepare finger foods to allow her to retain some independence. Ask the dietician to question the family about Mrs. Lewis's favorite foods. She is more likely to eat foods that are familiar to her.

❑ Ask the occupational therapist to suggest interventions that may utilize Mrs. Lewis's ability to feed herself.

❑ If Mrs. Lewis develops swallowing problems, the speech pathologist may need to complete an assessment to determine effective interventions.

Outcome

Mrs. Lewis will
❑ Maintain her usual body weight
❑ Retain adequate nutritional and hydration status
❑ Avoid aspiration
❑ Self-feed as long as possible

Interdisciplinary Assessment

Nursing and Physical Therapy.

Mrs. Lewis is able to transfer and ambulate independently but is occasionally unsteady. Her mobility skills will gradually deteriorate due to a shuffling gait, lack of coordination, and problems with balance, until she is unable to transfer or to stand and bear weight. The potential for impaired mobility exists early in the course of the disease if caregivers, out of the concern for safety, confine her to chair or bed.

Nursing Diagnosis

High risk for impaired physical mobility related to alterations in gait pattern and cognitive-perceptual impairments.

Nursing Interventions

❑ Allow Mrs. Lewis to wander in a safe environment. This is an essential component in the care of individuals with Alzheimer's disease or other dementias. The use of restraints to prevent wandering imposes physical and psychological risks.
❑ Intervene when necessary to prevent Mrs. Lewis from becoming exhausted. Clients with memory loss may wander endlessly because they have forgotten how to sit down. If this happens with Mrs. Lewis, gently lead her to a chair and ask her to sit down. At the same time, apply light pressure to her thighs. Demonstrate by sitting down on another chair in front of her.
❑ Avoid the use of restraints. Wandering does not usually justify the application of restraints.
❑ Observe Mrs. Lewis if there are patterned carpets or floors with alternating colors of tile. These are confusing and Mrs. Lewis may attempt to walk around or jump over the perceived barriers.
❑ Avoid the use of a cane or walker. This creates additional hazards for the person who is unable to understand the use of the equipment.
❑ Plan for intermittent periods of ambulation each day when Mrs. Lewis is no longer able to safely ambulate by herself. Place a transfer belt around her waist and walk beside her with one hand in the belt and your other hand in hers. Avoid crowding when you walk with her. If Mrs. Lewis's condition requires two people to walk with her, have the other person remain slightly in back instead of at her side.
❑ Seat Mrs. Lewis in a wheelchair for regular, brief periods throughout the day. With the pedals off, she can continue to move about and exercise her lower

extremities. An Alzheimer's chair will be useful later on. It is "tip over" proof and will allow Mrs. Lewis to safely rock, providing leg exercise as well as creating soothing sensations of movement. When her abilities have regressed to the point where she is unable to stand and bear weight, alternate periods of bed rest with sitting in a recliner that can be placed in varying positions. A lifting device may be needed for transferring.

❏ When mobility skills deteriorate, place Mrs. Lewis on a positioning schedule and carry out passive range-of-motion exercises at least twice a day. Arrange for her participation in activities that include physical movement. Clients with dementia tend to acquire hip adduction and internal rotation. This complicates ambulation or may make it impossible. Try to avoid this by placing pillows between her legs when she is on her side or in the supine position. Do this also when she is sitting in a chair.

Collaboration: Interdisciplinary Team

❏ Consult with the physical therapist for suggestions for maintaining Mrs. Lewis's mobility for as long as possible.

Outcome

Mrs. Lewis will
❏ Continue to participate in physical activity within the realm of her abilities
❏ Remain free of physical restraints
❏ Remain free of the complications associated with immobility

Interdisciplinary Assessment

Nursing.

Mrs. Lewis gets up once or twice almost every night and wanders in the hall. She is resistive to staff efforts to return her to bed. (It is unclear why sundowning occurs. Some investigators feel it is a result of a change in the individual's biological clock. It may be caused from a frightening dream or by a physical need.)

Nursing Diagnosis

Sleep pattern disturbance related to disorientation and characterized by sundowning.

Nursing Interventions

❏ Avoid stimulating activities prior to bedtime. Establish a consistent bedtime routine. Take Mrs. Lewis to the bathroom, allowing sufficient time for complete bladder emptying.
❏ Help her with a sponge bath and oral care; give her a back rub with warm lotion and slow, smooth strokes.
❏ Provide a light snack with a warm, noncaffeinated beverage and plain, easily digested cracker, cookie, or toast. Be patient and do not rush her through bedtime care.
❏ Question the family concerning previous bedtime routines and sleeping habits.

Perhaps she is used to wearing socks to bed or using two pillows or having a radio on.

□ Pull down the window shades and provide a night light. Eliminate shadows that can cause further confusion and agitation.

□ Repeat this routine when Mrs. Lewis awakens during the night. She may be hungry or need to void. Give her reassurance that she is safe. Let her sleep in the recliner in her room if she is agreeable to that.

□ Try a short nap early in the afternoon. Sundowning may be a result of overfatigue.

□ Avoid the use of sleeping medications. They are seldom effective and may contribute to further confusion and restlessness.

Outcome

Mrs. Lewis will

□ Experience fewer periods of wakefulness during the night. If she awakens she will remain calm and free of agitation.

Interdisciplinary Assessment

Nursing, Activities, Social Services.

Mrs. Lewis enjoys conversing but frequently stops in the middle of a sentence. She has made the comment that she is "losing her words" and forgets what she is saying. Mrs. Lewis appears embarrassed when this happens and occasionally becomes agitated.

Nursing Diagnosis

Impaired verbal communication related to brain damage and characterized by diminishing vocabulary and difficulty with verbal expression.

Nursing Interventions

□ Continue to engage Mrs. Lewis in conversation in a place free of noise and distractions. Place yourself at her eye level and not so close that she is uncomfortable.

□ Maintain eye contact and hold her hand. Touching gets through when words do not and it displays a sense of caring.

□ Be sure she can see and hear you. Speak slowly and softly, using short, uncomplicated sentences. Give her time to comprehend and respond.

□ Avoid topics she is unable to relate to. Mrs. Lewis is probably unaware and unconcerned with world affairs or the current institutional gossip.

□ If Mrs. Lewis consistently uses one word for another, use her substitution rather than trying to correct her. If she cannot think of a word, repeat the last few words she said or supply the word for her before she becomes agitated. As she loses verbal comprehension skills, rely on facial expressions and gestures to convey meanings.

□ Share humor with Mrs. Lewis. Persons with dementia frequently retain a keen sense of humor. Laughing together is wonderful therapy for both clients and staff.

□ Show respect for Mrs. Lewis's feelings. Never talk about her in her presence.

Watch for signs of restlessness or fatigue and bring the conversation to a close before she becomes agitated.

❑ As her verbal skills diminish, Mrs. Lewis may use other methods to relay her feelings. Biting, scratching, or other negative behaviors are often nonverbal means of expressing an unmet need. Rather than staff labeling her uncooperative, investigate possible reasons for the behavior.

❑ During the terminal stage of Alzheimer's disease, communication may be reduced to eye contact or a change in facial expression.

Collaboration: Interdisciplinary Team

❑ Ask all staff who have contact with Mrs. Lewis to follow the interventions suggested for nursing. Consistency in approach may prevent negative behaviors.

Outcome

Mrs. Lewis will
❑ Continue to communicate within her abilities
❑ Display fewer episodes of frustration related to impaired communication

Interdisciplinary Assessment

Nursing and Social Services.

It is a rare family that does not experience confusion, distress, frustration, anger, and guilt at some point in time when a family member is diagnosed with Alzheimer's disease. For the Lewises, their plans for retirement were shattered. Mr. Lewis has expressed feelings of loneliness as it becomes more difficult to share ideas and activities with his wife. The daughter is experiencing conflicts as a member of the "sandwich generation" as she tries to balance the needs of her own family with the needs of her parents.

Mr. Lewis and his daughter are physically tired and emotionally stressed from the years of coping with Mrs. Lewis's illness and her nursing home admission. They continue to visit her regularly and wish to participate in her care.

Mr. Lewis is concerned with finances. His wife may live for several more years in the nursing home. Medicare does not pay for the care of persons with Alzheimer's disease and private insurance rarely pays for nursing home care. The newer policies written specifically for long-term care may provide for these services. Mrs. Lewis's monthly Social Security check goes to the nursing home for her care, but Mr. Lewis still has to provide another twenty-one hundred dollars a month. By selling the business, he can afford several years of care for his wife, but will have nothing left for his own healthcare, should the need for long-term care arise.

Nursing Diagnosis

Altered family processes related to Mrs. Lewis's impaired cognitive abilities and subsequent disruption in family relationships.

Nursing Interventions

- ❑ Families are important members of the interdisciplinary team. Mr. Lewis and his daughter have had a long period of working with Mrs. Lewis. Invite and encourage their participation in the care plan conference so they can share their ideas, giving the other members valuable information.
- ❑ Allow them to participate in the care to the extent they wish to be involved. Either of them may enjoy helping Mrs. Lewis at mealtime or walking with her when they visit.
- ❑ Assure Mr. Lewis and his daughter that the staff is not judging Mrs. Lewis by her behavior. The family needs to know that comments made by the client should not be taken personally, that these are a result of the disease process.
- ❑ If physical expression of affection was important before, let the family know that it is beneficial to continue. Hugging and touching are positive methods of communication and indicate caring.

Collaboration: Interdisciplinary Team

- ❑ The family needs comfort, support, and information. The social worker is an important liaison with the family. This person can provide invaluable assistance in counseling the family regarding additional services and resources. This may include referring Mr. Lewis and his daughter to an Alzheimer's support group and introducing them to other families with loved ones in the facility. The social worker may invite their participation in nursing home activities, but accept their choice if they choose not to do so. Encourage them to maintain friendships and associations that were previously important.
- ❑ As Mrs. Lewis becomes more disoriented, she may eventually fail to recognize or respond to her husband and daughter. All staff must avoid being judgmental if their visits become less frequent. Sometimes it is too painful for the family to visit when this happens.

Outcome

Family members will
- ❑ Be actively involved in Mrs. Lewis's care, if not directly, by giving information and participating in the planning of care
- ❑ Express their feelings to the nurse or social worker
- ❑ Express accurate knowledge of the disease process and its prognosis.

COMMENTS

A truly interdisciplinary effort is utilized in planning and delivering care for persons with Alzheimer's disease or a related dementia. The needs of the client change as the disease progresses. The responsibilities of the team evolve with these changes.

Although Medicare does not consider the care of persons with dementia as skilled nursing, complex nursing care must be provided if these clients are to experience any quality of life. Experience alone is not sufficient to prepare employees for rendering this care. Education is a necessary prerequisite for all nursing staff and other caregivers involved with the clients.

Successful care is not based on the use of physical and chemical restraints but rather on what we give of ourselves. Caring for persons with a dementia can be a demanding, frustrating process. However, it can also be a satisfying, challenging assignment when the client responds to the care.

The greatest test of nursing is to care for those who are sometimes the most "unlovable." If the client is seen as a person who was young and healthy with dreams and desires, then the symptoms of dementia recede and the client will receive the loving care that he/she deserves. Clients like Mrs. Lewis must be assisted to retain their dignity and worth as a human being.

QUESTIONS AND DISCUSSION

1. Observe your clients with dementia. What behaviors identify the presence of perceptual deficits: apraxia, agnosia, perseveration, hyperorality, and sundowning?
2. How do these deficits affect the ability of the client to complete activities of daily living: eating, dressing, toileting, grooming, and hygiene?
3. Think of situations where you witnessed a client having a catastrophic reaction. Were there events preceding this that may have triggered the behavior? If so, how could the reaction have been prevented?
4. How can you preserve the dignity of clients with dementia?
5. Evaluate the nursing unit environment and staff in regard to the care of clients with a dementia. What environmental alterations would benefit the clients? Do staff interactions with clients indicate a need for staff education?
6. What resources are available in your community that might benefit individuals with dementia and/or their families?
7. Discuss other interventions by members of the interdisciplinary team that may be beneficial to Mrs. Lewis.

REFERENCES

Alzheimer's Association. 1990. *Alzheimer's Disease Fact Sheet*. Alzheimer's Association.

American Psychiatric Association. 1987. *Quick Reference to the Diagnostic Criteria from DSM-III-R*. Washington, DC: American Psychiatric Association.

Chipps, E., N. Clanin, and V. Campbell. 1992. *Neurologic Disorders*. St. Louis: Mosby-Year Book, Inc.

Garbarino, K.A. and P.R. Katz. 1992. Infectious Causes of Dementia. *Geriatric Focus on Infectious Diseases* 2(1): 1–3, 10, 14.

Gordon, M. 1991. *Manual of Nursing Diagnosis: 1991–1992*. St. Louis: Mosby-Year Book, Inc.

Gwyther, L.P. 1985. *Care of Alzheimer's Patients: A Manual for Nursing Home Staff*. Washington DC: American Health Care Association; and Chicago: Alzheimer's Disease and Related Disorders Association, Inc.

Hogstel, M.O. 1990. *Geropsychiatric Nursing*. St. Louis: The C.V. Mosby Company.

SUGGESTED READINGS

Allen, M.E., V.A. Yanchick, J.B. Cook, and S. Foss. 1990. Do Drugs Affect Social Behavior in the Confused Elderly? *Journal of Gerontological Nursing* 16(12): 34–39.

Aske, D. 1990. The Correlation between Mini-Mental State Examination Scores and Katz ADL Status among Dementia Patients. *Rehabilitation Nursing* 15(3): 140–42.

Beisgen, B.A. 1989. *Life-Enhancing Activities for Mentally Impaired Elders*. New York: Springer Publishing Company.

Blodgett, H.E., E. Deno, and V. Hathaway. 1987. For the Caregivers: Caring for Someone with Loss of Brain Function. *Clinical Report on Aging* 1(2): 16–19.

Chiverton, P. 1990. Dementia Is Not a Diagnosis. *Geriatric Nursing* 11(1): 24–25.

Goldman, L.S. and L.W. Lazarus. 1988. Assessment and Management of Dementia in the Nursing Home. *Clinics in Geriatric Medicine* 4(3): 589–600.

Gomez, G. and E.A. Gomez. 1989. Dementia? Or Delirium? *Geriatric Nursing* 10(3): 141–42.

Gropper-Katz, E.I. 1987. Reality Orientation Research. *Journal of Gerontological Nursing* 13(8): 13–18.

Hamdy, R.C., J.M. Turnbull, L.D. Norman, and M.M. Lancaster. 1990. *Alzheimer's Disease. Handbook for Caregivers*. St. Louis: The C.V. Mosby Company.

Harvis, K.A. 1990. Care Plan Approach to Dementia. *Geriatric Nursing* 11(2): 76–80.

Jacques, J.E. 1991. Working with Persons Who Have Alzheimer's Disease. *Nursing Homes* 40(1): 16–17.

Lee, V.K. 1991. Language Changes and Alzheimer's Disease. *Journal of Gerontological Nursing* 17(1): 16–20.

Lynch-Sauer, J. 1990. When a Family Member Has Alzheimer's Disease: A Phenomenological Description of Caregiving. *Journal of Gerontological Nursing* 16(9): 8–11.

Mace, N.L. and P.V. Rabins. 1981. *The 36-Hour Day*. Baltimore: Johns Hopkins University Press.

Marzinski, L.R. 1991. The Tragedy of Dementia: Clinically Assessing Pain in the Confused, Nonverbal Elderly. *Journal of Gerontological Nursing* 17(6): 25–28.

Mayers, K.S. 1991. A Sensitive Approach to the Demented Resident. *Nursing Homes* 40(1): 21–22.

McCahon, C.P. 1991. Why Did Martha Want Her Husband to Deteriorate? *Nursing 91* 21(4): 44–46.

Meddaugh, D.I. 1990. Reactance: Understanding Aggressive Behavior in Long Term Care. *Journal of Psychological Nursing* 28(4): 28–33.

Newbern, V.B. 1991. Is It Really Alzheimer's? *American Journal of Nursing* 91(2): 50–54.

Roper, J.M., J. Shapira, and B.L. Chang. 1991. Agitation in the Demented Patient: A Framework for Management. *Journal of Gerontological Nursing* 17(3): 17–21.

Taft, L.B. and R.L. Barkin. 1990. Drug Abuse? Use and Misuse of Psychotropic Drugs in Alzheimer's Care. *Journal of Gerontological Nursing* 16(8): 4–10.

Strome, T. and T. Howell. 1991. How Antipsychotics Affect Elders. *American Journal of Nursing* 91(5): 46–49.

A Restorative Approach to Caring for the Client with Lower Extremity Amputation

OBJECTIVES

❑ Assist the client who has undergone an amputation to cope with phantom sensations.
❑ Prevent infection in the residual limb.
❑ Prevent contractures and prepare the limb for a prosthesis.
❑ Teach the client mobility skills.
❑ Describe how to assist the client to work through the grieving process associated with loss of a body part.
❑ Identify the role of the interdisciplinary health care team in the management of the client with lower extremity amputation.

DESCRIPTION OF THE PROBLEM

There are a number of reasons that necessitate surgical removal of a lower extremity. Trauma, circulatory disturbances, malignant tumors, long-standing bone infections, and thermal injuries from heat or cold can result in amputation. There are thirty-thousand new amputations a year. About 85 percent of these are done on older adults. For the elderly diabetic client, insufficient tissue perfusion due to peripheral vascular disease is the most common reason (Swearingen 1992). Either the arteries or veins may be affected and either type can be acute or chronic. Left untreated, ulcers will usually appear on the lower extremities. Whether arterial or venous, the ulcers heal with difficulty due to impaired blood flow to the area. In some cases, chronic infection prevents healing. Amputation often follows a long period of unsuccessful treatment and discomfort.

Following amputation, the elderly person may require long-term health care.

Some clients remain independent with minimal assistance and others spend their remaining years in a nursing home. The outcome depends on the prior abilities of the client, postoperative mobility and motivation, general health status, living arrangements, community, family, and financial resources.

The client may or may not be fitted for a prosthesis after surgery. The use of a prosthetic device is not beneficial for all persons, especially the elderly. This decision should be made by the client in consultation with the physician after a thorough evaluation. Many clients without prostheses are confined to wheelchairs but can learn transfer techniques, thus managing to be reasonably independent and mobile. If the client is a good candidate for a prosthesis on all other counts, age should not be a barrier. Some amputees are fitted for the prosthesis before leaving the hospital. Most clients are discharged before fitting because they need more healing time. Adequate postoperative shrinkage and shaping of the residual limb increases circulation, thereby decreasing healing time. The prosthesis can be fitted earlier and independence regained sooner.

Phantom sensation is a common feeling that the missing body part is still there. This phenomenon has been reported following amputation of almost every external body part. It is experienced as a pain, an ache, as an itching, or a twisting, burning, or pulling sensation that may be intermittent or continuous. Phantom pain occurs in more than 80 percent of amputees. Even though the nerve endings have been severed, the brain is still receiving garbled messages (Marianjoy 1989). Certain areas called trigger zones may develop that cause the phenomenon to occur when the area is touched. Trigger zones are tender areas in skeletal muscle tissue that may initiate referred pain when the areas are compressed (McCaffery and Beebe 1989). These zones are sometimes on the opposite limb. Phantom sensation does not usually occur until several days or weeks postoperatively and tends to subside within several months. Some amputees report persistent, severe pain for many years. Individuals who experience pain prior to surgery seem to experience this sensation more often than those who lose a limb suddenly as a result of trauma (Marianjoy 1989).

Deformity will occur if the residual limb is not shaped correctly. Wrapping of the residual limb serves to control edema, minimize pain, support the soft tissue, and shrink and shape the limb. A firm conical shape facilitates the fitting and use of a prosthesis.

Flexion contracture of the knee can develop almost immediately in below-the-knee amputation because the flexor strength of the hamstrings is more powerful than the extensor strength of the quadriceps. For clients who are not candidates for a prosthesis, the surgeon may consider an above-the-knee amputation to avoid this problem. A residual limb with a knee flexion contracture is a severe hindrance to the client's mobility.

Some clients are discharged from the hospital to a nursing home. These individuals do not usually have a prosthesis but may be fitted for one later. They will require instruction in the care of the residual limb and mobility techniques.

Care is directed toward

❑ preventing infection of the surgical incision
❑ healing and shaping of the residual limb
❑ increasing general physical endurance and the strength of the client's arms and legs
❑ instructing in mobility skills and in the application, removal, and care of the prosthesis
❑ assisting the client to psychosocial adaptation and adjustment to life-style changes

CASE STUDY

Mr. Kelly, eighty-six years old, was admitted to the nursing home after a below-the-knee amputation (BKA) on his left leg. Mr. Kelly had a history of recurring stasis ulcers related to vascular insufficiency. Widespread infection and subsequent gangrene preceded the decision to amputate. Mr. Kelly lives in a retirement center and hopes to return there after he learns to manage his prosthesis and regains his mobility skills. Mr. Kelly has been widowed for several years. He had one son who died of a myocardial infarction two years ago at the age of fifty-four. He sees his daughter-in-law and grandchildren occasionally and has a close, supportive female friend at the retirement center.

Strengths

- Free of cognitive impairments
- Has satisfactory living facilities to return to after discharge from the nursing home
- Has positive outlook on life
- Has a significant other and support system

Interdisciplinary Assessment

Nursing.

The severity of pain following amputation is variable. Pain is what the person experiencing the pain thinks it is. Mr. Kelly does not readily complain, so the nursing staff will need to question him about the presence of pain and observe his body language for indications of discomfort. Pain may be reflected in his posture, facial expression, and mood. Tenseness, diaphoresis, and increased pulse rate are also signs of pain.

Social Services.

Mr. Kelly's female friend has had contact with the social worker and has indicated that she is eager to help him achieve comfort and to recover from the surgery.

Nursing Diagnosis

Pain related to surgery and phantom sensations related to the loss of a body part.

Nursing Interventions

- Administer oral medication for surgical pain as ordered by the physician. Offer the medication before dressing changes and whenever it is anticipated that he may experience pain. Reposition and massage the residual limb to enhance comfort. If Mr. Kelly complains of severe pain, notify the physician and investigate for impaired sensation, movement, or circulation.
- Acknowledge and treat the presence of phantom sensations. Medication is not effective, so other interventions need to be implemented. Opinion is divided as to whether or not preoperative teaching should include the information that these sensations may occur postoperatively. Some experts feel that clients with no knowledge of this phenomenon may neglect to report it, lest they be judged mentally unbalanced. The opinion of others is that this may create the

power of suggestion, programming the client to expend energies anticipating the sensation.

❑ If he experiences this phenomenon, assure Mr. Kelly that the feeling does exist and that he is not hallucinating or imagining the sensations. Tell him that learning to control it is part of the healing process and that you will help him to deal with it. Suggested interventions follow.

❑ Counter irritation may alleviate phantom sensations by using a painful stimulus to relieve another painful stimulus (Swearingen 1992). The stimulation can be provided with cold, warmth, rubbing, or pressure (McCaffery and Beebe 1989).

❑ Warm baths and massage are relaxing and may relieve triggering.

❑ Relaxation techniques (see chapter 18), guided imagery, hypnosis, and diversional activities are also useful.

Collaboration: Interdisciplinary Team

❑ The social worker, with Mr. Kelly's permission, will ask his friend to help in providing support for Mr. Kelly. They will ask her to participate in sessions when Mr. Kelly is learning how to control his pain. The friend can be a positive influence for Mr. Kelly when he returns to the retirement center.

Outcome

Mr. Kelly will
❑ Experience relief from pain related to surgery
❑ Demonstrate techniques to effectively manage phantom sensations

Interdisciplinary Assessment

Nursing.

Upon admission to the nursing home, Mr. Kelly's surgical incision was clean, with no signs of infection. Infection delays healing and prevents proper shaping, which in turn delays and affects the use of a prosthesis. Client teaching is an integral aspect of self-care to avoid infection and other complications. However, Mr. Kelly is eighty-six years old. Individuals who have previously functioned independently may be unable to resume their former self-sufficiency. The stress of major surgery and loss of a body part have a tremendous impact on the postoperative recovery of elderly clients. This can affect the ability to remember instructions. The teaching will need to be frequently reinforced. The presence of arthritis will also hamper motor skills, affecting the client's ability to carry out procedures.

Dietician.

The nutritional assessment indicates that Mr. Kelly's nutritional status is adequate at this time.

Nursing Diagnosis

High risk for infection related to interruption in skin integrity.

Nursing Interventions

- ❏ Instruct Mr. Kelly in the care of the residual limb when he is psychologically ready to participate in his care and after the sutures are removed. Teach him how to wash the residual limb twice a day with warm water and mild soap. Tell him to avoid soaking since it can increase edema and cause skin maceration. Have him rinse the area thoroughly to remove all traces of soap and then pat dry with a clean towel. The residual limb should air dry for thirty to forty minutes before rewrapping. (Moist skin becomes macerated, predisposing to infection.)
- ❏ Tell Mr. Kelly he should not use ointments, lotions, or other emollients on the residual limb.
- ❏ Inspect the incision area for inflammation, breaks in the skin, drainage, edema, increased pain, and hypersensitivity to touch. If he still has a dressing, change this after each washing. If drainage is present, more frequent changes are necessary. Avoid the use of tape since it may irritate the skin, causing excoriation. For incontinent clients, cover the area with plastic to prevent contamination.
- ❏ Advise Mr. Kelly to inspect his other leg at the same time that he checks the residual limb. The remaining leg must be protected against trauma, pressure, or temperature extremes. A well-fitting shoe and socks are essential, as well as cleanliness of the foot and leg. (See chapter 14 for further information on foot care.)
- ❏ Teach him to toughen the skin and prepare the limb for the use of a prosthesis so the chances of infection related to skin breakdown are decreased. Massaging the area will lessen the tenderness and improve vascularity. Brushing gently with a washcloth for three or four minutes three times a day also serves to toughen the skin (Swager 1991).

Collaboration: Interdisciplinary Team

- ❏ The dietician will monitor his nutritional status closely to assure sufficient protein intake, which is necessary for healing. Additional fluids of his choice will be provided to maintain his hydration status. (Elderly people do not always experience thirst. Inadequate fluid intake may lead to signs of confusion and hamper Mr. Kelly's ability to learn.)

Outcome

Mr. Kelly will
- ❏ Remain free of infection

Interdisciplinary Assessment

Nursing.

Without the weight of the lower leg, Mr. Kelly has a poor sense of proprioception with the residual limb. He has a tendency to flex the knee to ease pain and discomfort. In this position, the end of the limb rests on the bed, impeding the healing process and predisposing to pressure ulcers and knee flexion contractures. Flexion and abduction of the hip joint on the affected side encourages the formation of hip contractures. Mr. Kelly needs to be out of bed as much as possible in order to avoid the complications of inactivity.

Physical Therapist.

Mr. Kelly is a candidate for a prosthesis because of his positive outlook on life, the support of his significant other, his potential for discharge from the facility, and his alert mental status. After he receives his prosthesis, he will need practice and self-confidence to accomplish the goal of ambulation. Mr. Kelly will need physical and psychological support to accomplish this.

Nursing Diagnosis

Impaired physical mobility related to changes in balance and loss of the lower extremity.

Nursing Interventions

❏ Shrinking and Shaping
   —The first step is to teach Mr. Kelly how to rewrap the residual limb to promote shrinking and shaping. Provide him with four-inch elastic bandages and demonstrate a figure-eight wrapping technique, exerting the greatest amount of pressure over the end of the limb. Tell him to keep his knee straight and wrap until the bandage is three or four inches above the knee. Secure the bandage on the front of the thigh. Take off the bandage and reapply every four hours during the day and anytime it becomes loose (Harmarville 1983).
   —A shrinker made of elasticized fabric is sometimes used in place of the elastic bandage. This is applied like a stocking and goes three to four inches above the knee. The top may be folded (never rolled) down over the upper edge. Be sure the seam stays in a straight line over the end of the residual limb. Reapply the shrinker every four hours during the day (Harmarville 1983).
   —Either the elastic bandage or the shrinker is worn constantly except during bathing, after bathing when the residual limb is air drying, and when the prosthesis is worn. This procedure to shape the residual limb is maintained until the residual limb maintains its shape. This is usually after the prosthesis has been worn for about six months.
❏ Positioning (Refer to chapter 3, "Exercise and Activity," for additional information on positioning and mobility procedures.)
   —Incorrect positioning hastens the formation of flexion and abduction contractures. Explain to Mr. Kelly why maintaining extension of the knee is essential (Hill 1985). Tell him he should not prop the affected knee with pillows or blankets. Show him how to maintain his hips in a position of extension and adduction.
   —Encourage Mr. Kelly to lie prone (Alexander 1990) for thirty minutes a day to facilitate extension of the joints of the lower extremities.
   —When Mr. Kelly sits in a chair, instruct him to support the residual limb on another chair or footstool of the same height as the chair seat to maintain extension of the knee. Advise him to sit upright, with his weight equally distributed on both hips. Tell him to sit for no more than two hours at a time (Alexander 1990).
   —After he has his prosthesis, instruct Mr. Kelly to sit with the prosthetic foot forward with the heel on the floor and the knee only partially flexed.
❏ Exercises
   —Exercises are done to prevent contractures and to strengthen and condition the residual limb, the intact leg, and the upper extremities. Range-of-mo-

tion exercises for all joints are done at least twice a day. (A physician's orders are needed.)

❑ Teach Mr. Kelly safe transfer techniques. A pivot transfer with a transfer belt and one person assisting is a good choice for Mr. Kelly because of his small size. This will allow him to receive the benefits of weight bearing on his strong side. Remember to transfer him to the side of strength (his right side). After Mr. Kelly has his prosthesis, teach him independent transfer techniques.

❑ After Mr. Kelly has developed a tolerance for wearing the prosthesis, instruct him to apply it as soon as he gets up. Inspect the skin frequently and thoroughly for signs of undue pressure or breakdown.

❑ Stump Socks are worn with most prostheses to increase comfort and prevent friction with the prosthesis. The socks are made of cotton or wool and come in three weights: single ply, three ply, and five ply. Tell Mr. Kelly that as the residual limb shrinks with the use of the prosthesis, he will need to increase the number of socks or the weight of the socks. If there is swelling, he should decrease the weight of the socks. Advise Mr. Kelly to change socks daily and to wash them with warm water and mild soap, rinsing well to remove all traces of soap. He should lay the socks flat to air dry.

❑ Advise Mr. Kelly to maintain his current weight. A weight gain or loss of ten or more pounds can change the fit of the prosthesis.

❑ Advise Mr. Kelly to avoid situations that may cause him to fall. He is not used to being limbless and may forget his limitations. Provide him with instructions in case he does fall. If he falls when he is not wearing the prosthesis, tell him to walk on his knees to the closest sturdy object for support before attempting to stand. If he is wearing the prosthesis, tell him to try and fall toward the unaffected side. To get up, instruct him to get on his hands and knees and then place the unaffected foot flat on the floor. As he pushes upward with his hand and foot, he should bring the prosthesis forward. Afterwards, tell him to examine both limbs for signs of trauma (Hill 1985).

Collaboration: Interdisciplinary Team

❑ The physician and physical therapist will determine additional exercises appropriate for Mr. Kelly. These generally include isometric, active, active assistive, or active resistive range-of-motion techniques. Here are some examples that might be selected.

— Gluteal sets: Tell Mr. Kelly to lie on his back and tighten his buttocks. Have him hold for a count of five, relax, and repeat (Harmarville 1983).

— This exercise for hip adduction is also done while lying on the back. Place a towel or small pillow between Mr. Kelly's thighs. With his legs flat, tell him to squeeze the towel or pillow, hold for a count of five, and then repeat (Gandy and Veigh 1984).

— Advise Mr. Kelly to lie prone and hyperextend his hips several times (Gandy and Veigh 1984).

— To strengthen his upper body, teach Mr. Kelly sitting push-ups. While he is sitting up, have him do flexion of the elbows and shoulders while holding a book or weight in each hand.

— To condition the arms, have him sit up straight and raise his arms straight out at his sides at shoulder height with elbows straight. Then tell him to make small circles with both arms, going forward and then backward (Harmarville 1983).

— Additional exercises of the lower extremities can be done while Mr. Kelly is still sitting in the chair. Instruct him to do leg lifts with his knees flexed and then with his knees extended.

—Mr. Kelly's balance can be improved by this exercise: While sitting in the chair, have him use both arms to reach over his head, to the right, to the left, and toward the floor (Harmarville 1983).

❏ Prosthetic ambulation is preceded by building tolerance to weight bearing. Mr. Kelly will not be taught to walk until he can bear the amount of weight determined by the physician. This is usually five to fifteen pounds initially. In consultation with the physical therapist, have Mr. Kelly stand between the parallel bars with the prosthetic foot on a scale so he feels the sensation of the prescribed amount of weight. As the physician increases the amount of weight, repeat this procedure
so Mr. Kelly can again feel the change.

❏ Walking begins with the use of parallel bars or a walker. Teach Mr. Kelly to use a foot-over-foot, heel-strike gait. With progress, Mr. Kelly may be able to change to the use of a cane, holding it on his intact side (DiDomenico and Ziegler 1989).

❏ Consult with the prosthetist before, during, and after the fitting of the artificial leg.

Outcome

Mr. Kelly will
❏ Be free of contractures
❏ Transfer with assistance before obtaining the prosthesis
❏ Transfer independently with the prosthesis
❏ Ambulate with the prosthesis and an assistive device

Interdisciplinary Assessment

Nursing and Social Services.

Mr. Kelly frequently makes the comment that he "isn't much of a man any more" and he is concerned that his friend will no longer desire his companionship. Although he indicates readiness to learn self-care, he often makes negative comments about the appearance of the residual limb when it is exposed.

Nursing Diagnosis

Body image disturbance related to loss of body part.

Nursing Interventions

❏ Assist Mr. Kelly to work through his grief to facilitate acceptance of his changed body. Amputation of a body part drastically affects one's body image. Grieving for the lost part is a natural response and must be worked through to successful resolution.

❏ Assign Mr. Kelly consistent caregivers. This will establish a therapeutic nurse-client relationship. Actively listen to his comments and encourage verbalization of his feelings. Clarify areas of misunderstanding.

❏ Include Mr. Kelly in care planning. Allow him to make as many decisions as possible regarding his care. Reinforce the instruction given by other health care professionals and use a positive approach for exercises and activities. Make positive comments regarding his progress.

Collaboration: Interdisciplinary Team

- ❑ The social worker will encourage the female friend to visit and provide emotional support to Mr. Kelly. Her acceptance and continuing love for Mr. Kelly will reassure him of his worthiness. She needs to avoid overprotecting Mr. Kelly and she can encourage his independence. When she visits, they can leave the nursing unit for a more private area of the facility so they can talk together without interruption.
- ❑ The social worker will talk to Mr. Kelly's family when they visit and explain to them that he is not an invalid. It is important that he be treated as a competent adult.
- ❑ Mr. Kelly's daughter-in-law states that he always took great pride in his clothing and appearance. The social worker will ask his friend to bring in clothes from the retirement center. Staff can provide the assistance he needs to complete grooming and hygiene tasks every day. Mr. Kelly's appearance is important and enhances his sexuality and identity as a male. Acknowledging him as an attractive person reaffirms this identity.
- ❑ Ask the Activities Director to involve Mr. Kelly in purposeful activities as soon as it is psychologically appropriate. His desire to resume previous interests may be assessed for planning diversional activities during his stay at the nursing home.
- ❑ Consult with the mental health therapist if there is evidence that Mr. Kelly is not resolving his grief or developing acceptance of his body.

Outcome

Mr. Kelly will
- ❑ Verbalize his feelings about the amputation and himself
- ❑ Willingly participate in the care of the residual limb to the extent that he is able
- ❑ Express acceptance of his changed body
- ❑ Seek information regarding the ways and means of regaining his independence

COMMENTS

The same care is rendered to the amputee whether or not the use of a prosthesis is planned. Preventing deformities and contractures will prevent additional complications in the future.

There are many amputees living in nursing homes who will never be candidates for discharge. These clients need to be taught the same procedures so they will attain optimal functional levels, thereby reducing the risk of psychosocial impairments.

At age eighty-six, Mr. Kelly's remaining years are limited. Regardless of age, he can be assisted to live these remaining years with dignity and self-worth.

Monitor Mr. Kelly's progress and avoid unrealistic expectations. He may not regain the physical independence that he previously enjoyed. In that case, reassess the situation and plan for optimal function at a lower level. The elderly client needs to be carefully evaluated and aware of the time, effort, and energy that will need to be invested with an above-knee prosthesis. A prosthesis is expensive and does little good sitting in the closet.

QUESTIONS AND DISCUSSION

1. For clients who choose not to wear a prosthesis, or for those who cannot, what interventions can you implement to help them remain as independent as possible?
2. What techniques can you teach the client who has phantom sensations? Research one of the suggestions given in this chapter.
3. What actions presented by the client would indicate successful resolution of the grieving process?
4. Demonstrate wrapping of the residual limb.
5. Which members of the interdisciplinary health care team (in addition to those mentioned) could also provide assistance in managing Mr. Kelly's care?

REFERENCES

Alexander, T.T. 1990. In C.E. Carlson, W.P. Griggs, and R.B. King, eds. *Rehabilitation Nursing Procedures Manual*. Rockville, MD: Aspen Publishers, Inc.

DiDomenico, R.L. and W.Z. Ziegler. 1989. *Rehabilitation Techniques for Geriatric Aides*. Rockville, MD: Aspen Publishers, Inc.

Gandy, E.D. and G. Veigh. 1984. Help the Amputee Stand on His Own Again. *Nursing 84* 14(17): 46–49.

Harmarville Rehabilitation Center, Inc. 1983. *Learning and Living after Your Leg Amputation*. Pittsburgh: Harmarville Rehabilitation Center, Inc.

Hill, S.L. 1985. Interventions for the Elderly Amputee. *Rehabilitation Nursing* 10(3): 23–25.

Marianjoy Rehabilitation Center. 1989. Training Can Ease Phantom Pain. *PhysiCare* (September/October): 4.

McCaffery, M. and A. Beebe. 1989. *Pain Clinical Manual for Nursing Practice*. St. Louis: The C.V. Mosby Company.

Swager, J. 1991. In M. Shaw, ed. *Illustrated Manual of Nursing Practice*. Springhouse, PA: Springhouse Corporation.

Swearingen, P.L. 1992. *Pocket Guide to Medical-Surgical Nursing*. St. Louis: Mosby-Year Book, Inc.

10 A Restorative Approach to Caring for the Client with Joint Disease

---

OBJECTIVES

❑ Distinguish between rheumatoid arthritis and osteoarthritis.
❑ Develop a daily routine for a client with arthritis.
❑ Discuss nursing interventions that will prevent contractures.
❑ Identify joint-preserving adaptations for activities of daily living.
❑ Implement nursing interventions to alleviate the discomfort and potential complications of Sjögren's syndrome.
❑ Identify the role of the interdisciplinary health care team in the management of the client with joint disease.

DESCRIPTIONS OF THE DISEASES

Arthritis is one of more than one hundred rheumatic conditions that include all diseases in which tissues, joints, tendons, ligaments, and muscles are involved. Thirty-seven million people have been diagnosed with one or more of these processes (Arthritis Foundation 1987). Chronic pain is a significant factor in the lives of these people. Some individuals are hesitant to make any plans for fear that pain will prevent participation. Others overextend themselves in an effort to "be tough." A few people use the pain to evade responsibilities or to receive attention. The physical effects of arthritis are unpredictable, changing from day to day and even hour to hour. As with most chronic diseases, people with arthritis must learn to take charge of their lives and make the adaptations that are necessary to live fully and comfortably. Osteoarthritis (degenerative joint disease or degenerative arthritis) and rheumatoid arthritis are two of the most common rheumatic joint diseases. It is possible for more than one joint disease to occur in the same person at the same time.

TABLE 10–1	Comparison of Rheumatoid Arthritis and Osteoarthritis	
	Rheumatoid Arthritis	Osteoarthritis
Description	❑ Autoimmune reaction ❑ Joint inflammation ❑ Systemic disease	❑ Degeneration of cartilage and other joint tissues ❑ No inflammation ❑ Localized
Cause	❑ Most people with R.A. have genetic marker. ❑ Family history	❑ Wear and tear, injury of joints
Incidence	❑ 3% of adult population ❑ 7 million in U.S. ❑ ¾ are women. ❑ 35 years, average age of onset	❑ 17 million people. ❑ Twice as many women as men. ❑ Onset, over age 40
Characteristics of the Disease	❑ Swelling, heat, redness ❑ Limitation of function ❑ Bilateral, symmetrical ❑ Starts in hands, feet, then larger joints ❑ Rheumatoid nodules on scalp, ear, ulna, olecranon, heels ❑ Sjögren's syndrome may be present. ❑ Pain worse in a.m. ❑ Exacerbations/remissions or only few attacks or slowly progressive ❑ Ankylosis occurs in severe cases.	❑ No heat or redness ❑ No limitation of function unless degeneration is severe ❑ No constant symptoms of any specific joint ❑ Heberden's nodes, Bouchard's nodes ❑ Morning stiffness is brief, alleviated with shower, exercise. ❑ Pain alleviated with rest, but stiffness sets in with rest. ❑ Pain is affected by weather. ❑ Ankylosis does not occur.
Diagnosis	❑ -C reactive protein, positive ❑ Sed. rate increased ❑ Latex fixation and antinuclear antibody tests are positive. ❑ X ray shows erosion of bone, tissue swelling	❑ No definitive lab test ❑ History
Treatment	❑ NSAIDs ❑ Aspirin ❑ Corticosteroids ❑ Gold treatment ❑ Penicillamine ❑ Cytotoxic drugs ❑ Heat/cold treatments ❑ Balance of rest/exercise ❑ Joint-protection techniques	❑ NSAIDs ❑ Aspirin ❑ Heat and cold treatments ❑ Exercise/rest ❑ Joint-protection techniques

Assessment of the client with arthritic involvement includes inspection and palpation of the joints, observing for swelling, warmth, tenderness, erythema, and crepitation. Compare the extremities for symmetry and range of motion, noting any deformity, atrophy, or weakness.

Osteoarthritis

Osteoarthritis is the most common joint disease occurring as a primary (idiopathic) process or as a secondary one, resulting from previous injury to a joint. Almost 90 percent of persons over age forty show evidence of osteoarthritis. It affects the weight-bearing joints including the hips, knees, feet, and spine. It can also affect the hands (Newman and Smith 1991). Although it is seldom disabling. osteoarthritis can cause degeneration of the affected joints resulting in severe pain and impaired mobility. The cartilage surface softens, becomes pitted and frayed and loses elasticity. The cartilage eventually wears away completely. Shooting pain may occur as bony spurs form next to joints, pinching nerves (Newman and Smith 1991).

Osteoarthritis is not a systemic disease. It affects only the joints and surrounding tissues, usually with little or no inflammation. Pieces of bone and cartilage may float in the joint space, causing irritation, leading to inflammation. Symptoms are insidious, with morning stiffness upon arising as one of the first symptoms noted. It is generally of briefer duration than that associated with rheumatoid arthritis and improves with exercise or activity. Pain results from overuse of the joints and subsides with rest, although long periods of inactivity also cause joint stiffness (Swager 1991).

Examination may reveal bony enlargement and tenderness of the affected joints. Crepitus (crunching, grating noise) is often heard when the joint is moved and joint movement may be limited. Warmth and erythema are rarely noted. Heberden's nodes, Figure 10–1, are bony growths of the distal interphalangeal

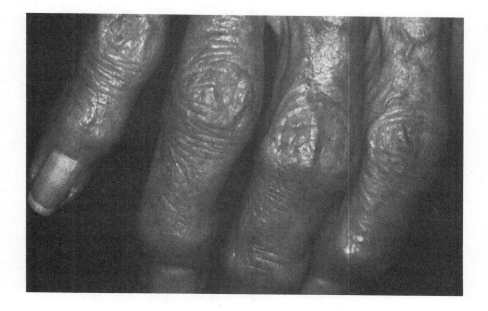

Figure 10–1 Proximal interphalangeal joint — Bouchard's nodes; distal interphalangeal joint — Heberden's nodes *(From AHPA Arthritis Teaching Slide Collection, 2d ed. © 1988. Used by permission of the Arthritis Foundation.)*

joints of the fingers. Erythema, swelling, tenderness, and aching may be present in the nodes. Bony growths of the proximal interphalangeal joints of the fingers are called Bouchard's nodes (Newman and Smith 1991), Figure 10–1. These may or may not be painful.

Diagnosis of osteoarthritis is based on X rays, history, and clinical findings. Examination of synovial fluid and erythrocyte sedimentation rate (ESR) may be done to rule out an inflammatory process. X rays may show bony destruction (Swager 1991).

A large number of older adults have a diagnosis of osteoarthritis. Although in most cases it is a primary form of the disease, it is usually a secondary diagnosis, with another medical problem as the primary health care problem. Because it is so common, health care professionals sometimes tend to dismiss it as a natural result of aging. It deserves attention with treatment of the presenting symptoms. A regular exercise program preserves joint mobility by strengthening the bones and surrounding structures. Joints should be put through the full range of motion several times a day. Low-impact aerobics, swimming, bicycling, and walking are effective forms of exercise. Aspirin or acetaminophen is helpful in controlling pain. Corticosteroids are sometimes injected into arthritic joints, but are usually not helpful in the absence of inflammation. Joint replacement surgery is effective for persons with severe involvement of the hips and knees, bringing freedom from pain and restored mobility.

Rheumatoid Arthritis

Rheumatoid arthritis affects 6.5 million people in this country. It is three times more common in women than men and has a familial tendency. The cause is unknown, but it is thought to develop as a result of an autoimmune reaction (Newman and Smith 1991). Onset is insidious and the prognosis is uncertain.

Joint soreness, aching, and fatigue are noted early in the disease. Stiffness is common upon arising and after long periods of inactivity. In the morning, this lasts anywhere from thirty minutes to two hours. Inflammation of the synovial membranes is followed by destruction of the cartilage, bone, and ligaments, Figure 10–2. Fibrotic tissue and calcification causes subluxation of the affected joint.

Joint involvement is usually symmetrical. The joints of the hands and feet are affected first. The cervical spine, temporomandibular joint, shoulders, elbows, hips, and knees may also be affected. Painless, moveable, rheumatoid nodules are often found over pressure points on the elbows, extensor arm surfaces, knuckles, knees, and heels (Swager 1991).

Rheumatoid arthritis may be chronic and disabling, and because of the systemic manifestations, can even cause death. There is an increase in infections and sepsis in persons with rheumatoid arthritis. Anorexia, slight loss of weight, low-grade fever, anemia, fatigue, and tachycardia are indications of systemic involvement. Carpal tunnel syndrome and Sjögren's syndrome are frequently associated with rheumatoid arthritis, Figure 10–3.

Deformities occur in a small percentage of people with rheumatoid arthritis. Early in the disease, spindling of the fingers results from swelling and inflammation of the interphalangeal joints. Deformities involving the hands include swan neck deformity, Figure 10–4, boutonniere deformity, Figure 10–5, and ulnar deviation with or without subluxation. Flexion deformities of the knees, hips, elbows, and toes may also occur.

Laboratory studies are helpful but not necessarily diagnostic. Erythrocyte sedimentation rate (ESR), platelet counts, and c-reactive protein may be elevated. The rheumatoid factor and antinuclear antibody (ANA) tests are positive in most

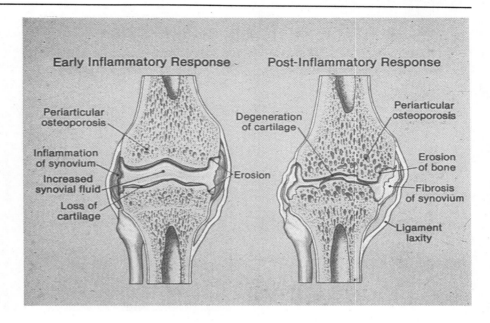

Figure 10–2 Inflammatory and postinflammatory response *(From* AHPA Arthritis Teaching Slide Collection, *2d ed. © 1988. Used by permission of the Arthritis Foundation.)*

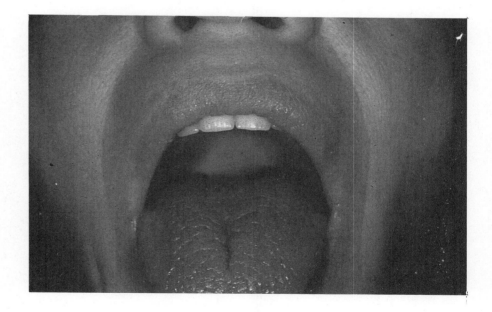

Figure 10–3 Sjögren's syndrome *(From* AHPA Arthritis Teaching Slide Collection, *2d ed. © 1988. Used by permission of the Arthritis Foundation.)*

cases, especially in the later stages of the disease (Pagana and Pagana 1986). Synovial fluid is opaque, with increased white blood cells and decreased viscosity (Swager 1991). X rays taken over a period of time will show the progressive deteriorating changes of the bone and cartilage.

Rheumatoid arthritis is classified according to the presence and degree of joint inflammation. In the acute form, the joints are painful and inflamed. They are boggy, hot, and swollen to palpation. The erythrocyte sedimentation rate is

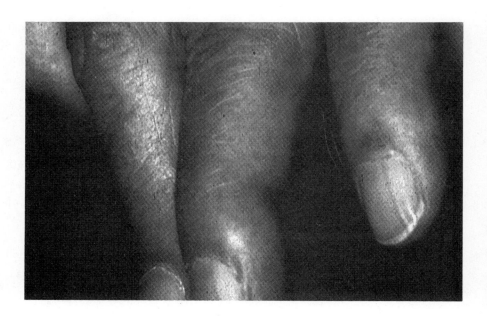

Figure 10–4 Swan neck deformity *(From* AHPA *Arthritis Teaching Slide Collection, 2d ed. © 1988. Used by permission of the Arthritis Foundation.)*

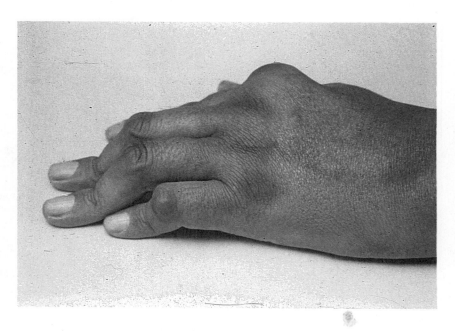

Figure 10–5 Boutonniere deformity *(From* AHPA *Arthritis Teaching Slide Collection, 2d ed. © 1988. Used by permission of the Arthritis Foundation.)*

elevated and there is severe anemia. During the subacute phase, inflammation has subsided, the sedimentation rate returns to normal, and the anemia is resolving. The pain and swelling remain. During chronic rheumatoid arthritis, the laboratory tests are normal and there is no sign of active inflammation in the joints (Mirabelli 1990).

CASE STUDY

Mr. Franklin, seventy-nine years old, was admitted to the nursing home with diagnoses of rheumatoid arthritis and Sjögren's syndrome. Rheumatoid arthritis was diagnosed several years ago and the Sjögren's syndrome a few years later. Mr. Franklin and his wife were living at home, but Mrs. Franklin has become very forgetful, disoriented much of the time, and is suspicious of her husband. She is dependent on her husband and he has found it increasingly difficult to care for her, himself, and the household. They have two children, neither of whom lives in the area. Mr. Franklin decided that admission to the nursing home was the best choice for both of them. He would like to have meals with his wife, but has chosen not to share a room with her at the nursing home.

Strengths

- ❑ Alert and oriented to all three spheres
- ❑ Skin condition is good
- ❑ Continent of bowel and bladder
- ❑ Ambulates without assistance for short distances
- ❑ Capable of completing own activities of daily living with minimal assistance
- ❑ Adequate communication skills
- ❑ Successfully adapted to physical limitations imposed by the rheumatoid arthritis
- ❑ Had a satisfying relationship with his wife until she became markedly disoriented
- ❑ Participates in self-care by making decisions and accepting responsibilities for decisions

Interdisciplinary Assessment

Nursing and Physical Therapy.

Mr. Franklin states that most of the time he has some degree of pain in his hands, shoulders, hips, knees, and feet. Moderate flexion of the elbows, hips, and knees is noted when he is standing. Ulnar deviation without subluxation is observed in both hands. The joints of the hands, knees, and feet are edematous. Morning stiffness lasts about an hour.

Nursing Diagnosis

Alterations in comfort (painful joints) related to arthritis.

Nursing Interventions

- ❑ Continue the medication regime as ordered by the physician — Ibuprofen 300 mg four times daily. In the treatment of arthritis, better results are obtained if the drug is taken routinely rather than prn. Ibuprofen, like most nonsteroidal anti-inflammatory drugs (NSAIDs), should be administered with food or antacids to prevent stomach irritation. Renal and hepatic function should be checked periodically. Tell Mr. Franklin to report any signs of gastrointestinal bleeding (blood in stools or black, tarry stools), visual disturbances, edema, or weight gain (Loeb 1992).
- ❑ Teach Mr. Franklin to use a scale of 0–10 to rate his pain and to evaluate the effectiveness of the medication: 0 is no pain and 10 is the most severe pain (Swearingen 1992).

❏ Allow Mr. Franklin to rest for thirty minutes after he takes the medication. Establish a routine that alternates exercise with rest to help prevent pain from overuse and the stiffness that results from prolonged periods of inactivity. Have Mr. Franklin assist with setting up the routine.

TABLE 10–2	Sample Daily Schedule for Mr. Franklin
	❏ Toileting upon awakening; medication with milk
	❏ Range-of-motion exercises, with gentle stretching
	❏ Rest
	❏ Morning care, including light lotion massage and oral care
	❏ Rest
	❏ Breakfast, followed with oral care
	❏ To therapy for heat treatments
	❏ Rest and relaxation techniques in his room
	❏ Ambulation to tolerance, in hall
	❏ Rest
	❏ Activity of his choice: crossword puzzle, checkers, or other solitary activity; 1:1 activity if he chooses
	❏ Lunch, followed with oral care; medication with lunch
	❏ Rest
	❏ To therapy for heat treatments
	❏ Rest
	❏ Exercise: range of motion and gentle stretching; isometrics
	❏ Rest
	❏ Dinner, followed with oral care; medication with dinner
	❏ Rest
	❏ Ambulation to tolerance, in hall
	❏ Rest
	❏ Activity of his choice: musical presentation, group speaker; medication at bedtime

❏ Suggest the use of relaxation techniques to enhance the effects of the medication and heat treatments (Swearingen 1992). Pain, anxiety, and muscle tension perpetuate each other. The use of skeletal muscle relaxation techniques interrupts this cycle and may diminish pain by easing muscle tension (McCaffery and Beebe 1989). A quiet, undisturbed environment is required, so ask the roommate if he minds being out of the room during this time. Provide Mr. Franklin with the equipment to play a tape recording that takes him through a progressive relaxation technique. Work with him for the first few sessions. By using this technique, he will be able to recognize and locate the involuntary muscle tension in his body and learn to let go. Schedule sessions for twenty minutes, twice a day. Place a sign on his door to avoid interruptions by staff or visitors.

Note: Alert staff to avoid pulling or grabbing Mr. Franklin's joints and extremities. To do so can trigger severe pain.

Collaboration: Interdisciplinary Team

❑ The physical therapist has prescribed paraffin baths to both hands and moist heat applications to the knees and feet twice a day. Both heat and cold are used for temporary relief of arthritis pain. It is better to use either modality intermittently for short periods than for longer periods only once a day. Cool compresses are usually more effective for acute pain resulting from hot, inflamed joints; heat is more often used for subacute or chronic joint problems. Moist heat is preferable since it penetrates the joints deeper. Use both heat and cold treatments with caution. Either may be contraindicated in the presence of vascular, neurological, or dermal disorders. Temperature manipulation relieves pain by altering the pain threshold, decreasing muscle spasm, and increasing the range of motion, thereby alleviating stiffness (Newman and Smith 1991).

Outcome

Mr. Franklin will
❑ Verbalize a decrease in or relief from pain thirty minutes after medication is given
❑ Successfully demonstrate relaxation skills
(See also the section on alterations in family processes.)

Interdisciplinary Assessment

Nursing.

Sjögren's syndrome (also called Sicca's syndrome) is a chronic, inflammatory, autoimmune disorder frequently associated with connective tissue diseases such as rheumatoid arthritis. Mr. Franklin has dry eyes (keratoconjunctivitis) and dry mouth (xerostomia) due to diminished lacrimal and salivary secretions (Shannon-Bodnar 1991). This is caused by the infiltration of the lacrimal and salivary glands with lymphocytes and plasma cells (Tarail 1987). Mr. Franklin's speech is strained, which he says is due to the "dry mouth syndrome." He has been using a spray to help produce saliva and artificial tears to keep his eyes moist. His eyes frequently feel burning and gritty. If dry spots develop on the cornea, they become sclerosed and fibrinous, leading to blindness if not treated (Tarail 1987).

Dietician.

Mr. Franklin has had no problems with choking, but has difficulty swallowing dry foods and drinks large amounts of fluids while eating.

Dental Hygienist.

Routine oral examination revealed the presence of soreness of the lips and oral mucosa and enlarged parotid and submaxillary glands.

Nursing Diagnosis

Alterations in comfort related to decreased salivation and diminished lacrimal secretion due to Sjögren's syndrome.

Nursing Interventions

- ❑ Observe Mr. Franklin's ability to administer his own eye drops. If he has the dexterity to do this, leave the artificial tears at the bedside so Mr. Franklin can administer them four or five times a day. After instilling the drops, teach him to apply a small amount of ophthalmic ointment to the wet eyelids to help retain moisture (Teutsch and Hill 1987). Mr. Franklin is mentally competent and physically able to do this, but provide any assistance that he needs. Ask him to record the time of each treatment.
- ❑ Assess his eyes frequently for signs of infection. Remind Mr. Franklin to wear tinted glasses with side shields when he is in bright light. Advise him to avoid air contact from fans or outdoor breezes (Teutsch and Hill 1987).
- ❑ Monitor for the presence of pain in the eye upon awakening. This may be due to the eyelid adhering to the cornea. The corneal epithelium may be disrupted, causing erosion of the cornea. Place a wet washcloth over the closed eye and call an ophthalmologist immediately. An ophthalmic ointment applied to each eye at bedtime helps prevent this. Place a cool, mist humidifier in the room (Tarail 1987).
- ❑ Keep artificial saliva at his bedside for dry mouth, allowing him to use it as necessary. He may find a mouthwash helpful, but avoid those with alcohol.
- ❑ Instruct Mr. Franklin to do thorough oral care after each meal. Using a Water Pic® helps to dislodge food particles. Inspect his mouth frequently for signs of infection or other dental problems (Teutsch and Hill 1987).
- ❑ Keep a pitcher of fresh water available to him. Suggest to Mr. Franklin that he try saliva-stimulating agents such as hard, sugarless candy and gum.
- ❑ Leave a saline-solution spray or applicators with a container of saline at the bedside and instruct Mr. Franklin to use these to moisten his nasal passages once or twice a day (Shannon-Bodnar 1991).
- ❑ Mr. Franklin has dry skin as a result of Sjögren's syndrome and the aging process. Use a glycerin or superfatted soap for his personal hygiene. Help him apply a water-miscible ointment to the damp skin after he bathes. Watch for cracks or ulcers at the corners of his mouth and around fingernails and toenails (Teutsch and Hill 1987).

Collaboration: Interdisciplinary Team

- ❑ The dietician will provide thickened fluids, such as fruit nectars or juices with a commercial thickener, which are often more manageable. Beverages that contain caffeine will be omitted. Adequate amounts of liquids will be provided with his meals. Spicy, salty, and highly acidic foods that irritate the mouth will be avoided.
- ❑ The dentist or dental hygienist will see Mr. Franklin every three months, more often if necessary.
- ❑ Arrange for the ophthalmologist to examine Mr. Franklin regularly.

Outcome

Mr. Franklin will
- ❑ Experience decreased discomfort related to decreased salivary and lacrimal secretions
- ❑ Remain free of complications resulting from dryness of the eyes, mouth, upper respiratory tract, and skin

Interdisciplinary Assessment _____

Successful management of rheumatoid arthritis is dependent upon a balance of rest and activity. This includes physical and mental activity interwoven with physical rest of the joints, adequate sleep for systemic rest, and emotional rest by learning to handle psychological stress.

Nursing and Occupational Therapy.

At the time of admission, it was evident from the condition of his clothes and body that Mr. Franklin had developed poor hygiene habits. The functional assessment indicates that he is capable of carrying out routine activities of daily living with minimal or moderate assistance.

Physical Therapy.

The effects of arthritis (pain, stiffness, and fatigue) place Mr. Franklin at risk for complications resulting from musculoskeletal inactivity. He is able to walk without assistance in his room and for short distances on the nursing unit. But he prefers to use a wheelchair for longer distances.

Nursing Diagnosis _____

High risk for disuse syndrome related to joint stiffness and pain due to disease process.

Nursing Interventions _____

❏ Check Mr. Franklin frequently around the clock and assist him to change his position at least every two hours. Avoid positions of flexion. Keep the bed flat and, if Mr. Franklin can tolerate it, help him to lie in the prone position for fifteen minutes four times a day. Have his feet hang over the end of the bed while he is prone. This avoids forcing the feet into plantar flexion. It also avoids knee flexion that occurs when a pillow is placed under the ankles. The prone position decreases the risk of knee and hip flexion contractures. When Mr. Franklin is in the supine position, avoid the use of pillows under his knees. Place one flat pillow under his head. Place a rolled towel under his neck to support the cervical spine. This prevents neck flexion. Make sure the covers are loose over his feet to avoid forcing the feet into plantar flexion (Mirabelli 1990).
❏ Note Mr. Franklin's position when he is sitting in the chair. Provide positioning devices as necessary to maintain body alignment. (See chapter 3.)
❏ Assist Mr. Franklin with activities of daily living, encouraging him to do as much as possible by himself. Be sure he has everything he needs within reach. His performance will vary from day to day, so instruct staff to monitor for signs of fatigue and pain and give him help as necessary. Observe him while he is completing these activities.

Collaboration: Interdisciplinary Team _____

The physical therapist has suggested exercises that can be carried out by the nursing staff. Range-of-motion and stretching exercises maintain joint mobility, thus decreasing pain and deformity. *During an acute phase of rheumatoid arthritis, adaptations must be made to these interventions. Rest plays a major role in reducing inflammation.* Strengthening exercises lend stability to affected joints. Endurance exercises promote cardiovascular fitness. Swimming is excellent exercise for persons with access to a heated pool. Isometric exercises are good for strengthening because little stress is placed on the joint and a few repetitions are adequate, thereby avoiding fatigue.

❑ Help Mr. Franklin carry out active assistive range-of-motion exercises twice a day. Teach him to start with a slow, general stretch. Next have him move each joint through its full range of motion. It is important that he control the movement with assistance being given only as needed to support the extremity. Inflamed joints can be gently moved through range of motion twice a day, but only to the point of pain. Other exercises are avoided during these flare-ups.

❑ Suggest to Mr. Franklin that he ambulate within his room and for short distances in the hall, gradually increasing the distance. Teach him to swing his arms while walking and to keep his arms and legs in rhythm. Tell him to alternate periods of brisk walking with periods of leisurely pacing. Have him coordinate deep breathing with the walking pace. Walk with him to monitor his performance and to lend encouragement. (See chapter 3, "Exercise and Activity," for additional information.) Persons with arthritis should avoid high-tension exercises. If pain persists after exercise, advise cutting back but not stopping the exercise.

❑ Consult with the occupational therapist for modifying techniques to avoid placing excessive stress on the joints and for adaptive aids to help him maintain independence. The occupational therapist may suggest the use of resting splints during periods of acute inflammation. These will keep Mr. Franklin's hands and wrists in a natural position to prevent deformities. During a subacute phase, the splints should be worn only at night and for one or two periods during the day.

Outcome

Mr. Franklin will
❑ Maintain current levels of range of motion in all joints
❑ Gradually increase ambulation distances in the hall with a long-range goal of walking to and from the dining room
❑ Carry out activities of daily living with minimal assistance

Interdisciplinary Assessment

Nursing and Social Services.

Mr. Franklin has made many statements concerning his present family status. In the past, he has maintained control of his life, even with the adaptations he has had to make because of the arthritis. It is upsetting to him to be in a situation that he perceives as demeaning. He expresses feelings of guilt because he is unable to care for his wife and because he finds it distressful to be around her for long periods of time. They enjoyed a solid and satisfying relationship for more than fifty years before Mrs. Franklin's cognitive abilities began to deteriorate. Mr. Franklin is worried about their financial status, fearful that they will not have sufficient funds to cover their nursing home costs unless they sell their home. While he understands the need for this and realizes they will probably never live in the home again, it represents to Mr. Franklin another loss in his life that he finds difficult to accept. The family problems are compounded by the fact that they have no support systems available to them. At different times, the two children each visit their parents every six months for a week. Mr. Franklin speaks highly of his children and states that they were a very close family. Because Mr. Franklin does not like to "bother them" with his problems, the children were unaware of their parents' anticipated move to the nursing home until the day before they were admitted.

Age brings with it a succession of losses, each creating a need for change and adaptation. Whether an event or change is perceived as stressful depends on the meaning of that event to the individual. Stress, depression, and pain are closely related. Stress causes muscle tension, increasing the pain of arthritis. Moving to a nursing home is a crisis situation for most people because of the cascading effect associated with the move. It represents a drastic change in the marital relationship and intimacy, loss of health, loss of home and independence, and financial losses. Being thrust among strangers to care for one's most personal needs is overwhelming for most people.

Although Mr. Franklin's wife is living, he is probably experiencing a form of bereavement brought about by the changes in his wife's cognitive status. She is not the same person; the wife he knew no longer exists. Watching one's spouse slowly deteriorate is a most devastating experience.

Mr. Franklin needs to regain a sense of control over his current situation by directing his own financial affairs and health care. After discussion with the social worker, he made the decision to appoint a former business associate to serve as his durable power of attorney for property. This will allow Mr. Franklin to make decisions now that may need to be implemented at a later time when he may not be capable of making decisions. The individual agreed to this and will meet with Mr. Franklin to review his financial status and listen to Mr. Franklin's long-range plans. Mr. Franklin consulted with his children and they agreed this is an appropriate decision. Both Mr. and Mrs. Franklin have living wills that were drawn up previous to Mrs. Franklin's illness. The business associate has been appointed by Mr. Franklin to also serve as his durable power of attorney for health care. In the event of Mr. Franklin's incapacitation, the business associate will legally serve as Mr. Franklin's agent (House of Representatives 1990). Because Mrs. Franklin is not mentally competent to appoint someone as her durable power of attorney for health care, Mr. Franklin will serve as her surrogate as stipulated by state regulations. Should Mr. Franklin predecease his wife, the children will then be appointed surrogates for their mother's health care planning. (See chapter 1 and chapter 11 for additional information.) These forms are attached to their medical records. The physician, business associate, and each child have copies. Mr. Franklin is concerned that his wife will survive him and he is anxious that the terms of this document be carried out.

Nursing Diagnosis

Altered family processes related to diminished physical functional capacities of Mr. Franklin, the increased cognitive impairment of Mrs. Franklin, and change of residence to the nursing home.

Nursing Interventions

❑ Assist Mr. Franklin to direct all activities to the extent that he wishes to do so. His children have made arrangements to visit their parents and to participate in a group meeting with their father and his business associate. While they are here, they will take their father home and help him dispose of household furnishings. Work with Mr. Franklin to help him plan these activities to make optimal use of his available energies.

❑ Make arrangements for the Franklins to have lunch and dinner together every day as Mr. Franklin desires. They are both able to go to the dining room. Let him know that you will help him if he wishes to visit his wife at any other time, but do not be judgmental of his choices. Discuss his wife's condition with him and invite him to attend her care plan conference. Do not place too much emphasis on this if he does not appear interested in attending. At this point, he may not have the emotional energies to deal with decisions regarding her care.

❑ Allow Mr. Franklin to ventilate his feelings, releasing any anger that he may be turning inward.

Collaboration: Interdisciplinary Team

❑ The social worker, in conjunction with the mental health consultant, will visit Mr. Franklin regularly to help him work through his feelings. An understanding of the relationship between stress, pain, and depression will help him deal with it by sharing these feelings with others. While it is beneficial to strive for independence, Mr. Franklin also needs to be aware that it is necessary and natural for everyone to need help from others at various times. To seek help when it is needed is just as important as seeking independence.

❑ A support group for Alzheimer's disease and related disorders meets regularly in the nursing home. The social worker will provide Mr. Franklin with this information and encourage his attendance. He may find it beneficial to meet spouses of nursing home clients with dementia.

Outcome

Mr. Franklin will
❑ Express his feelings regarding nursing home residence and his wife's condition
❑ Verbalize acceptance of his wife's condition
❑ Continue to direct his own financial affairs as long as he desires to make these decisions
❑ Communicate with his children on a regular basis by letter or telephone with the help of the staff if necessary

Interdisciplinary Assessment

Nursing and Activities.

Mr. Franklin expresses little interest in attending any activities and since admission has spent most of the time in his room. He leaves his room only for meals and physical therapy. He has commented that "activities are for kids."

Nursing Diagnosis

Diversional activity deficit related to physical discomfort, previous life-style, and current family situation.

Nursing Interventions

❏ Consult with the activities director and arrange Mr. Franklin's schedule so that he can participate in the activities of his choice.

Collaboration: Interdisciplinary Team

❏ The activities director will talk to Mr. Franklin about individualized activities. He enjoys board games (like checkers) and likes to do crossword puzzles. Puzzles with large squares and a built-up pencil can compensate for his loss of finger and hand dexterity.
❏ Mr. Franklin may enjoy group activities that do not require active participation, such as musical programs, guest speakers, or travelogue presentations.

Outcome

Mr. Franklin will
❏ Participate in activities within his physical capabilities and personal choice.

COMMENTS

Mr. and Mrs. Franklin are faced with a number of serious physical and psychosocial problems. It is difficult to experience the loss of independence due to physical deterioration. To have to witness the deterioration of the spouse at the same time is an additional burden. This situation will become more and more common as the number of elderly persons increases. When one of the couple has a dementia, the other one is usually concerned that the cognitively impaired person will outlive the other. It is imperative that health care staff be aware of the issues involved in each case and be prepared to assist the family to cope with the ongoing situation and any crises that occur. The staff need to allow clients to make decisions. Staff should support those decisions even if/when they seem inappropriate.

A creative interdisciplinary approach can assist both Mr. and Mrs. Franklin to experience a quality of life and peace of mind in their remaining time together.

QUESTIONS AND DISCUSSION

1. Assess a client with rheumatoid arthritis and a client with osteoarthritis. What differences do you note in the clients' descriptions of pain and in the changes in life-style that have resulted from the diseases?
2. What adaptations would you suggest to the client at home for completing activities of daily living and for completing household tasks?
3. Develop a schedule for a client with either form of arthritis. Alternate periods of rest and activity. Evaluate the client after one week to determine whether or not the schedule is effective.
4. Evaluate the positioning programs of clients with arthritis in your facility. Do the positions avoid the use of flexion?
5. Discuss additional interventions by the interdisciplinary health care team that may be beneficial to Mr. Franklin.

REFERENCES

Arthritis Foundation. 1987. *Arthritis: A Serious Look At The Facts*. Atlanta: Arthritis Foundation.

Loeb, S., ed. 1992. *Nursing 92 Drug Handbook*. Springhouse, PA: Springhouse Corporation.

McCaffery, M. and A. Beebe. 1989. *Pain Clinical Manual for Nursing Practice*. St. Louis: The C.V. Mosby Company.

Mirabelli, L. 1990. Caring for Patients with Rheumatoid Arthritis. *Nursing 90* 20(9): 67–68, 70, 72.

Newman, D.K. and D.J. Smith. 1991. *Geriatric Careplans*. Springhouse, PA: Springhouse Corporation.

Pagana, K.D. and T.J. Pagana 1986. *Pocket Guide to Laboratory and Diagnostic Tests*. St. Louis: The C.V. Mosby Company.

Shannon-Bodnar, R. 1991. In M. Shaw, ed. *Illustrated Manual of Nursing Practice*. Springhouse, PA: Springhouse Corporation.

Swager, J. 1991. In M. Shaw, ed. *Illustrated Manual of Nursing Practice*. Springhouse, PA: Springhouse Corporation.

Swearingen, P.L. 1992. *Pocket Guide to Medical-Surgical Nursing*. St. Louis: Mosby-Year Book, Inc.

Tarail, J. 1987. Sjögren's Syndrome, A Dry-Eyed Diary. *American Journal of Nursing* 87(3): 324–26.

Teutsch, E. and M. Hill. 1987. Sjögren's Syndrome, Adding Moisture to Your Life. *American Journal of Nursing* 87(3): 326–29.

U.S. Congress. House. Conference Report. *Omnibus Budget Reconciliation Act of 1990*. 101st Congress, 2nd Session.

CHAPTER 11

A Restorative Approach to Caring for the Client with Terminal Illness

CONTENT OUTLINE

OBJECTIVES

- ❑ Identify effective pain-relieving techniques.
- ❑ Describe methods to provide adequate nourishment for the terminally ill client.
- ❑ List nursing interventions that will prevent respiratory complications in the client with lung cancer.
- ❑ Plan a schedule for the client with cancer that will avoid fatigue.
- ❑ Discuss how to establish a trusting relationship with a dying client that will facilitate the client's comfort and serenity.
- ❑ Identify the role of the interdisciplinary health care team in the management of the client with terminal illness.

DESCRIPTION OF THE DISEASE

Cancer includes a large group of diseases characterized by the uncontrolled growth of abnormal cells that invade and destroy normal tissue, causing metastases and death if not controlled. Cancer is the second leading cause of death, with heart disease as the first and cerebrovascular diseases as the third leading cause of death. In 1990, approximately 1,040,000 people were diagnosed as having cancer. Four of 10 persons who have cancer will be alive five years after diagnosis. The American Cancer Society estimates that 42,500 cancer deaths in 1989 could have been prevented with early detection and treatment (American Cancer Society 1990).

Cancer is a common cause of disability and death in the elderly population. As with all diseases, the risk of acquiring cancer increases as the individual ages. The increase in cancer with age is thought to be due to the combined effects of age-associated changes and longer exposure to carcinogens. Fifty percent of all cancers occur in the group of persons sixty-five years of age and older. Currently, 60 percent of all cancer deaths are in the age group of persons sixty-five years and over (Rosen 1991). With the current growth of this age group and the current incidence of cancer, it is predicted that cases will double by the year 2030. Lung, colon and rectum, prostate, pancreas, and stomach are the leading cancer sites for males age fifty-five to seventy-four. Lung, breast, colon and rectum, ovary, and pancreas are the leading cancer sites for females in this age group. In the age group of seventy-five years and over, lung, prostate, colon and rectum, pancreas, and bladder cancer are the major sites for males. Colon and rectum, breast, lung, pancreas, and ovary are the major sites for females over age seventy-five (Mirand and Knopp 1991).

Decisions regarding treatment and management of older persons with cancer should not be based solely on chronological age, nor should the older person be excluded from the decision process. Many issues, while not unique to the elderly, are often more complicated in this age group. The geriatric client requires special consideration in regard to treatment, pain control, compliance, nutrition, sexual concerns, hospice, and home care (Rosen 1991). A thorough nursing assessment and investigation of the client's history are essential to developing the plan of care. Depression is a common psychiatric disorder in the elderly population and may present symptoms similar to those of advanced cancer. It is important to distinguish reactive depression related to the situation from depression associated with an organic state (D'Agostino, Gray, and Scanlon 1990).

TABLE 11–1	Cancer Detection for People Over Age 40
	The Seven Warning Signs Of Cancer ❑ Change in bowel or bladder habits ❑ A sore that does not heal ❑ Unusual bleeding or discharge ❑ Thickening or lump in breast or elsewhere ❑ Indigestion or difficulty in swallowing ❑ Obvious change in wart or mole ❑ Nagging cough or hoarseness
	Screening Guidelines ❑ Digital rectal exam every year after age forty ❑ Sigmoidoscopy every three to five years beginning at age fifty, based on the recommendation of a physician ❑ Stool Guaiac Slide Test every year beginning at age fifty. ❑ Health counseling and cancer checkup every year after age forty ❑ Breast self-examination monthly for women ❑ Breast examination by physician every year after age forty ❑ Mammogram every one to two years beginning at age forty and annually beginning at age fifty. ❑ Women generally should continue having Pap tests periodically into their sixties. Physicians may recommend stopping tests after age sixty following two consecutive normal tests or if the client has had a hysterectomy.

Continues

❏ Endometrial tissue samples should be taken for women at high risk at the time of menopause. (History of infertility, obesity, failure to ovulate, abnormal uterine bleeding, or estrogen therapy.) (Knopp and Croghan 1991)

The elderly client with cancer who requires long-term health care is often in the advanced stages of the disease. Care may be rendered in the client's home or in a long-term-care facility. The client may have previously undergone treatment in the form of surgery, radiation, chemotherapy, or a combination of these. Treatment may or may not be continuing in an effort to halt the progression of the disease.

Some clients in long-term care have had a chronic form of cancer. They require services to help them adapt to functional losses occurring as a result of cancer therapy as well as age-related changes. Still others in long-term care may be cured of the disease, but need further care, rehabilitation, and teaching after hospital discharge.

The planning of care is dependent upon the reasons for the client's admission to long-term care. For the person in advanced stages, care is directed toward symptom control, psychological support, and the prevention of painful and distressing complications. An acceptance of a hospice philosophy of care is fundamental to giving the client and family a role in the client's care, providing assistance for the client to die in peace and with dignity.

CASE STUDY

Mr. Thomas, age seventy-two, was diagnosed with cancer of the lung two years ago. He had a cough accompanied by shortness of breath for several months. But when he began to expectorate blood-streaked sputum, he sought medical attention. A chest X ray and bronchoscopy with biopsy confirmed the diagnosis of cancer. Symptoms of lung cancer often do not appear until an advanced stage of the disease. After a right lower lobectomy, Mr. Thomas was treated with radiation therapy. He had smoked twenty to thirty cigarettes a day for over fifty years. He stopped after his surgery.

TABLE 11–2	Facts and Figures — Lung Cancer
Incidence	Approximately 157,000/year. Incidence for men is declining while incidence for women continues to increase.
Mortality	92,000 deaths/males (1990 estimate) 50,000 deaths/females (1990 estimate)
Risk Factors	80–90 percent of lung cancer cases are attributable to the carcinogens in tobacco smoke. Risk is related to the age when smoking started, degree of inhalation, number of packs/day, and number of years smoking. In smokers who stop at the time of early, precancerous, cellular changes, damaged bronchial lining tissues often return to normal. New research shows a positive correlation between the occurrence of lung disease and exposure to secondary or passive smoke in the environment (White 1991).
Symptoms	Persistent cough, blood-streaked sputum, chest pain, recurring pneumonia or bronchitis

Continues

Pathology	*Epidermoid* — Usually starts in the periphery of a lung and is usually not detected until the bronchi are invaded *Adenocarcinoma* — Usually starts in the periphery, frequently arising in areas of previous pulmonary damage *Oat-cell* — Centrally located tumor that has usually metastasized at the time of diagnosis *Large-cell, undifferentiated* — Appears most frequently in the peripheral lung, with pleural and regional node involvement
Treatment	Surgery, radiation therapy, chemotherapy — determined by the type and stage of cancer
Survival	13 percent 5-year survival rate in all persons, regardless of the cancer stage at diagnosis (White 1991)

Mr. Thomas has a wife, five children, twelve grandchildren, and two great-grandchildren. He worked in a factory for many years, retiring at the age of sixty-five. His wife retired as a domestic worker two years ago when Mr. Thomas had surgery. He has been at home since the surgery, in relatively good health until six months ago, when his condition began to deteriorate. His wife was diagnosed with congestive heart failure two months ago and is now unable to continue providing the care Mr. Thomas needs. Because of this, he was admitted to the nursing home. The nursing care of older clients with cancer is no different than that of younger persons. However, age-associated changes predispose Mr. Thomas to complications associated with the cancer and inactivity, such as pneumonia, skin breakdown, joint stiffness, and constipation.

Strengths

❑ Cognitively unimpaired
❑ Continent of bowel and bladder
❑ Able to ambulate for short distances with assistance
❑ Three children live in the area and have been supportive of their parents throughout Mr. Thomas's illness

Interdisciplinary Assessment

Nursing.

Mr. Thomas complains of pain in the lower back. Cancer pain can be related to the tumor, the cancer therapy, or may stem from a preexisting or concurrent condition. The goal for treatment of pain is pain relief without marked sedation or serious side effects from the medication.

Nursing Diagnosis

Chronic pain related to progression of the disease state.

Nursing Interventions

❑ Give acetaminophen 325 mg with 60 mg codeine (Tylenol with Codeine No.

4®) every four hours around the clock. As the cancer metastasizes and the pain increases, Mr. Thomas will be started on morphine 15–20 mg p.o., titrated at increments until adequate pain relief is achieved. Pain is a subjective, personal experience and Mr. Thomas is the best judge of the severity of the pain. To assess the need for beginning the morphine, ask him to rate his pain on a scale of 0–10, with 0 being no pain and 10 being severe pain.

❏ Monitor Mr. Thomas for signs of sudden, acute, temporary pain. This is breakthrough pain that requires adjusted doses of medication or a supplemental medication. Breakthrough pain may be precipitated by something the client does or by a treatment or procedure. If the precipitating factor is known, give medication thirty to sixty minutes before the event. For unpredictable breakthrough pain, give the medication as soon as possible. Administer a supplemental analgesic dose — a rapid-acting drug with a short half-life (Nursing 90 1990).

❏ Use nonpharmacologic techniques with the medication. Build a trusting relationship with Mr. Thomas and assure him that you will help him manage the pain and keep it under control. Give back massages and reposition as necessary for comfort. Mr. Thomas may wish to learn progressive relaxation techniques. If he agrees to this, provide him with a tape player and tape that can be utilized at his discretion.

❏ Monitor bowel elimination. Constipation is a common side effect of analgesia. If irregularity becomes a problem, ask Mr. Thomas what has worked in the past.

TABLE 11–3	Pseudo-Addiction
	It is important to know that if short-acting opiates are given at ineffective dosing intervals, pseudo-addiction can occur. As a result of inadequate pain treatment, the client may exhibit signs of psychological dependency and resort to bizarre behavior to prove that medication is needed. This can be prevented by giving adequate doses around the clock, using oral drugs if possible and frequently assessing the client's pain level (Nursing 90 1990).

Outcome

Mr. Thomas will
❏ Verbalize relief of pain

Interdisciplinary Assessment

Nursing.

Alterations in breathing rate and depth and pulse rate are noted during increased physical activity. Mr. Thomas reports shortness of breath during increased physical activity. Infection, inflammation, or the tumor can cause coughing. Persistent coughing can cause chest pain and hemoptysis, interferes with rest, and can even cause pathologic rib fractures.

Activities.

Mr. Thomas occasionally chooses to attend an activity but during participation exhibits discomfort related to the shortness of breath.

Nursing Diagnosis

Ineffective breathing patterns related to diminished lung function.

Nursing Interventions

- ❑ Teach Mr. Thomas breathing exercises and effective coughing techniques to enhance the gas exchange in the alveoli. (See chapter 18.) He is at risk for pneumonia because of the diminished lung function.
- ❑ Allow Mr. Thomas plenty of time for the physical activities. For example, a.m. and p.m. care may need to be given at intervals instead of all at one time. Provide as much assistance as he needs. If he is having difficulty breathing, postpone the activity.
- ❑ Mr. Thomas may require low-flow oxygen. This will not be effective if his blood gases are normal.
- ❑ Encourage him to drink eight to ten glasses of fluid each day to liquify respiratory secretions and promote hydration.
- ❑ Humidify the air with a cold-water vaporizer.
- ❑ Assess for signs of respiratory tract infection. (See chapter 18 for additional information.) Request an order for antibiotics, antipyretics, and cough suppressants if signs of respiratory infection occur.

Collaboration: Interdisciplinary Team

- ❑ Caution all staff to allow Mr. Thomas adequate time for activities or to postpone them if necessary in order to avoid causing shortness of breath.

Outcome

Mr. Thomas will
- ❑ Not experience moderate or severe dyspnea
- ❑ Remain free of respiratory tract infections

Interdisciplinary Assessment

Nursing.

Mr. Thomas has little interest in eating and has obvious difficulty swallowing. Anorexia is a common problem among people with cancer and can be caused by the disease or by treatments. In Mr. Thomas's case, impaired swallowing is a result of the effects of radiation on the esophagus. Problems associated with appetite, taste, and eating are major causes of protein-calorie malnutrition in persons with cancer. Ingestion of adequate nutrients aids in preventing skin breakdown and constipation, maintains optimal function of the immune system, repairs normal cells, and increases the client's energy levels.

Dietician.

Mr. Thomas has lost 15 pounds in the last six months. His usual body weight is 170 pounds.

Nursing Diagnosis

Alterations in nutrition, less than body requirements, related to loss of appetite and impaired swallowing.

Nursing Interventions

☐ Advise Mr. Thomas that drinking milk and eating milk products coats the mucous membrane, making eating more comfortable. Suggest that he avoid foods with temperature extremes, foods that are spicy or acidic, and foods that are hard, crunchy, or coarse.

☐ Talk with the family to see if there are special foods they can bring in that Mr. Thomas likes.

☐ Prepare Mr. Thomas for mealtime and provide an appetite-stimulating environment. (See chapter 5.) Arrange for pain medication to be administered thirty to sixty minutes before meals.

☐ Protein malnutrition can cause stomatitis, resulting in painful ulcerations. Assess Mr. Thomas's oral mucosa daily and assist him with careful and thorough mouth care at least twice daily. Use a soft-bristle toothbrush and nonirritating toothpaste. Instruct Mr. Thomas to rinse with a solution of 500 ml water, ½ teaspoon salt, and ½ teaspoon sodium bicarbonate every four hours. Use Toothettes® if the brush causes bleeding. Avoid the use of glycerine and lemon-juice swabs. They could irritate the oral tissues (Kelly 1990). Avoid commercial mouthwashes containing alcohol. Lubricate Mr. Thomas's lips with cocoa butter or lip balm.

☐ Constipation can become a problem as a result of the codeine and inactivity. Include high-fiber foods in Mr. Thomas's diet that are easy to swallow, such as cooked prunes, prune juice, and whole-grain cereals with milk.

☐ Weigh Mr. Thomas weekly.

Collaboration: Interdisciplinary Team

☐ Ask the dietician to complete a nutritional assessment.

☐ Ask the dietician to give Mr. Thomas suggestions for food preparation that may facilitate swallowing. Have Mr. Thomas assist with the development of diet plans. Liquids such as gravies, sauces, or mayonnaise can be added to solid foods for easier swallowing.

☐ The dietary department can increase the calorie and protein value of foods without increasing quantity. Prepare double-strength milk by mixing dry skim milk with liquid milk instead of water; mix instant breakfast drinks with the double-strength milk. Evaporated, condensed, or double-strength milk can be used to make casseroles, puddings, milk shakes, and soups. Cheese, cream cheese, and whipped cream can be added to appropriate foods. Margarine added to sandwiches and cooked vegetables increases calories. Additional protein can be served by adding eggs, meat, poultry, and fish to salads, casseroles, and sandwiches. Commercially prepared protein-rich supplements can be given between meals. Include foods that need chewing in each meal since chewing promotes circulation in gum tissues.

❑ Consult with the speech pathologist for additional interventions to facilitate swallowing.
(See chapter 5, "Alterations in Nutrition," for additional information.)

Outcome

Mr. Thomas will
❑ Participate in meal planning
❑ Gain two pounds within the next month
❑ Establish a regular pattern of defecation

Interdisciplinary Assessment

All Disciplines.

Mr. Thomas reports feelings of exhaustion and tiredness. He is frustrated when he is unable to enjoy his family's visits because of the fatigue. Fatigue is another common problem associated with cancer. In Mr. Thomas's case, nutritional alterations, chronic pain, anxiety, depression, chronic pain, and altered sleeping patterns all contribute to fatigue.

Nursing Diagnosis

Fatigue related to multiple factors due to cancer.

Nursing Interventions

❑ Monitor comments and behaviors indicative of fatigue by observing Mr. Thomas's physical appearance, breathing patterns, level of activity, food and fluid intake, and mental status. Observe for aggravating factors and associated symptoms, such as pain.
❑ Assess and correct environmental factors, such as noise and excessive heat, that can contribute to fatigue.
❑ Assist Mr. Thomas to pace his activities according to his energy level by establishing a structured schedule of alternating rest periods and activity. Help him with active assistive range-of-motion exercises at least twice daily. Assist him to ambulate once or twice a day within the limits of his tolerance. Suggest he sit up in a comfortable chair for several short periods during the day.
❑ Rearrange Mr. Thomas's schedule when he has special activities planned, giving priorities to such activities as family visits.
❑ Schedule night procedures, such as repositioning and skin care, to be done when his medication is administered.

Collaboration: Interdisciplinary Team

❑ Ask all staff to be knowledgeable and considerate of Mr. Thomas's schedule and the activities that are his priorities for the day.

Outcome

Mr. Thomas will
❑ Participate in planning a routine that balances his energy level

❑ Verbalize alleviation of fatigue

Interdisciplinary Assessment _____

Nursing and Dietary.

Assessment for pressure-ulcer potential places Mr. Thomas in the high-risk category. (See chapter 4.)

Nursing Diagnosis _____

High risk for impaired skin integrity related to alterations in nutrition, inactivity, and radiation therapy.

Nursing Interventions _____

Establish protocol for pressure-ulcer prevention. (See chapter 4.)

Outcome _____

Mr. Thomas will
❑ Be free of impaired skin integrity

Interdisciplinary Assessment _____

Nursing and Social Services.

It is difficult to determine whether some of the symptoms (lack of appetite and fatigue) exhibited by Mr. Thomas are a result of the physiological aspects of cancer or whether they are related to depression. Researchers have noted that the client's fears of cancer and death are often subordinate to fears of abandonment, unacceptability, and isolation (National Cancer Institute 1982). Family members and close friends may withdraw from the dying client as they mourn the loss before it occurs. This is a self-protective mechanism to ease grieving when death actually occurs.

Mr. Thomas has expressed his inability to deal with dying and death but occasionally makes comments that he just wants to get it over with and die. He is often irritable with his wife when she visits, ignoring her offers for assistance and criticizing her efforts to help him. When his children visit, he is less irritable, but is uncommunicative at times. Throughout his adult life, Mr. Thomas has been the patriarch of the family, making all major decisions. Efforts of Mrs. Thomas to discuss any legal matters with her husband have been unsuccessful. She understands his reaction and is willing to listen to suggestions that can help her assist her husband. She is sad that he will not be getting better but has accepted his death and wishes to make the rest of his life as pleasant as possible.

Nursing Diagnosis _____

Ineffective individual coping related to prognosis.

Nursing Interventions

- Consult with Mr. Thomas on all aspects of his care, giving him information he can use to make wise decisions. He needs to be in control of his care as long as he wishes and as long as he is able to make decisions.
- Establish a trusting relationship with Mr. Thomas and provide him with opportunities to express his feelings. Acknowledge his feelings and let him know that crying and grieving are not reflections of a lack of masculinity.
- Observe his potential for self-destructive behavior.
- Arrange for him and Mrs. Thomas to have uninterrupted privacy when she visits so they may share intimacy and affection. Suggest that she seek her husband's input for decisions related to their home and finances. Let them know that their grandchildren are welcome to visit at any time and that arrangements can be made for a dining room if the family wishes to share a meal with Mr. Thomas.
- Suggest that progressive relaxation techniques used for breathing may assist him to cope when he is feeling anxious.
- Listen for clues indicating that Mr. Thomas may have "unfinished" business that needs attention. There may be something in his past that needs to be resolved before he can successfully cope with the business of dying. Encourage the process of life review. All older persons confront the task of what Erikson calls *ego integrity*: "a basic acceptance of one's life as having been inevitable, appropriate, and meaningful" (Erikson 1963).

Collaboration: Interdisciplinary Team

- Ask for a mental health evaluation if these interventions are not effective. The physician may prescribe an antidepressant. Tricyclics are the agents most frequently used in cancer-related depression. If a tricyclic is ordered, monitor Mr. Thomas for anticholinergic side effects common with these medications.
- Although Mr. Thomas has never been a religious person in the usual sense of the word, inquire as to whether he would like to talk to a clergyperson.
- Discuss with Mr. Thomas and his family whether they would like a representative from the local hospice agency to meet with them. Let the family know that hospice also provides bereavement counseling when it is needed.
- If weather permits, ask a volunteer to take Mr. Thomas outdoors for a wheelchair walk and a change of environment. Ask activities staff to invite him to participate in pet therapy or musical presentations.
- Refer the Thomas family to a support group for families of clients with cancer.
- If Mr. Thomas is unable to discuss issues concerning his care, Social Services can offer to discuss with Mrs. Thomas the kinds of decisions that may need to be made regarding her husband's health care. It is beneficial to clients and their families to look ahead and devise plans that will affect health care decisions and financial arrangements. The federal government legislated the Self-Determination Act in 1990 so that competent adults would have the right to make decisions regarding their health care. Each state has interpreted and implemented this law within the realm of state legislation.

TABLE 11–4	Legal Considerations for Decision Making
Living Will	This document, drawn and signed while the client is competent, expresses the client's decisions concerning the administration of life-prolonging medical procedures when there is no chance of regaining a meaningful life. In order for the living will to work, the client must be in a terminal condition. This document should be reinforced with the Durable Power of Attorney for Health Care document (Illinois Department of Public Health 1991).
Do-Not-Resuscitate Orders (DNR)	Physicians' orders tell nursing and facility staff that certain measures designed to keep the client alive are not to be done if the client suffers cardiopulmonary arrest. In most states, CPR must be started unless there is an order to the contrary in the client's chart. DNR orders are consistent with other advance directives, but are not substitutes for them.
Durable Power of Attorney for Health Care	The client (principal) can delegate to a person of his choice (agent) the power to become his agent for any health care decision he is unable to make. The agent, not necessarily an attorney, will speak for the client and make decisions according to the client's wishes even during periods of physical or mental incapacity. The client can specify the time which the Durable Powers of Attorney will begin and terminate. Unless stated otherwise, the document continues until death (Illinois Department of Public Health 1991).
Durable Power of Attorney for Property	The client (principal) can delegate to a person of his choice (agent) the power to become his agent for financial decisions when the client becomes incapacitated.
Health Care Surrogate	If the client lacks decisional capacity, has a "qualifying condition," and does not have an operative living will or durable power of attorney for health care, a surrogate is selected from a statutory hierarchy to make decisions regarding life-sustaining treatment. *Note:* This varies among states and not all states have health care surrogate legislation (Illinois Department of Public Health 1991).
Guardianship	Guardianship is initiated when an individual (other than the client) petitions the civil court. The allegedly incompetent person, the petitioner, and anyone who would be entitled to be an heir of the estate attend a competency hearing. After hearing evidence, the judge decides incompetency based on the criteria of that state. If the individual is declared incompetent, the judge assigns a guardian to oversee the person and/or that person's estate. The guardian may be a family member, attorney, government agency, or a professional specializing in this work. If plenary guardianship is assigned, the guardian has total legal authority over estate and person. The incapacitated person no longer has the rights of an adult (Stevenson and Capezuti 1991).

Outcome

Mr. Thomas will
❑ Identify and demonstrate positive coping mechanisms
❑ Maintain a satisfying relationship with his wife and family, accepting their support
❑ Express his feelings openly

COMMENTS

Mr. Thomas and his family would prefer to have him at home for the remainder of the time he has left to live. Because of Mrs. Thomas's health and other circumstances, this is not possible. It is imperative that nursing home staff plan his care around his needs rather than around facility routine and procedures. Everyone caring for Mr. Thomas must be able to provide the spiritual and emotional help that he needs. When people like Mr. Thomas are terminally ill, death is not something to resist, but a natural rite of passage with spiritual significance for him and his family. Acceptance of death does not imply hopelessness. Rather, it extends hope — hope for comfort, for pleasure in whatever time is left, and when the time comes, a dignified death.

Gerontological nurses must accept the responsibility of serving as advocates for clients and their families. There are a myriad of ethical issues today that require knowledge so that the caregivers may contribute to the welfare of those in their care.

The elderly population has a need for education in terms of cancer prevention and detection. Health care professionals need to be aware of their role in providing this education and in assisting the frail elderly in this matter.

The elderly are a heterogeneous group. Age should not be the sole criterion for determining the course of treatment for cancer. The physiological and functional status of the individual also needs to be considered. Caregivers need to help their clients live well and die well.

QUESTIONS AND DISCUSSION

1. Evaluate your clients' knowledge of cancer prevention, risk reduction, screening, and detection.
2. Examine your personal feelings regarding terminal illness and the Self-Determination Act.
3. What nonpharmacologic interventions can you implement that will facilitate the effectiveness of the pain medication?
4. What actions can the nursing staff take to provide support to clients with cancer and to their families?
5. What other interventions by the interdisciplinary team would be beneficial to Mr. Thomas?

REFERENCES

American Cancer Society. 1990. *Cancer Facts and Figures – 1990*. Atlanta: American Cancer Society.

D'Agostino, N.S., G. Gray, and C. Scanlon. 1990. Cancer in the Older Adult: Understanding Age-Related Changes. *Journal of Gerontological Nursing* 16(6): 12–15.

Erikson, E. 1963. *Childhood and Society*. 2d ed. New York: W.W. Norton and Company, Inc.

Illinois Department of Public Health. 1991. *Advance Directives and the Health Care Surrogate Act*. Springfield, IL: Illinois Department of Public Health.

Kelly, F.M. 1990. Preventing Oral Infection. *Nursing 90* 20(8): 88.

Knopp, J.M. and I.T. Croghan. 1991. In S.B. Baird, M.G. Donehower, V.L. Stalsbroten, and T.B. Ades, eds. *A Cancer Source Book for Nurses*. 6th ed. Atlanta: American Cancer Society, Inc.

Mirand, A.L. and J.M. Knopp. 1991. In S.B. Baird, M.G. Donehower, V.L. Stalsbroten, and T.B. Ades, eds. *A Cancer Source Book for Nurses.* 6th ed. Atlanta: American Cancer Society, Inc.

National Cancer Institute. 1982. *Coping with Cancer.* Bethesda, MD: U.S. Department of Health and Human Services.

Rosen, S.T. 1991. Cancer and the Aged. *Center on Aging* 6(3): 1–2.

Staff. 1990. Cancer Update 90. *Nursing 90* 20(4): 61–64.

Stevenson, C. and E. Capezuti. 1991. Guardianship: Protection vs. Peril. *Geriatric Nursing* 12(1): 10–13.

White, E.J. 1991. In S.B. Baird, M.G. Donehower, V.L. Stalsbroten, and T.B. Ades, eds. *A Cancer Source Book for Nurses.* 6th ed. Atlanta: American Cancer Society.

White, E.J. and J.M. Knopp. 1991. In S.B. Baird, M.G. Donehower, V.L. Stalsbroten, and T.B. Ades, eds. *A Cancer Source Book for Nurses.* 6th ed. Atlanta: American Cancer Society.

CHAPTER ![12] A Restorative Approach to Caring for the Client with Impaired Communication

---

OBJECTIVES

❑ Distinguish between aphasia, verbal apraxia, and dysarthria.
❑ Describe effective nursing interventions for the client with aphasia and dysarthria.
❑ Identify the role of the interdisciplinary health care team in the management of the client with impaired communication.

DESCRIPTION OF THE PROBLEM

Communication is a process used for sending and receiving messages. It provides a means for utilizing information and facilitates social interaction. Information is received by the brain through auditory, visual, and tactile channels. The brain integrates and processes this information so it can be expressed by means of speaking, writing, gesturing, or body movements. Impairments in the auditory, visual, or tactile senses, in the brain, or in the muscles used for speech can interfere with the process of communication. Communication requires the use of language and speech. Language consists of a set of symbols used to receive and transmit messages (Adkins 1991). Letters, numbers, signs, and gestures are utilized for language. To use language, one must know what the symbols mean before the information can be interpreted and understood. Speech is a motor act involving coordinated movements of the muscles of respiration, the lips, tongue, jaw, palate, and larynx. Aphasia is a language impairment and apraxia of speech (verbal apraxia) and dysarthria are speech impairments due to neuropathology.

Aphasia involves all language modalities. It affects speaking, reading, writing, comprehension, object recognition, and arithmetic. It is secondary to brain damage in the left (dominant) hemisphere of the brain resulting from stroke, trauma, infection, tumors, or dementia. A stroke involving the left hemisphere of the brain is the cause of aphasia. Major speech centers are located in the nondominant (right) hemisphere in about 25 percent of left-handed clients. In these cases, aphasia results from damage to the right hemisphere (Newman and Smith 1991).

Aphasia is categorized by the location of the brain damage and the resulting deficits. There are a number of adjectives used to describe each category. The nurse needs to understand the classifications of aphasia to interpret the progress notes of the speech pathologist and to know what to expect of the client.

Broca's aphasia is also referred to as verbal, motor, expressive, and nonfluent aphasia. Individuals with Broca's aphasia use flat sounding, slow, hesitant speech. They may grimace and use hand gestures in their efforts to communicate (Chipps, Clanin, and Campbell 1992). The ability to write language is often more impaired than verbal communication. Because it is a problem of expression, these individuals can comprehend spoken and written language better than they can speak or write. However, comprehension is also impaired. A client with Broca's aphasia is often aware of the errors made while trying to communicate and will try to correct them, but usually without success. The client becomes very frustrated with the deficits (Adkins 1991).

Wernicke's aphasia is also described as sensory, receptive, acoustic, and fluent aphasia. Clients with Wernicke's aphasia can produce fluent speech, but it is usually lacking in content. They are generally unaware of their errors and may talk endlessly. Language is circumlocutory, i.e., long sentences and meaningless words are used when a few, specific words would suffice (Chipps et al. 1992).

Global aphasia is nonfluent and is a result of a lesion that affects a major portion of the language area of the brain. Individuals with global aphasia are unable to communicate by speech, gestures, or writing. This type is very difficult to treat.

Speech

Most clients with aphasia also have apraxia of speech. This impairment is not due to muscle weakness or paralysis. The problem is that the brain is not sending the information to the muscles that enable the client to articulate speech. It is characterized by the partial or complete inability to produce speech voluntarily. The client knows what to say, but is unable to produce the movements necessary for speech. Clients with mild verbal apraxia may have intelligible speech, but use inconsistent sound substitutions. For example, pencil may be fensil or bed may be led. The client with severe apraxia may be unable to produce any meaningful sounds. The following guidelines may enhance communication with clients with verbal apraxia.

❑ Encourage the use of gestures.
❑ Provide a notebook of pictures of objects that relate to the client's immediate needs — a toilet, bed, glass of water, etc., Figure 12–1. The client can point to the correct object.
❑ Provide a magic slate if the client can write.
❑ Provide a notebook of common, frequently used words, if the client can read.
❑ If the client acquires a new word in speech therapy, reinforce the use of the new word.

(Larson 1988)

Dysarthria is a speech disorder, usually secondary to brain damage resulting

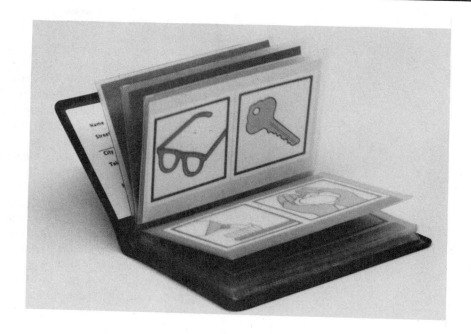

Figure 12–1 Communications notebook (*Provided by Fred Sammons Inc. © 1991 by Bissell Health Care Company*)

from trauma, stroke, or neurological disorders such as Parkinson's disease, multiple sclerosis, cerebral palsy, and amyotrophic lateral sclerosis. Clients with dysarthria rarely have language problems unless there has been diffuse bilateral brain damage due to stroke or trauma. In these cases, aphasia, apraxia of speech, and dysarthria may all be present. Dysarthria is due to a weakness or paralysis of one or more of the muscles used in speaking. There may be a combination of disorders characterized by difficulties with phonation, articulation, resonance, and the rate and rhythm of speech. Clients with dysarthria generally have associated problems with swallowing and/or breathing. Follow these guidelines when the client has dysarthria:

❑ Listen very carefully to the client and concentrate on what is being said because the problem is often one of volume. Be sure the environment is quiet.

❑ Listen for consistency, as errors in sounds may be predictable. This can help you interpret what the client is saying.

❑ Remember that dysarthria does not affect comprehension. Do not simplify your communication. Ask questions that do not require lengthy answers that cause the client to become fatigued.

❑ Ask the client to think about the movements of the tongue, lips, and cheeks when speaking.

❑ Consider a communication board for the client who is extremely unintelligible.

Evaluation and Treatment of Language and Speech Disorders

The skills and knowledge of the speech pathologist are required for the evaluation and treatment of language and speech disorders. This person is a member of the interdisciplinary team and should participate in care plan conferences for clients utilizing these services. Communication among caregivers is maintained by including the client-therapist goals and interventions on the care plan.

Through evaluation, the speech pathologist makes a diagnosis and determines the strengths and deficits of the client. Psychosocial status is taken into consideration by evaluating the client's previous coping patterns, motivation, presence of emotional stressors, and self-concept. The client is assessed for the presence of sensory deficits (such as hemianopsia). Treatment may be provided on an individual basis or in group sessions.

The goals of speech therapy are usually directed toward developing an effective means of communication. Goals are geared to the special needs of the client. These are partially determined by the environment in which the client will be living.

The prognosis of the client depends upon the type and severity of the aphasia. The damaged brain cells will not recover, so the healthy cells that are left must be trained to take over the areas that are lost. The client left with little speech and language will therefore not regain as much as the client with minimal impairment. Although the client with minimal impairment may not appear to need therapy, the individual may be aware of the problem and become frustrated in trying to deal with it. These clients can benefit greatly from therapy.

Health care professionals may feel that speech therapy is not necessary for older clients, particularly those living in nursing homes. The longer treatment is delayed, the less chance there is of improvement. However, success has been attained in many cases with the initiation of late treatment.

Although the evaluation and treatment of speech disorders is not within the realm of the professional nurse, it is the nurse who may need to suggest an evaluation to the physician. The nurse is the liaison between physician, speech pathologist, and staff. The speech pathologist may or may not involve the nursing staff in the implementation of specific interventions. All members of the interdisciplinary team need to have an understanding of communication impairments and the techniques to use during ongoing contacts with the client. In-services presented by the speech pathologist can be very beneficial in stimulating interest and enhancing the communication skills of staff.

CASE STUDY

Mr. Baker, seventy-six years old, was admitted to the nursing home from the hospital after treatment for a stroke involving the left hemisphere of the brain. He has right hemiplegia and communication deficits. Mr. Baker requires assistance in all activities of daily living. Nursing home placement is regarded as permanent at this time. His wife is in poor health and has been staying with her son and his family since Mr. Baker's hospitalization. Before the stroke, Mr. and Mrs. Baker lived together in a small home in the city. He was a foreman in a factory for several years before retirement and Mrs. Baker was a homemaker. His care at the nursing home will be directed toward improving his skills in activities of daily living, preventing complications, establishing a means of communication, and facilitating his adaptation to the nursing home. (See chapter 21, "A Restorative Approach to Stroke," for additional information.)

Strengths _____

- ❑ Adequate hearing and vision; to be assessed for hemianopsia
- ❑ Nutritional status adequate
- ❑ Skin intact
- ❑ Continent of bowel and bladder if assistance is given
- ❑ Active in a number of associations previous to stroke

Interdisciplinary Assessment

Nursing and All Disciplines.

Both the staff and Mr. Baker are frustrated over the inability to communicate effectively. Mr. Baker has difficulty initiating speech and talks very slowly. He is frequently unable to find the correct words to use. He often tries to correct his mistakes and becomes very frustrated when he cannot. Mr. Baker responds to "How are you, Mr. Baker?" with "fine, fine, fine." Sentences with just two or three words dominate his speech pattern. He may say "go bed" or "want drink" or "to bathroom." This is referred to as telegraphic speech. Sometimes these words are not understood by staff due to awkwardness with articulation. Some of the staff do not understand how Mr. Baker can sing old Sunday school songs but is unable to talk. This is an example of automatic speech — the retrieval of overlearned words, phrases, or sentences that can be uttered without thought. It is the use of information that was previously learned by rote memory. Swearing is another example of automatic speech that Mr. Baker sometimes uses. This annoys some of the caregivers who do not understand the reasons for his behavior. Mr. Baker's family is embarrassed by the swearing. They too have difficulty talking with Mr. Baker. When they visit, they often talk over him rather than to him.

Nursing Diagnosis

Impaired verbal communication related to left brain damage.

Nursing Interventions

- Suggest to Mr. Baker's physician that he be evaluated by the speech pathologist.
- Provide the staff and Mr. Baker's family with information on Mr. Baker's condition and the ramifications of left-side brain damage. Provide them with general guidelines for communicating with aphasic persons. These guidelines should be used by nursing staff and all members of the interdisciplinary team.

Collaboration: Interdisciplinary Team

Ask all staff members to follow these guidelines when communicating with Mr. Baker:

- Be relaxed and calm when you are working with Mr. Baker.
- Eliminate environmental distractions and noise when communicating.
- Treat Mr. Baker as an adult. Do not talk down to him or use baby talk. His intellect is not impaired.
- Avoid the temptation to talk louder — he is not deaf. Shouting may confuse him or he may think you are angry.
- Accept him as he is at his speech and language level. Make every effort to understand his efforts whether they are verbal or gestures.
- Avoid showing disapproval or shock when Mr. Baker swears. He may retreat, refusing to attempt speech entirely.
- Get his attention before communicating by calling him by his name.
- Talk to Mr. Baker while doing other procedures with him.
- Speak slowly and distinctly without dragging out the words or overarticulating. He needs time to process the information.

❑ Talk about concrete topics since he may have difficulty comprehending abstract ideas. Use short, complete phrases, especially if he will need to respond or if you are giving him instructions.

❑ Name objects as you work with him, e.g., "Here is your fork," "I will wash your legs now." Talk in a sequential, organized manner, keeping related topics together. Randomly presented ideas may cause confusion. Check his comprehension by asking a question based on a previous statement. Ask questions that require short answers or yes and no answers. Comprehension may be noted by other than verbal means, such as facial expression.

❑ Check the accuracy of his yes and no answers by asking a question with a no answer that is within the realm of his comprehension, e.g., "Are you under fifty years of age?"

❑ Be an active listener. Maintain eye contact, stop the activity for a moment, reflect on his words, and ask questions that flow from his comments. Be patient and give him time to prepare and deliver his message.

❑ Acknowledge Mr. Baker's frustration. "You're having a hard time with that word. Let's talk about something else and then you can try it again later."

❑ Give Mr. Baker opportunities to use automatic speech, such as greetings and other social exchanges. These increase his feelings of confidence.

❑ Do not pressure Mr. Baker to say things he has said before. Just because he said something yesterday, does not mean he will be able to say it today.

❑ Allow Mr. Baker to speak for himself. Anticipating his comments and voicing them for him can impede his progress. If he communicates a desire for help in finding a word, pronounce it slowly and distinctly.

❑ Try to maintain a consistent routine, consistent caregivers, and a consistent environment. Mr. Baker will feel more secure with the familiar.

❑ Allow Mr. Baker to make decisions commensurate with his abilities and encourage him to do as much as possible for himself. As with all clients, remember to draw on his residual abilities and avoid dwelling on disabilities.

❑ Provide appropriate opportunities for socialization.

❑ Laughter is sometimes the best medicine. Use appropriate humor and encourage staff and clients to laugh together. Laughter is conducive to a relaxed environment and facilitates interaction. Everyone will benefit.

Outcome

Mr. Baker will
❑ Experience fewer periods of frustration due to impaired communication
❑ Develop successful techniques for communication

Interdisciplinary Assessment

Nursing and Physical Therapy.

Functional assessment reveals that Mr. Baker has minimal use of his right arm and moderate use of his right leg.

Nursing Diagnosis

Impaired physical mobility related to right hemiplegia.

Nursing Interventions

- ❏ Initiate a range-of-motion program and begin a progressive mobilization program.
- ❏ Use a one-person assist and a transfer belt to transfer Mr. Baker. Remember to move toward the side of strength, the left side. Begin teaching self-transfer techniques.
- ❏ Obtain a lap board or arm trough for Mr. Baker's wheelchair to avoid injury and contracture to the right arm. Because his right hemisphere is intact, Mr. Baker may benefit by observing others walking and transferring. (See chapter 3 for additional information.)

Collaboration: Interdisciplinary Team

- ❏ Consult with the physical therapist for suggestions for teaching Mr. Baker self-transfers.
- ❏ Ask the physical therapist about starting Mr. Baker on a gait training program. With the ability remaining in his right leg, he will probably do well with a quad cane.

Outcome

Mr. Baker will
- ❏ Remain free of contractures
- ❏ Transfer independently within three months
- ❏ Walk safely with the assistance of a quad cane

Interdisciplinary Assessment

Nursing and Occupational Therapy.

Mr. Baker is able to carry out the basic activities of daily living with some assistance. He is very slow and cautious and somewhat disorganized when he attempts to carry out a task.

Nursing Diagnosis

Self-care deficit (total) related to right hemiplegia.

Nursing Interventions

- ❏ Assess Mr. Baker for right hemianopsia before establishing a restorative program.
- ❏ Set up restorative programs for only one or two activities of daily living. Mr. Baker may become very frustrated if too many goals are established at one time.
- ❏ If verbal instructions are used, follow the guidelines for communication. Remember that real situations are used for restorative programs. Provide instruction during mealtimes, bathing, etc.
- ❏ Mr. Baker may learn more effectively if demonstrations, gestures, or pantomime are used for instruction.
- ❏ Divide tasks into small steps and work on just a few steps at a time. Give Mr.

Baker prompt, frequent, and accurate feedback with each step. Use facial expression, a nod, or a pat on the back with short, simple phrases. If errors are made, wait for Mr. Baker to correct the mistake without saying anything. If he seems unaware of the error, tactfully point out the error and give him a clue so he can self-correct the problem. Praise him when he is successful.

❑ Do not overestimate Mr. Baker's understanding of speech. Conversely, do not underestimate his ability to learn and communicate. (See chapter 2 and chapter 21 for additional information.)

Collaboration: Interdisciplinary Team

❑ If Mr. Baker does not progress in the restorative programs, consult with the occupational therapist for further assessment of sensory-perceptual deficits that may be impeding his performance.

Outcome

Mr. Baker will
❑ Improve his self-care skills, requiring only minimal assistance

Interdisciplinary Assessment

Nursing.
Mr. Baker spends most of the day in his room except for meals and therapy.

Activities.
He consistently refuses invitations to attend any activities.

Social Services.
His family visits a few times a week but they converse very little with Mr. Baker because of the frustration he usually exhibits when they are unable to understand his comments. Mr. Baker frequently cries, upsetting the family even more.

He and his family are beginning to comprehend the many changes and residual damage caused by the stroke. Depression is a common reaction as the full impact of the stroke is realized. Social withdrawal and dependency of the client are frequently responses to this phase of mourning. Although Mr. Baker's learning readiness for restorative programs may be delayed during this time, it is important that the staff avoid encouraging dependency. To do so will create a situation of learned helplessness, continuing social isolation and dysfunctional grieving.

Nursing Diagnosis

Social isolation related to impaired communication and emotional lability.

Nursing Interventions

❑ Mr. Baker needs the support and understanding of the staff to successfully resolve the issues of grieving. Establish a trusting relationship with Mr. Baker. Learn his body language and be sensitive to his moods and feelings. Acknowledge and accept his feelings, allowing him to mourn his losses.

❑ Provide positive reinforcement toward progress no matter how limited. Avoid dwelling on his inabilities.

❑ Continue with the restorative programs. Do not set goals that are too comprehensive or unrealistic. Monitor staff performance when they are working with Mr. Baker to ensure that programs are carried out consistently with appropriate approaches.

❑ Give the family guidance in learning how to communicate with Mr. Baker and stress the importance of including him in the conversations. Invite them to the care plan conference and encourage their support, but avoid expecting too much from the family.

❑ As Mr. Baker's mobility skills improve, talk with the family about taking him home for a few hours. If this proves successful, he may enjoy community activities sponsored by the nursing home.

Collaboration: Interdisciplinary Team

❑ Ask the social worker to visit Mr. Baker regularly to facilitate a satisfactory resolution to his grieving.

❑ Mrs. Baker depends on her son to drive her to the nursing home. She has not been alone with her husband since his stroke. The social worker may suggest to the son that he arrange for his parents to spend time together alone. Provide them with privacy and avoid interrupting their visit. They need the opportunity to express affection and to reaffirm their feelings and commitment to each other.

❑ Monitor Mr. Baker for signs of regression, increased dependency and withdrawal, and feelings of hopelessness. Consultation with a mental health therapist may be necessary.

❑ Ask the activities department to involve Mr. Baker in individual activities outside of his room. Ask the activity aide to invite him to play checkers or other board games that do not rely on verbal input for success. Although his comprehension is impaired due to the aphasia, he may enjoy small group activities such as musical presentations or movies. Mr. Baker may enjoy attending the Residents' Council meetings. Assure him that he is welcome to attend as an observer if he chooses not to actively participate. Because of his previous community involvement, he may eventually find this a rewarding activity.

❑ Implement these interventions gradually. To attempt them all at once would be overwhelming and detrimental to Mr. Baker. Use a positive approach in seeking his participation but always give him a choice.

❑ The Baker family is undergoing a time of stress and change. They too are grieving and need support in dealing with the issues at hand. Ask the social worker to talk with the family and, if necessary, make referrals to appropriate resources.

Outcome

Mr. Baker will
❑ Openly and honestly ventilate his feelings verbally or through body language
❑ Express interest and progress in increasing his self-care skills
❑ Enjoy the visits of his family, evidenced through verbal expression or body language
❑ Participate in activities of his choice

COMMENTS

Maintain open communications with the family. There are many variables in their lives at this time. Mrs. Baker is unable to live alone and the family plans to continue with the present arrangements. However, if her health deteriorates, she may also require nursing home care. The family will need to make a decision regarding the Baker home. Mr. Baker needs to be a part of this process to the extent that he is able to participate.

There are a number of potential nursing diagnoses for Mr. Baker if the grieving process is not successfully resolved and if the family is unable to cope with the multiple changes they are experiencing. These are dysfunctional grieving, hopelessness, body image disturbance, any of the ineffective coping diagnoses including individual and family, and alterations in family processes. Through ongoing assessment and communication among the interdisciplinary team, a determination can be made as to whether the plan needs to be revised to include these diagnoses.

Mr. and Mrs. Baker are in a dilemma faced by thousands of elderly couples. These individuals cope satisfactorily with the deteriorating health of one of the partners. When the other becomes ill or disabled, they do not have the resources to manage. The death of a spouse is one of life's most devastating crises. Permanent separation because of poor health is also a crisis and can lead to total disintegration of the family structure if help is not provided. In long-term care, it is not only the client who needs our help and support; we must consider the entire family.

QUESTIONS AND DISCUSSION

1. What examples of automatic speech have you observed in your clients with aphasia?
2. Can you determine what type of aphasia your client has?
3. If a speech pathologist is not available, what communication adaptations can you devise for your aphasic clients?
4. What additional interventions by the interdisciplinary team may be beneficial to Mr. Baker?

REFERENCES

Adkins, E.R.H. 1991. Nursing Care of Clients with Impaired Communication. *Rehabilitation Nursing* 16(2): 74–76.

Chipps, E., N. Clanin, and V. Campbell. 1992. *Neurologic Disorders*. St. Louis: Mosby-Year Book, Inc.

Larson, L.J. 1988. In R.D. Sine, S.E. Liss, R.E. Roush, J.D. Holcomb, and G. Wilson, eds. *Basic Rehabilitation Techniques*. Rockville, MD: Aspen Publishers, Inc.

Newman, D.K. and D.A.J. Smith. 1991. *Geriatric Care Plans*. Springhouse, PA: Springhouse Corporation.

Swearingen, P.L. 1992. *Medical-Surgical Nursing*. St. Louis: Mosby-Year Book, Inc.

SUGGESTED READINGS

Cohen, L.K. 1985. *Communication Problems after a Stroke*. Minneapolis: Sister Kenny Institute.

Kumin, L. and N. Rysticken. 1985. Aids to Bridge the Communication Barrier. *Geriatric Nursing* 6(6): 348–51.

MacKay, S., D.W. Holmes, and A.T. Gersumky. 1988. Methods to Assess Aphasic Stroke Patients. *Geriatric Nursing* 9(3): 177–79.

Olson, D.A., ed. 1986. Communication and the Elderly. *Topics in Geriatric Rehabilitation*. Rockville, MD: Aspen Publishers, Inc.

CHAPTER 13   A Restorative Approach to Caring for the Client with Decreased Cardiac Output

OBJECTIVES

- Identify nursing interventions to prevent complications associated with decreased cardiac output through ongoing evaluation of the client with chronic congestive heart failure.
- Identify the signs of digitalis toxicity.
- List the signs of side effects of furosemide and nitroglycerin.
- Describe nursing interventions to avoid dyspnea and fatigue.
- Discuss the client's decision to forego life-saving measures in the event of cardiac arrest.
- Identify the role of the interdisciplinary health care team members in the management of the client with decreased cardiac output.

DESCRIPTION OF THE DISEASE

Congestive heart failure is one cause of decreased cardiac output. The presence of myocardial dysfunction causes abnormal circulatory congestion and impaired pump performance (Bass and Meissner 1991). The heart is unable to pump sufficient blood to meet the metabolic needs of the body. The most common causes of congestive heart failure in the elderly are hypertension, cardiomyopathy, valvular disease, and ischemic heart disease. The resulting changes affect preload, afterload, contractility, and heart rate. Cardiac output is the heart rate multiplied by stroke volume. Stroke volume depends on preload, afterload, and contractility (Dennison 1990). *Preload* is the force that stretches the heart muscle during diastole. With increased preload, too much stretching diminishes the heart's ability to contract. Preload decreases as a result of hypovolemia. *Afterload* is the pressure the ventricles must overcome to open the aortic and pulmonic valves and pump blood out of the heart. Afterload may be increased in the left or right ventricle and decreased in both ventricles. *Contractility* is the intensity with which the heart muscle contracts. Cardiac output may be decreased by both increased and decreased contractility (Dennison 1990).

In some cases, there may be no apparent clinical cause for the heart disease. Congestive heart failure can be acute or chronic and either left-sided or right-sided or both. Left-side failure due to a damaged left ventricle is more common; but failure in the right ventricle may occur either as a primary condition, secondary to left-side failure, or simultaneously with left-side failure. Most clients with this medical diagnosis have a chronic form associated with sodium and water retention (Bass & Meissner 1991).

TABLE 13–1	Distinguishing Between Left-Side and Right-Side Cardiac Failure
Left-Side Failure	Right-Side Failure
❑ Increased preload	❑ Increased preload
❑ Decreased contractility in left ventricle	❑ Decreased contractility in right ventricle
❑ Decreased cardiac output	❑ Decreased cardiac output
❑ Increased heart rate	❑ Increased heart rate
❑ Exertional dyspnea, possibly paroxysmal nocturnal dyspnea, Cheyne-Stokes respirations, orthopnea	❑ Edema
❑ Pale, cool skin	❑ Distended, rigid neck veins
❑ Dysrhythmias	❑ Hepatomegaly
❑ Fatigue	❑ Occasional ascites
❑ Shortened attention span, restlessness, irritability	❑ Cyanosis
	❑ Dysrhythmias
	❑ Dyspnea

Dyspnea is the major symptom associated with decreased cardiac output due to left-side failure. Initially it occurs with moderate to severe exertion due to increased physical activity. As cardiac reserve decreases, less exertion triggers increased dyspnea. As heart failure progresses, paroxysmal nocturnal dyspnea occurs — the client wakes up suddenly, out of breath. The client eventually finds it necessary to sleep propped up in bed or sitting in a chair (orthopnea) (Van Parys 1987). Fatigue is an inevitable symptom of left-side failure. In some cases, dyspnea is the only sign noted by the client who may not seek treatment, blaming the symptoms on aging or other causes.

When congestive heart failure is secondary to another medical problem, treatment is directed to the primary problem. If there is a correctable underlying cause, such as hypertension, that problem is treated. In all cases, treatment is directed at controlling the heart failure. Digitalis, diuretics, and low-sodium diets remain the standard form of treatment.

CASE STUDY

Mrs. Wells, age ninety-four, was admitted from the hospital to the nursing home with diagnoses of congestive heart failure secondary to cardiomyopathy and a secondary diagnosis of osteoarthritis. The purpose of the hospitalization was to investigate the cause of increased pain in her right hip. The findings were essentially negative except for the arthritis, which she has had for several years. Before the hospitalization, Mrs. Wells was living in a retirement center. She was experiencing increasing functional incapacity as a result of the fatigue related to the heart problem and pain and stiffness due to the arthritis.

Damaged myocardial muscle fibers result in dilated cardiomyopathy. In this condition, the ventricles are dilated, causing the heart to contract poorly during systole. The disease is frequently not diagnosed until advanced stages. The primary cause of cardiomyopathy is unknown. There are several secondary mechanisms that may induce cardiac damage, but there is no direct evidence to support a cause-and-effect relationship. Included in these secondary mechanisms are muscle disorders, viral infections, alcoholism, endocrine disorders, and nutritional disorders (Gyetvan & McCann 1988).

Mrs. Wells has a living will and has assigned her daughter-in-law to be her agent as durable power of attorney for health care. Her physician has written an order not to resuscitate in the event of cardiac arrest. Mrs. Wells has been widowed twice, the last time thirty years ago. She has one son, a daughter-in-law, and three grandchildren. Her son recently had a stroke and is recovering at home. He has not been able to visit his mother since his illness. The daughter-in-law is supportive and visits often.

Strengths

- ❏ Free of cognitive impairment
- ❏ Continent of bowel and bladder
- ❏ History of healthy life-style and is compliant with medical regime
- ❏ Supportive family
- ❏ Finds solace in spiritual beliefs
- ❏ Although she is "happy to be alive," she is "ready to die."

Interdisciplinary Assessment

Nursing.

Mrs. Wells is experiencing exertional dyspnea. At the present time, Mrs. Wells is not displaying the signs of fluid volume excess.

Nursing Diagnosis

Decreased cardiac output related to decreased cardiac contractility due to cardiac muscle changes.

Nursing Interventions

- ❏ Administer digoxin as ordered. Digoxin strengthens the heart muscle, thus increasing cardiac output and reducing the risk of fluid volume excess. Take Mrs. Wells's apical pulse for one minute and notify physician if her pulse is under sixty. Because of her age, Mrs. Wells is especially prone to digitalis toxicity. The therapeutic plasma level is 0.5–2.0 mg/ml. Tell Mrs. Wells to report signs of toxicity — anorexia, nausea, vomiting, visual disturbances, weakness, fatigue, mood alterations, and decreased pulse rate (Loeb 1992).
- ❏ Administer furosemide (Lasix®) as ordered. Furosemide increases water excretion by increasing sodium ion excretion. Tell Mrs. Wells to report signs of side effects — weakness, dizziness, nausea, vomiting, diarrhea, muscle cramps, confusion. This is a potassium-deleting diuretic, so monitor potassium levels and for indications of hypokalemia — irregular heart rate, hypoactive reflexes, paresthesia, and twitching. Low serum potassium levels predispose to digitalis toxicity (Loeb 1992).

❑ Mrs. Wells is on a 2-Gm sodium diet (see alterations in nutrition). Assess diet and monitor for compliance.

❑ Observe lower extremities, back, and hips for signs of edema.

❑ Measure and record fluid intake and output every eight hours.

❑ Weigh Mrs. Wells daily and notify physician of weight gain over one kilogram (2.2 pounds). This equals one liter of fluid retention. Weigh her in the morning, after she has voided and before breakfast, on the same scale and at the same time every day (Swearingen 1992).

❑ Take blood pressure, pulse, and respirations daily. Monitor for signs of orthostatic hypotension. Take her blood pressure while she is supine and immediately after she stands up.

❑ Monitor for signs and symptoms of left-side heart failure (see Table 13–1).

Collaboration: Interdisciplinary Team

❑ Alert all the staff to Mrs. Wells's inability to deal with exertion due to cardiac disease.

Outcome

Mrs. Wells will
❑ Report any signs of side effects from furosemide and digoxin
❑ Maintain fluid volume intake and output at optimal level without fluid retention

Interdisciplinary Assessment

Nursing.

Mrs. Wells is able to complete basic activities of daily living if she takes her time. Walking causes exertional dyspnea and causes her heart rate to increase. She complains of shortness of breath after walking more than a few feet.

Activities.

Mrs. Wells has expressed interest in activities but has not participated due to shortness of breath.

Social Services.

Although Mrs. Wells would like to attend worship services, she is fearful that she does not have the stamina to do so.

Pharmacy.

The physician ordered Nitro-Dur® patches to deliver the nitroglycerin consistently over a twenty-four-hour period. The medication dilates coronary arterioles, increasing the oxygen supply to the heart. Nitroglycerin dilates peripheral vessels, reducing blood pressure and the work load of the heart (Clark, Queener, and Karb 1986).

Nursing Diagnosis

Activity intolerance related to alterations in oxygen delivery to body tissues.

Nursing Interventions

❑ Apply Mrs. Wells's Nitro-Dur patch as ordered. Apply to a site free of hair and change daily to a new site, preferably on the chest or back. Remove excess ointment from previous site before applying the next dose. Do not apply to the hands or feet. Squeeze the prescribed dose onto the measuring applicator included in the package. Apply ointment in a thin, uniform layer over an area of three to six square inches. Cover site with transparent dressing. Avoid massaging or rubbing the ointment into the skin. Observe for side effects of flushing, headache, dizziness, hypotension, and tachycardia. *Note:* Do not use your fingers to apply the ointment because your skin will absorb it (McConnell 1990).

❑ Assess Mrs. Wells's pulse before and after she gets out of bed. Note any complaints she has of weakness, fatigue, shortness of breath or chest pain. If she has chest pain, take her blood pressure, auscultate her lungs and heart, and note the duration, intensity, location, quality of pain, and presence of diuresis.

❑ Place a commode at the bedside for use during the night.

❑ Plan for a gradual increase of activity within her ability.

❑ Use a positive approach and encourage her independence while acknowledging her problem.

Collaboration: Interdisciplinary Team

❑ Ask activities staff to invite Mrs. Wells to passive activities. They can assure her that they will transport her in her wheelchair to and from the activity and that they will return her to her room if she experiences shortness of breath. Ask the activities staff to notify the nurse on the unit before the time of the activity so that Mrs. Wells's schedule can be adapted to allow her to rest first. Allow her to take as much time as she needs to complete activities. Plan her schedule so she has rest periods alternating with periods of exertion.

❑ Ask Social Services to arrange for the priest to visit Mrs. Wells (with her approval). They may also approach her to attend worship services (see suggestions above for activities).

Outcome

Mrs. Wells will
❑ Pace herself to avoid fatigue and shortness of breath
❑ Enjoy an increase in activity tolerance
❑ Report any increase in fatigue, shortness of breath, chest pain, headache, or dizziness
❑ Be able to participate in the activities of her choice

Interdisciplinary Assessment

Nursing and Physical Therapy.

Mrs. Wells's level of musculoskeletal activity has decreased in the last year. She is able to transfer from bed to chair with assistance. Due to dyspnea and fatigue, she is transported in a wheelchair when she wishes to go elsewhere in the building. Because her joints have been more painful and stiff due to arthritis, she avoids movement. Mrs. Wells needs increased physical activity to avoid the complications associated with immobility. She is potentially at risk for contractures, pressure ulcers, infections, and cardiovascular complications.

Nursing Diagnosis

High risk for disuse syndrome related to inactivity.

Nursing Interventions

□ Teach Mrs. Wells why activity is necessary and how you plan to help her. She may think that because she is elderly exercise is not necessary. The challenge here is to increase her activity to a tolerable level without causing dyspnea.

□ Do active assistive range-of-motion exercises with Mrs. Wells two times a day with all extremities. Monitor for signs of activity intolerance.

□ Begin a walking program with Mrs. Wells. Start by having her walk four or five steps from the bed to the chair. Gradually increase the number of steps if possible. This may be as much activity as she will be able to tolerate. Monitor for signs of dyspnea and discomfort. Take her pulse before and after the activity. If the pulse increases thirty or more beats per minute from the preactivity level, have her sit down. If the pulse remains elevated five to ten minutes after stopping the activity, do not start another one until the pulse returns to preactivity levels (Van Parys 1987).

□ Anticoagulants are sometimes ordered for inactive clients with cardiomyopathy. If the physician orders an anticoagulant, monitor Mrs. Wells for bleeding and occult blood in the stool. Monitor blood coagulation studies.

Collaboration: Interdisciplinary Team

□ Consult with the physical therapist about Mrs. Wells using the fitness trail once a day after she has made progress with walking. She can do this from her wheelchair, doing only those exercises that are tolerable and safe.

Outcome

Mrs. Wells will
□ Remain free of the complications associated with inactivity

Interdisciplinary Assessment

Nursing and Dietary.

Mrs. Wells finds the 2-gm sodium diet tasteless and frequently does not finish her meals. Her weight is currently ninety-four pounds, five pounds less than six months ago. Her laboratory values for nutritional status are within normal limits. (See chapter 5.)

Nursing Diagnosis

Alterations in nutrition, potential for less than body requirements.

Nursing Interventions

❑ Fatigue may be another reason why she does not complete her meals and may also contribute to her anorexia. Arrange for her to rest before each meal. Going to the dining room, even per wheelchair, may be too exhausting, particularly for the evening meal. Suggest she remain on the nursing unit for dinner. Prepare her tray so this task will not wear her out before she eats. Encourage her to take her time. Offer light snacks in between meals and at bedtime.

Collaboration: Interdisciplinary Team

❑ Ask the dietician to talk with Mrs. Wells about her likes and dislikes. Suggest that she try a salt substitute and consider the use of other spices to add flavor. Foods that are easy to chew will require less energy.
❑ The dietician may need to consider three smaller meals a day and high-protein snacks in between meals. Mrs. Wells's appetite may increase with her activity.

Outcome

Mrs. Wells will
❑ Maintain adequate nutritional status as evidenced through body weight, laboratory values, and physical signs
❑ Verbalize satisfaction with her diet

Interdisciplinary Assessment

Nursing and Social Services.

Throughout her long life, Mrs. Wells has utilized effective coping mechanisms and, as she says, "rolled with the punches." Her son's illness has caused her a great deal of worry and concern. She has not seen him since he had the stroke. Mrs. Wells is fearful that her daughter-in-law may be hiding the truth from her in regard to the son's condition so Mrs. Wells "won't worry." She says she hopes she does not outlive her son. Mrs. Wells, her son, and his wife have had a close, satisfying relationship throughout the years. In the last few years, she has depended on her son to give her advice and manage her financial affairs.

Nursing Diagnosis

Altered family processes related to son's illness.

Nursing Interventions

❑ Listen to and acknowledge Mrs. Wells's concerns for her son.

Collaboration: Interdisciplinary Team

❑ Ask social services to talk with the daughter-in-law and encourage open communications between her and Mrs. Wells. They may be able to arrange for the son to visit his mother as soon as he is able. It is better for her to see him with the impairments resulting from the stroke than to imagine a far worse situation. If his speech is understandable, Mrs. Wells may wish to talk to her son on the telephone.

❑ Ask Mrs. Wells if she would like her priest to visit. The family has attended the same church for several years and the priest is well acquainted with all the family members.

Outcome

Mrs. Wells will

❑ Express her concerns openly
❑ Continue a satisfying relationship with her daughter-in-law and son
❑ Communicate with her son in person or by telephone

COMMENTS

Mrs. Wells is typical of many clients residing in a nursing home. She has a long-standing health problem that, over the years, has diminished her functional abilities. She is oriented, has excellent communication skills, and is capable of making decisions regarding her care. Her choice not to be involved in most of the activities offered by the staff should be honored. She is content to socialize while dining. Otherwise, she prefers to spend most of the time in her room reading and occasionally watching television.

Mrs. Wells, like many elderly persons, is ready to die. Staff needs to acknowledge and respect her feelings about this. It may be necessary to discuss this with staff if Mrs. Wells's comments make them uncomfortable. Mrs. Wells has taken responsibility for her life by completing a living will and appointing an agent (her daughter-in-law) as durable power of attorney for health care. As per her wishes, the physician has written a do-not-resuscitate order in the medical record. This relieves the family and physician of making the decision and provides direction for the staff.

We can learn much from clients like Mrs. Wells. She has survived the deaths of two husbands, her parents, and her siblings. She has lived through the depression, numerous wars, and witnessed years of social upheaval. She deserves our respect and admiration.

QUESTIONS AND DISCUSSION

1. What nursing interventions can be implemented to maintain a high quality of life for Mrs. Wells?
2. How can you communicate Mrs. Wells's wishes regarding no resuscitation to the staff?
3. What role does the interdisciplinary health care team play in the management of clients with chronic, congestive heart failure?

REFERENCES

Bass, L.S. and J.E. Meissner. 1991. In M. Shaw, ed. *Illustrated Manual of Nursing Practice*. Springhouse, PA: Springhouse Corporation.

Clark, J.B., S.E. Queener, and V.B. Karb. 1986. *Pocket Guide to Drugs*. St. Louis: The C.V. Mosby Company.

Dennison, R.D. 1990. Understanding the Four Determinants of Cardiac Output. *Nursing 90* 20(7): 35–41.

Gyetvan, M.C. and J.A.S. McCann, eds. 1988. *Diseases And Disorders Handbook*. Springhouse, PA: Springhouse Corporation.

Loeb, S., ed. 1992. *Nursing 92 Drug Handbook*. Springhouse, PA: Springhouse Corporation.

McConnell, E.A. 1990. Applying Nitroglycerin Ointment Correctly. *Nursing 90* 20(8): 70.

Swearingen, P.L. 1992. *Pocket Guide to Medical-Surgical Nursing*. St. Louis: Mosby-Year Book, Inc.

Van Parys, E. 1987. Assessing the Failing State of the Heart. *Nursing 87* 17(2): 42–49.

CHAPTER ▮14▮ A Restorative Approach to Caring for the Client with Knowledge Deficit (Diabetes Mellitus)

OBJECTIVES

❑ Distinguish between Type I Diabetes Mellitus (IDDM) and Type II Diabetes Mellitus (NIDDM).
❑ Recognize the symptoms of both Type I and Type II Diabetes Mellitus.
❑ Identify the signs and symptoms of potential complications of diabetes mellitus.
❑ Describe nursing interventions that will prevent the onset of diabetic complications.
❑ Recognize the signs and symptoms of diabetic emergencies.
❑ Render the appropriate nursing care during diabetic emergencies.
❑ Identify the responsibilities of the interdisciplinary health care team members in the management of the client with diabetes mellitus.

DESCRIPTION OF THE DISEASE

A knowledge deficit occurs when the individual lacks the ability to explain or demonstrate the necessary information or skill to manage self-care in the presence of a specific health problem (Gordon 1991). The satisfactory self-management of diabetes mellitus requires extensive knowledge. At the time of diagnosis, most clients lack this information.

Diabetes mellitus is a disease of varying severity with many serious complications if not managed properly. Type I, insulin dependent diabetes mellitus (IDDM), occurs most often in thin people under thirty years of age. Little or no insulin is produced in the islets of Langerhans, which are smaller in size or fewer in number, requiring exogenous insulin injections for survival (Hass 1991). Ketoacidosis is a major complication in cases of uncontrolled or undiagnosed

IDDM. Without insulin to metabolize the glucose, the body gets its energy from fats. This results in the formation of ketone bodies that accumulate in the blood, eventually resulting in diabetic coma.

About 80 percent of all diabetic persons have Type II, non-insulin dependent diabetes mellitus (NIDDM). It is more common in people over forty years of age, who rarely have the classic symptoms (Newman and Smith 1991). In people with Type II diabetes, the islets of Langerhans are present but either do not produce insulin in sufficient quantities or secretion is delayed. There may be diminished insulin sensitivity in receptor cells, or the excess fat causes cells to become insulin resistant. NIDDM has a more insidious onset than IDDM. It is frequently diagnosed when the individual is being treated for another medical problem or for complications from the untreated diabetes. Blood sugar levels tend to rise with age as a result of renal and pancreatic changes. Reference ranges for older adults may therefore be higher than for younger people (Newman and Smith 1991).

NIDDM is managed by diet and exercise, with weight control a major goal of therapy. If this regime fails to bring the disease under control, oral agents may be added to the treatment plan. Under certain circumstances, the person with NIDDM may need temporary or permanent injections of insulin. In both types of diabetes mellitus, client teaching is a crucial component of disease management. Unfortunately, clients and health care professionals alike may not consider NIDDM a serious disease. However, the same long-term complications can occur with either type.

TABLE 14–1	Warning Signs of Diabetes Mellitus
	Insulin Dependent Diabetes Mellitus (IDDM)
	❑ Frequent urination (polyuria)
	❑ Excessive thirst (polydipsia)
	❑ Unusual hunger (polyphagia)
	❑ Rapid loss of weight
	❑ Irritability
	❑ Weakness and fatigue
	❑ Nausea and vomiting
	Non-Insulin Dependent Diabetes Mellitus (NIDDM)
	❑ Family history of diabetes
	❑ Overweight
	❑ Fatigue and drowsiness
	❑ Skin infections, slow healing
	❑ Pruritus
	❑ Blurred vision
	❑ Tingling and numbness in feet

(American Diabetes Association, Inc. 1990)

CASE STUDY

Mrs. Sara Burns, seventy-three years old, was recently diagnosed with Type II NIDDM on a visit to her physician for complaints of fatigue. The diagnosis was based on the results of fasting blood sugar levels on two occasions of 152 mg/dl and 149 mg/dl respectively. Mrs. Burns has had osteoarthritis for several years but otherwise has enjoyed relatively good health throughout her life. She has no other medical problems at this time. She lives alone in an apartment since her husband died two years ago and has no children. Learning about diet, exercise, and the prevention of complications related to diabetes is a top priority for Mrs. Burns.

Strengths

❑ Cognitively alert
❑ Needs reading glasses, but has adequate vision and hearing
❑ Physical mobility is satisfactory, although Mrs. Burns states that she occasionally has stiffness and aching in her hips and knees.
❑ Mrs. Burns is interested in learning how to manage the diabetes and indicates a willingness to make the necessary changes in her life.
❑ Mrs. Burns does not use tobacco or drink alcoholic beverages.

Interdisciplinary Assessment

Nursing.

Mrs. Burns reveals she has developed a pattern of weight gain over the past fifteen years and presently is 25 pounds over her ideal body weight of 125 pounds. She has not enjoyed cooking since the death of her husband. She often snacks throughout the day on pastries, cold meat sandwiches, and soup. Mrs. Burns has never exercised consistently because she feels that doing housework is adequate activity for a person her age.

Nursing Diagnosis

Alterations in nutrition, more than body requirements related to decreased activity and lack of basic nutritional knowledge.

Nursing Interventions

❑ Discuss with Mrs. Burns the basics of healthy eating, pointing out the need to include items from each of the four different food groups each day.
❑ Advise her to avoid sugars and foods high in cholesterol and saturated fats, and to limit her salt intake. Increasing fiber content will help maintain bowel regularity and help control blood glucose and lipid concentrations. Over half of the daily food intake should consist of complex carbohydrates, with the remainder divided between fats and proteins (Byrnes 1987).
❑ Find out what foods are important to Mrs. Burns and how often she eats away from home. Compliance is more likely if a food plan is tailored to her personal preferences. Simplify menu planning as much as possible to avoid overwhelming Mrs. Burns with too many changes. Give her a list of foods to avoid and stress the variety of items from which she can choose.

TABLE 14–2	Dietary Management of Diabetes Mellitus
	Avoid high-sugar foods: ❑ Sugar, syrups, honey, candy, candy-coated gum, jelly, jam, marmalade, soft drinks, condensed milk, pie, cake, pastries, cookies, rich desserts **Avoid high-sodium foods:** ❑ Processed meats (ham, bacon, sausage, lunch meats), tuna, cheese, pickles, olives, sauerkraut, most canned vegetables and soups, some frozen dinners **Avoid high-cholesterol foods:** ❑ Cream, butter, egg yolks, organ meats, meat fat, poultry skin, rich pastries, puddings, custards **Avoid foods high in saturated fat:** ❑ Some cheeses, cream, ice cream, shortening, lard, rich pastries, pudding, custards

❑ Instruct her to divide each day's intake fairly evenly into three meals, so that any one meal does not raise her blood sugar level too high. Since she is used to eating throughout the day, allowing for a light snack mid-morning and evening may increase her motivation to follow the plan. A period of four to five hours between the main meals allows the blood sugar to return to normal. Mrs. Burns may need additional instruction in food purchasing and preparation. Assist Mrs. Burns to plan a week's menus at a time, suggesting changes only if needed.

TABLE 14–3	Dietary Recommendations for Diabetes Mellitus
	The American Diabetic Association recommends: ❑ 55–60 percent of calories from complex carbohydrates and natural sugars such as fruits, vegetables, grains ❑ Protein intake of 0.8 grams per kilogram of body weight ❑ Less than 30 percent of calories from fat, preferably unsaturated ❑ Less than 1,000 milligrams of sodium per 1,000 calories, not to exceed 3,000 milligrams of sodium per day ❑ Less than 300 milligrams of cholesterol per day (Diabetes Forecast 1988)
	Suggested Dietary Adaptations
	❑ Replace butter with margarine. ❑ Limit egg consumption to 1–2 a week. Consider "hidden" eggs in baked goods, puddings, and custards. ❑ Trim all fat from meats, including skin from poultry. ❑ Avoid organ meats. ❑ Limit ice cream or switch to low-fat frozen yogurt. ❑ Replace whole milk with skim milk. ❑ Avoid fried foods.

❑ Diabetes experts now consider exercise as important as diet in the management of NIDDM. It is not enough to simply tell a client who has never exercised to "try and get some exercise." Help Mrs. Burns develop a personal plan, taking into account her resources, interests, and abilities. Regular exercise and endurance training lowers triglycerides and blood glucose. After five to ten minutes of exercise, glucose uptake from the blood is seven to twenty times the resting rate, depending on how strenuous the exercise is (Gavin 1988). With regular exercise, weight loss will occur without severe caloric restrictions. In addition, the risk of cardiovascular disease is lowered and Mrs. Burns will enjoy an overall feeling of well-being.

❑ Mrs. Burns has decided to implement a walking program. She plans to join other residents of her apartment building who walk regularly outdoors. During inclement weather, indoor hallways are used. Teach Mrs. Burns about target heart rate and show her how to take her pulse. Discuss with her the need for appropriate shoes and clothing. Stress the need to start slowly, gradually increasing distance and speed (see chapter 3). Advise her to begin with a five- to ten-minute warm-up session and end each session with a five- to ten-minute cool-down. She should walk at a brisk pace for twenty to forty-five minutes at least three days a week. Because Mrs. Burns is over thirty-five years old, she had a stress electrocardiogram before beginning the exercise program (Nursing 90). During her physical examination, no cardiovascular abnormalities were found that would interfere with her walking program. Mrs. Burns can monitor the effects from exercise on her arthritis. If an increase in pain is noted, she may need to cut back on the length of time she is walking.

❑ Mrs. Burns needs to keep track of her blood sugar levels. Because elderly people often have a high renal threshold, results of urine tests may be inaccurate. To determine the reliability of urine tests for Mrs. Burns, compare results of simultaneous urine and blood sugar tests. Her vision is adequate, so if comparison tests are valid, she can be taught to use one of the dipstick tests to monitor her urine for glucose and ketones. Tell her to use a double-voided specimen taken first thing upon arising (Crigler-Meringola 1984).

❑ If Mrs. Burns has difficulty controlling her diabetes, it may become necessary for her to monitor her blood glucose levels with a glucometer. At that time, determine if she has the dexterity and ability to use a home monitoring device.

Collaboration: Interdisciplinary Team

❑ Arrange for Mrs. Burns to receive instruction from a dietician if she fails to follow her diet plan.

Outcome

Mrs. Burns will
❑ Maintain a steady weight loss of one-half to one pound per week, striving to attain her ideal body weight
❑ Reach and maintain satisfactory blood sugar levels
❑ Exercise regularly on a daily basis and verbalize positive feelings about the effects of exercise

Interdisciplinary Assessment

Nursing.

In addition to planning a diet and exercise regime, Mrs. Burns needs information on preventing complications associated with diabetes mellitus and how to treat problems that may occur. By following her diet plan, she will significantly lower her risk factors for complications. The combination of diabetes with the usual aging changes creates special concerns. However, the better informed Mrs. Burns is, the more likely that she will avoid serious complications. High-risk problems include diabetic retinopathy that develops silently without symptoms. Cataracts are also common in diabetic persons. Peripheral vascular insufficiency, which is common in the elderly, poses special problems for diabetics. About 25 percent of people with diabetes will develop foot problems, and one in fifteen will require limb amputation. Foot ulcers are generally a result of neuropathy, ischemia, and infection (Lipsky 1992). Mrs. Burns also needs instruction on skin care, oral care, and diabetic emergencies.

Nursing Diagnosis

Altered health maintenance related to present life-style and recent diagnosis requiring life-style changes.

Nursing Interventions

❑ Eye care
— Advise Mrs. Burns to have an eye examination once a year with a funduscope, which requires that her pupils be dilated.
— Tell her to report to her physician at once symptoms of blurred vision, "cobwebs," "floaters," or sudden loss of vision.
❑ Foot care
— Teach the need for regular foot care. Instruct Mrs. Burns to wash her feet daily in lukewarm water and mild soap, to rinse thoroughly, and pat dry. She needs to give special attention to the areas between her toes.
— At the same time, she should inspect both feet, using a mirror and light for the soles if necessary. Tell her to look for signs of injury or infection — blisters, ulcers, fissures, or reddened areas, red or purple discolorations on the lower legs, temperature changes, absence of hair growth, or thick, deformed toenails. Advise Mrs. Burns to notify her physician if these signs appear.
— Moisturizer can be applied sparingly. Tell her to never cut or pick at corns, calluses, splinters, blisters, or abscesses. Chemicals and medications should not be used on the feet without a physician's order.
— Teach Mrs. Burns to trim and file her toenails after soaking in warm water for fifteen to twenty minutes or after a bath or shower. Tell her to use a toenail clipper, cutting a little at a time instead of cutting the entire nail with one clip. She should follow the curve of the toe. The nail length should be even with the ends of her toes.
— Exposure to moisture, cold, heating pads, or hot water bottles is an unsafe practice. A pillow placed at the end of the bed will keep the covers off the feet.
— Advise wearing seamless cotton or wool socks, changing daily. Well-fitting panty hose can be worn for short periods of time. Wearing round garters or tying knots to keep stockings up are forbidden practices. Shoes should be one-half inch longer than the longest toe and wide enough to avoid squeezing the toes. Leather or canvas shoes with firm soles and soft uppers are the best choice. Avoid sandals or open-toed shoes. Allow shoes to "rest" twelve to twenty-four hours between wearing. Going barefoot is not a wise

habit for persons with diabetes. Break new shoes in by wearing them for no more than two hours the first few times.

— Instruct Mrs. Burns to avoid sitting with legs crossed or standing in one position for a long time. If Mrs. Burns used tobacco, she would be referred to a smoking cessation program to further lower her risk for circulatory problems (Christensen, Funnell, Ehrlich, Fellows, and Floyd 1991).

❑ Skin care and prevention of problems

— Changes in the skin associated with aging cause the skin to break down easily. This risk in combination with diabetes increases the potential for infections and ulcerations. Advise Mrs. Burns to bathe or shower every other day, using superfatted soap and moisturizer to keep the skin lubricated. Advise her to avoid using bubble bath, feminine hygiene sprays, or scented soaps.

— Special attention must be given to skin folds and the genital area to prevent fungal infections caused by *Candida albicans*. These are detected by the presence of itching, moist, red areas surrounded by tiny blisters and scales. Bacterial infections of the skin, such as boils or carbuncles, need medical attention. When diabetes is not well controlled, the leukocytes lose some of their ability to destroy harmful bacteria. The presence of an infection further disturbs the disease control (American Diabetes Association 1988).

— Diabetic dermopathy is common in older diabetics and is caused by diabetic changes in the small blood vessels. These light brown, scaly patches may be mistaken for "age spots." They are usually noted on the lower legs but are not symmetrical. The patches do not hurt, itch, or ulcerate, and require no treatment (American Diabetes Association 1988).

❑ Oral care and prevention of problems

— Tell Mrs. Burns that it is important to continue her regular dental checkups. She needs to inform her dentist of her diagnosis and any changes in her medical condition. Brushing after every meal and daily flossing will help prevent dental problems.

❑ Diabetic emergencies

— Two life-threatening conditions can arise in people with NIDDM. Hypoglycemia most often occurs in people who take insulin, but it can also strike those who take oral agents. Hyperglycemic hyperosmolar nonketotic coma (HHNK) is a danger for the elderly Type II diabetic. Be sure that Mrs. Burns recognizes the signs of these complications and how to avoid them.

TABLE 14–4	Diabetic Emergencies	
Hypoglycemia		
Cause	Signs	Treatment
Overdoses of antidiabetic agents; reduced food intake and usual dosage of antidiabetic agent	Sweating, clamminess, tremors; rapid pulse and respirations; hunger, anxiety, headache; unusual behavior; poor coordination; unconsciousness (Loeb 1991)	Any of these: 4 oz orange juice or apple juice, 1 tbsp jelly, 3 oz nondiet cola, 2 packets sugar, 7–9 hard candies, 4 sugar cubes, OR commercial glucose products OR glycogen (Swearingen 1992)

Continues

This treatment brings only temporary improvement. Follow with longer-acting carbohydrates, such as crackers, milk, or high-fiber fruit to avoid recurrence.		
Hyperglycemic Hyperosmolar Non-Ketotic Coma		
Untreated or poorly controlled diabetes mellitus; can be triggered by infection, surgery, extreme emotional stress, myocardial infarction, blood-sugar-raising drugs.	Extreme dehydration with serum osmolarity elevated to 350 mOsm/liter or above; blood sugar greater than 600 mg/dl; lethargy, confusion, depressed sensorium, unconsciousness; rapid pulse and respirations; skin warm, flushed, dry, loose; eyeballs soft (Hass 1991)	Fluid replacement, insulin, electrolyte replacement

❏ Tell Mrs. Burns to report to her physician any signs of acute illness, such as fever, nausea, vomiting, or signs of respiratory tract infections. The other complications associated with diabetes discussed here probably will never affect Mrs. Burns as long as she complies with the medical regime. However, the nursing management of persons with diabetes includes monitoring for signs and symptoms indicating the onset of these problems.

❏ Cardiovascular complications
   —Diabetics are predisposed to cardiovascular problems. Discuss with Mrs. Burns the warning signs of heart attack, stroke, and hypertension.
   —Check available community resources to see if free blood pressure monitoring is available to the elderly on a regular basis.

❏ Kidney disease
   —Persons who become diabetics before age forty and who are insulin dependent are at special risk for developing kidney problems associated with diabetes. Mrs. Burns is not in this category, but she should be aware of the function of the kidneys and be able to recognize signs of urinary tract infections — burning and urgency of urination, fever, cloudy urine, and lower-back pain and tenderness. Since these signs may not be readily noticed in older adults, the physician may wish to do a routine urinalysis when Mrs. Burns has her blood sugar drawn.

❏ Diabetic neuropathy
   —Diabetes is the most common cause of neuropathy, a disorder of the peripheral nerves. The longer a person has diabetes, the greater the risk for developing neuropathy. The person with diabetes and diabetic neuropathy has increased risk for cardiovascular disease.
   —Clinical manifestations of peripheral neuropathy include dull, aching, burning, lancinating, or crushing pain, and paresthesia (tingling, burning, coldness, and numbness) (Mitchell, Hodges, Muwaswes, and Walleck 1988).

❏ In addition to the symptoms already mentioned, instruct Mrs. Burns to notify her physician if she notes signs of respiratory or urinary tract infections, vomiting or diarrhea, or other indications of acute illness.

❏ Assist Mrs. Burns to obtain a medical identification device that she can wear all of the time.

Collaboration: Interdisciplinary Team

Refer Mrs. Burns to
- An ophthalmologist for regular eye care
- A podiatrist for regular foot care
- A dentist for regular oral care

Outcome

Mrs. Burns will
- Describe the self-care procedures for eye care, foot care, skin care, and oral care
- List the signs of diabetic emergencies and precautions she can take to avoid these emergencies
- Recognize the signs of complications associated with diabetes and report these signs to the physician or nurse
- Remain free of complications

Interdisciplinary Assessment

Nursing.

Before Mr. Burns died, he and Mrs. Burns dined out regularly and took frequent motor trips around the country. They attended church sporadically and although they were acquainted with a number of people, they rarely socialized with them. To avoid the burden of household maintenance, Mrs. Burns moved to the apartment six months after her husband died. Mrs. Burns states she seldom leaves the apartment except to go shopping and have her hair done. She drives and owns a car, but prefers not to drive after dark. She comments on feeling lonely but is not sure how to change her situation. Her daily routine consists of household chores, watching television, and reading.

Nursing Diagnosis

Social isolation related to death of husband and subsequent move to apartment.

Nursing Interventions

- Discuss possibilities for socialization. The residents in her building have a monthly potluck supper that she might enjoy.
- Though she has never been an active church member, she has always enjoyed her contacts with the church. She feels that by attending regularly, she may eventually join one of the organizations in the church.
- Encourage her to meet the other single ladies living on her floor. This may provide her with opportunities for socializing.

Outcome

Mrs. Burns will
- Develop new interests and relationships, thereby decreasing her feelings of loneliness.

COMMENTS

Mrs. Burns will need much encouragement and support to make the necessary changes in her life-style. If she finds menu planning difficult, congregate eating sites for older adults may serve diabetic meals upon request. She would then have to plan only two meals each day. Dining out also provides additional opportunities for socialization. It's important for her to record her food intake so the nurse can review it and make suggestions as needed. By keeping a food diary, she can see the cause and effect between urine or blood glucose tests and her diet.

Reinforce the teaching so Mrs. Burns realizes this is a lifelong condition. The changes she is making must be continued if she is to avoid complications. If the diabetes is not controlled by diet and exercise, additional teaching will be required in regard to antidiabetic agents prescribed by the physician and glucose monitoring.

Explain to Mrs. Burns that severe stress can increase her blood sugar levels. The action of stress hormones goes unchecked because of lack of effective insulin. Advise her to notify her physician if events in her life cause her to feel stressful. Closer monitoring of her blood sugar levels may be indicated. Some diabetics need insulin injections temporarily until the crisis is resolved. If Mrs. Burns has problems coping with her diagnosis, she may benefit from learning stress management techniques.

Mrs. Burns is eager to comply with the regime advised by her physician and nurse. This positive approach improves her prognosis dramatically. Avoid overwhelming her with information or placing too much emphasis on the possibility of complications. She could become overcompliant, allowing the disease to manage her, thus diminishing the quality of her life. It is important for the person of any age with diabetes or other chronic illness to realize that life continues and it can be satisfying and fulfilling. Diabetes is no barrier to traveling, enjoyment of hobbies, socialization, and sexuality.

QUESTIONS AND DISCUSSION

1. What impact do cultural and psychological factors have in the management of diabetes? Why is it important to include these factors in assessment?
2. Evaluate the available teaching resources for clients with diabetes. Are there adequate materials for teaching self-care practices?
3. How can Mrs. Burns be taught about diabetic emergencies without becoming frightened?
4. How available are members of the interdisciplinary health care team to clients receiving home care?

REFERENCES

American Diabetes Association. 1988. *Diabetes A to Z*. Alexandria, VA: American Diabetes Association, Inc.

———— 1990. *Fact Sheet*. Alexandria, VA: American Diabetes Association, Inc.

Byrnes, C.A. 1987. What's New in the Diabetic Diet. *Nursing 87* 17(8): 58–59.

Christensen, M.H., M.M. Funnell, M.R. Ehrlich, E.P. Fellows, and J.C. Floyd. 1991. How to Care for the Diabetic Foot. *American Journal of Nursing* 91(3): 50–56.

Crigler-Meringola, E.D. 1984. Making Life Sweet Again for the Elderly Diabetic. *Nursing 84* 14(4): 61–64.

Diabetes Forecast. *Nutrition Notes*. January 1988.

Gavin, J.R. 1988. Diabetes and Exercise. *American Journal of Nursing* 88(2): 178–80.

Gordon, M. 1991. *Manual of Nursing Diagnosis 1991–1992*. St. Louis: Mosby-Year Book, Inc.

Hass, L.B. 1991. In M. Shaw, ed. *Illustrated Manual of Nursing Practice*. Springhouse, PA: Springhouse Corporation.

Lipsky, B.A. 1992. Diagnosis and Treatment of Foot Infections in Elderly Diabetic Patients. *Geriatric Focus on Infectious Diseases* 2(1): 4–5, 11, 14.

Mitchell, P.H., L.C. Hodges, M. Muwaswes, and C.A. Walleck. 1988. *AANN's Neuroscience Nursing*. Norwalk, CT: Appleton and Lange.

Newman, D.K. and D.A.J. Smith. 1991. *Geriatric Care Plans*. Springhouse, PA: Springhouse Corporation.

Staff. 1990. Diabetes Update 90. *Nursing 90* 20(10): 49–51.

Swearingen, P.L. 1992. *Pocket Guide to Medical-Surgical Nursing*. St. Louis: Mosby-Year Book, Inc.

A Restorative Approach to Caring for the Client Requiring Orthopedic Management

OBJECTIVES

❑ Describe the types of fractures common in the older adult.
❑ Recognize the factors that increase the risk of falls for older adults.
❑ Identify residents at risk for falling.
❑ List foods high in calcium.
❑ Describe nursing interventions that will prevent the incidence of falls.
❑ Describe emergency care for a person with a suspected fracture.
❑ Describe nursing care for the client with a hip prosthesis.
❑ Describe nursing care for the client with open reduction, internal fixation (ORIF).
❑ Identify the role of the interdisciplinary health care team in the management of the client with hip surgery.

DESCRIPTION OF THE PROBLEM

The incidence of fractures increases sharply with age, particularly among women. Each year, one-fourth to one-half of the elderly living in the community suffer a fracture. For persons in nursing homes, this figure rises to 61 percent (Daleiden 1990). The increase is due primarily to the elderly's predisposition to falling and to the progressive bone loss associated with osteoporosis. Accidents are the sixth leading cause of death in persons over seventy-five years of age, with falls being the leading contributor (Woollacott 1990). The elderly are at risk for falling due to a number of age-related changes. As people age, they tend to develop a stooped posture to see the pathway, and a shuffling, broad-based gait. This gait, slowed reflexes, and loss of muscle strength make it difficult to prevent a fall. Medications including antihypertensives, diuretics, psychotropics, and antiparkinsonism drugs have been associated with falling. Sensory impairments, orthostatic hypotension, cardiac arrhythmias, infections, occult blood loss, depression, syncope, and confusion are causes of falls. An unsafe environment with slippery, uneven walking surfaces, unstable railings, poorly marked stairs, loose rugs, barriers in the walkway, and inadequate lighting increase the risk of falling (Daleiden 1990).

Osteoporosis

Some researchers feel that osteoporosis rather than age itself is the primary reason for fractures among the elderly. A reduction in bone mass reflects an imbalance in the body's system for storing and using calcium in the bone. By the third and fourth decades, both men and women begin to lose bone mass. From birth to young adulthood, special cells called osteoblasts are active in bone formation, resulting in increased length and weight of the bones. During the twenties, bone mass reaches its peak due to the constant process of remodeling by osteoblasts and resorption by osteoclasts. This highly coordinated process is referred to as coupling. By the thirties, uncoupling occurs and resorption overtakes the amount of bone formation. The excessive absorption of calcium and phosphorus causes bones to become porous and brittle. The loss of bone mass increases rapidly in women at the time of menopause due to diminishing estrogen levels.

Osteoporosis occurs in both men and women of all races. However, white, small, fair-skinned, postmenopausal females of Northwestern European descent appear to be most at risk for osteoporosis. Estrogen deficiency is a primary causal factor in bone loss. Family history, sedentary life-style, and heavy use of tobacco and alcohol further increase the risk. Diseases such as rheumatoid arthritis, diabetes mellitus, hyperparathyroidism, hyperthyroidism, and kidney disease are associated with osteoporosis. Drugs including corticosteroids, tetracycline, thyroid supplements, furosemide, and aluminum-containing antacids may also contribute to osteoporosis.

The diagnosis of osteoporosis is often first made based on X rays taken of fractures resulting from minimal trauma. However, standard X rays do not accurately measure bone mass. Recent diagnostic advances are more precise. Bone density of the radius can be determined with single-photon absorptiometry. Dual-photon absorptiometry is used for the spine and femur. Quantitative digital radiography (QDR) and single- and dual-energy computed tomography are other noninvasive tests used to determine bone density (Palmieri 1988).

Preventing Falls and Fractures

It is clear that fractures are a common cause of disability among the elderly. Prevention of fractures is based on the identification of individual risk factors, maintaining mobility skills, provision of a safe environment, and the detection and prevention of osteoporosis (see chapter 3). Preventing or delaying osteoporosis will significantly reduce the risk of falling and subsequent fracture. Estrogen deficiency is the main cause of postmenopausal bone loss and also contributes to aging-associated bone loss. Estrogen therapy is the preferred treatment for preventing bone loss in menopausal women. Adequate calcium intake is necessary throughout life for normal bone growth. A daily minimum intake of 800 milligrams is recommended for all adults. Higher amounts are required during childhood, adolescence, pregnancy, lactation, and old age. Women who continue a high calcium intake after menopause suffer fewer fractures than those with low intake. The recommended daily intake of calcium for all postmenopausal women and for older men is 1000 milligrams (Dairy Council 1991). Adequate ingestion of dietary calcium can be maintained by including sufficient amounts of low-fat dairy products and dark, green, leafy vegetables in the nutritional plan. An eight-ounce glass of skim milk contains 275–300 milligrams of calcium. Salmon, tofu, and almonds are also calcium rich (Palmieri 1988). Foods high in calcium and fiber should not be eaten together because fiber prevents calcium absorption. The benefit of calcium supplements is unclear and the decision to use them should be made on an individual basis. Calcium carbonates or antacids without aluminum may be recommended if dietary intake is inadequate. Sufficient intake of protein is necessary for strong bones; however, excessively high levels can aggravate bone loss. Vitamin D is needed to facilitate calcium absorption, but megadoses of this vitamin are toxic.

Weight-bearing exercise contributes to the maintenance of bone mass. Exercise also maintains flexibility, agility, and muscular function, thus reducing the likelihood of falls. Walking three times a week for thirty minutes, swimming, back exercises, and abdominal isometrics are some of the recommended activities. The present degree of osteoporosis must be considered when planning a program so that activities that could cause fractures, such as jumping and twisting, are avoided.

Management of Falls

When an elderly person falls, it may be difficult to determine if the fracture resulted from the fall or if the individual fell after a spontaneous fracture resulting from osteoporosis. If a client falls, the correct response by the caregiver can minimize injury. Precautions must be taken to avoid injury to the caregiver.

- Maintain good body alignment with a broad base of support. Bend your knees and hips, keeping your back straight.
- Place your arms around the client's trunk, supporting the head and trunk. Support the client's body with the thigh of one leg. Gently ease the client to a supine position on the floor.
  After a fall, assess the individual carefully before moving.
- If the fall was unwitnessed and potential injuries are questionable, assess the ABCs: airway, breathing, and circulation. If the fall was caused by respiratory or cardiac arrest, proceed accordingly. If pulse and breathing are present, check blood pressure and pulse, determine level of consciousness, and check pupils for size, equality, and reaction to light.
- Examine the head and body for lacerations, abrasions, and deformities.
- Immobilize the head if cervical spine injury is suspected.
- In the presence of osteoporosis, a fall can fracture the ribs, sometimes causing a pneumothorax.
- Consider the possibility of a fractured pelvis. This is frequently associated with hip fracture but can also happen in the absence of hip fracture.
- Assess the limbs for strength and motion. *Do not perform full range-of-motion exercises, particularly if fracture is suspected.*
- If a hip fracture is present, localized pain is generally noted in the area of the greater trochanter or anterior pelvis. Occasionally, referred pain to the knee may be the only discomfort noted by the client with a fractured hip. Except for rare instances, the individual is unable to walk and prefers to lie down

rather than sit. The affected limb is usually shortened, abducted, and externally rotated. Crepitus may be present (DaCunha 1991).

❑ Immobilize fractured extremities to minimize swelling, bleeding, and pain and to prevent further damage to muscles, tendons, blood vessels, and nerves. A splint may not be needed if the client can follow directions and if the emergency medical system responds promptly. If a splint is necessary, it can be improvised from anything that is firm and large enough. Use a tie, belt, scarf, or elastic bandage to hold it in place. Support the joint above and below the fracture site while another person slides the splint in place. Do not try to straighten the injured limb, but maintain the extremity in the position it was found.

❑ Cover the client with a blanket if the client will remain on the floor until emergency medical services arrive. Do not place a pillow under the head if you suspect neck injuries.

❑ If no injuries are detected, return the client to bed. Provide first aid to minor injuries. Monitor the client closely for the next twenty-four hours. Check vital signs every four hours.

❑ Although most falls do not result in immediate life-threatening injuries, immediate attention is necessary. Surgery is more successful if completed within twenty-four to forty-eight hours.

❑ Make out an incident report, document the fall, and notify the family and the physician.

Whether or not a fracture occurs with a fall, the incident should be investigated to determine the cause.

❑ Check the environment and the activity of the client. Was the client attempting to transfer, using unsafe methods?

❑ Was the client suffering emotional stress or pain? Was the fall associated with voiding, defecating, or coughing?

❑ Were there any associated symptoms, such as palpitations or dyspnea?

❑ Does the client have an infection or a change in mental status?

❑ Is the client taking a new medication?

Once an elderly person falls, the individual becomes fearful of repeating the incident and may reduce physical activity in an effort to prevent further falls. This in turn decreases opportunities for socialization and may result in almost total isolation. Providing instruction and counseling on the prevention of falls can do much to allay the client's fears.

Types Of Fractures Common Among The Elderly _____

The most common and potentially most disabling fracture site is the upper third of the femur (hip). One million hip fractures occur every year in women over age forty-five. Forty percent of elderly women will have experienced a hip fracture before they die. Colle's fractures (distal end of radius) are also common and frequently occur as a result of a protective reflex action when the arm is extended as the person falls. There is a high incidence of vertebral compression fractures, which may be the earliest sign of osteoporosis. The lower thoracic or upper lumbar area is most often involved. Symptoms are first noted by a sudden onset of severe pain when the vertebral body collapses as a result of minimal trauma.

Femoral fractures are the most frequent type seen in the elderly and generally occur in one of three areas. Intertrochanteric fractures are most frequent, followed by transcervical (femoral neck) and subtrochanteric. Hip fractures are generally treated by surgical means. Open reduction and internal fixation (ORIF) is usually the preferred procedure, particularly for the elderly. Ambulation can be resumed relatively early in the course of healing. Internal fixation immobilizes fractures through the surgical insertion of metal pins, screws, or nails, sometimes in conjunction with a plate. If the femur head is badly damaged, a prosthesis may be inserted for a total hip procedure.

TABLE 15–1	Femoral Fractures	
LOCATION	DESCRIPTION	TREATMENT
Subtrochanteric	Fracture occurs below greater trochanter; usually caused by severe, direct trauma, such as falling out of bed	Usually treated with triflanged nail with side plate or with intermedullary rod
Femoral Neck	Most common in women over age sixty; fall follows the fracture of osteoporotic bone, which is caused by a rotational force	Femoral head is usually excised and is replaced with metal prosthesis.
Intertrochanter	Most common in older women, seventy-five to eighty years of age; swelling of thigh more evident than in other types	Repaired with triflanged and side plate and a thread-cutting screw attaching a sliding nail to the handle of the side plate

(DiDomenico and Ziegler 1989)

Arthroplasty replaces both joint components. The degenerated femoral head is removed and a prosthetic head and intermedullary stem are inserted. A plastic or metal cup replaces the acetabulum. The components are cemented in place. A prosthesis may be implanted following a femoral neck fracture or for degenerative disease of the hip characterized by severe, unrelenting pain not relieved by nonsteroidal anti-inflammatory drugs; loss of motion; and functional deficits. The surgery relieves the pain and restores motion, enabling the client to resume activities.

TABLE 15–2	Nursing Care for the Client with a Hip Prosthesis
	❏ Maintain hip abduction and avoid hip adduction when client is sitting, lying, or standing. Place abductor splint or pillows between legs at all times.
	❏ Avoid internal and external rotation. Maintain hip in neutral position, with toes pointing straight up when lying supine and toes straight ahead while client is sitting or walking. Advise client not to turn hip or knee inward or outward.
	❏ Turn client to back and unaffected side only. Keep the affected hip straight, with pillows to support affected limb when client is lying on the side.

Continues

□ *Instruct the client to not cross the legs at any time. Avoid more than ninety degrees flexion of the hip.*

□ Advise client to sit in a chair with arms. To come to a standing position from the chair, move to edge of chair and place unaffected leg back and affected leg forward. Use hands to push off the arms of the chair.

□ Use raised toilet seat to maintain proper position of hip.

□ Monitor affected hip for signs of dislocation — swelling, redness or discoloration, sudden or severe pain, or unusual positioning of affected extremity.

(Stevens 1990)

Skin traction with a Buck's extension device is occasionally used for persons who are poor surgical risks. The affected extremity is immobilized through direct application of a pulling force on the client's skin. Although limited activity of the affected limb and exercising of the other extremities are possible, the enforced confinement to bed places the client at risk for complications associated with immobility. The care of the elderly client with a fracture is a challenge. Regaining mobility without a loss of function is the major goal.

CASE STUDY

Miss Charlotte Adams was admitted to a long-term-care facility for further restorative care following an ORIF at the local hospital. Previous to hospitalization, she lived alone at a senior citizen complex. Miss Adams remembers falling but has no recollection of the events leading up to the fall. She had not seen a physician for four or five years yet says she is taking medication. She is eighty-one years old and her only family is an older brother who had a stroke two years ago. He is living in a nursing home in another state. Miss Adams was a school teacher and a principal for several years in the local school system. Admission information indicates that she had an intertrochanteric, comminuted fracture of the left femur. Osteoporosis is listed as a secondary diagnosis. The surgical report describes the insertion of a triflanged and side plate and a thread-cutting screw attached to a sliding nail to the handle of a side plate. This is anchored to the femoral shaft to produce compression of the intertrochanteric fracture.

Strengths

□ Cognitively alert
□ Continent of bowel and bladder
□ Adequate nutritional status
□ History of participation in many church and community activities

Interdisciplinary Assessment

Nursing and Physical Therapy.

Miss Adams has limited range of motion of the left lower extremity and is reluctant to move in bed without assistance. She is hesitant to get out of bed for fear she will fall again. Miss Adams is not to bear weight on the affected side. However, she can begin a program of progressive mobility to avoid complications and to enable her to eventually resume her preoperative level of activity.

Nursing Diagnosis

Impaired physical mobility related to recent surgery and physician's orders for no weight bearing.

Nursing Interventions

- Place Miss Adams on a two-hour positioning schedule. Instruct the staff to avoid positions of adduction, external rotation, or acute flexion of the left hip. Place the affected limb on a pillow in a position of mild abduction. Place a pillow between the legs to maintain alignment and use a trochanter roll to avoid external rotation (see chapter 3). Miss Adams can lie on either side but be sure a pillow is placed between her legs when she lies on the unaffected side to maintain abduction.
- Teach her how she can help turn herself onto her side. Avoid knee flexion in bed to prevent formation of knee and hip flexion contractures.
- Instruct the staff to perform skin inspections each shift over pressure areas, particularly the heels.
- Remove the support stockings for one hour out of every eight hours; wash and dry her legs before reapplying.
- Get Miss Adams up in a wheelchair for several short periods during the day. This will allow her to be out of her room, to go the dining room, and to attend other activities.
- Teach Miss Adams to help with a one-person pivot transfer using a transfer belt. Tell her to slightly extend the left leg and to place the right foot back. This will facilitate her ability to rise from the chair and to avoid placing weight on the left leg. Maintain body alignment with the hips and knees at ninety-degree angles. Remind Miss Adams that she should not bend forward or cross her legs.
- Teach Miss Adams to do active range-of-motion exercises twice each day, avoiding adduction, external rotation, and flexion of the left hip.

Collaboration: Interdisciplinary Team

- The physical therapist has recommended isometric exercises for the thigh, gluteal, and abdominal muscles to condition her extremities for later ambulation. Arm-strengthening exercises will prepare her to use the walker.
- When the surgeon allows her to begin ambulating, Miss Adams may begin by using the parallel bars in physical therapy or she may begin with a walker. When a compression screw is in place, the surgeon generally allows toe-touch-only weight bearing. This progresses to weight bearing to tolerance in four to six weeks if bony healing is taking place (DiDomenico and Ziegler 1989). After full weight bearing is allowed, Miss Adams may progress to a quad cane.

Outcome

Miss Adams will
- Remain free of contractures
- Move herself in bed
- Transfer in and out of bed safely
- Ambulate safely with a walker

Interdisciplinary Assessment _____

Nursing.

Miss Adams states that although she has never been injured before, she had fallen several times in the last year. She has no recollection of what may have caused her to fall.

Nursing Diagnosis _____

High risk for injury related to history of falling with unknown cause.

Nursing Interventions _____

❑ Leave Miss Adams's bed in the lowest position with the brakes on.
❑ Monitor her for orthostatic hypotension. Take her blood pressure while she is lying flat and again immediately after she stands. A drop of 20 mm Hg or more, either systolic or diastolic, may indicate slowed vasoactive reflexes, causing her to faint.
❑ Instruct her to come to a sitting position slowly and to sit on the edge of the bed for a while before attempting to stand. Then she should rise slowly. Tell her to avoid any sudden movements that involve turning her neck or twisting.
❑ Advise Miss Adams to wear shoes when she transfers and when she is ambulating to promote her stability. Check her shoes for proper fit and condition.
❑ Teach Miss Adams how to safely operate her wheelchair (see chapter 3).

Outcome _____

Miss Adams will
❑ Demonstrate safe wheelchair mobility
❑ Maintain/increase mobility without injury

Interdisciplinary Assessment _____

Nursing and Social Services.

Miss Adams has always been an independent person. She has lived alone all of her adult life, assuming responsibility for all aspects of her life. She is proud of the fact that she has never had to rely on others and states that she has never believed in airing one's problems to the world. She has had few adult relationships, utilizing most of her time for her career and volunteer work. The emergency hospital admission and subsequent nursing home placement occurred so rapidly that she has had little time to adjust to the changes in her life. She feels that she has had little control or influence over the situation. She is concerned about her home and possessions and the fact that she may never live in her home again.

Nursing Diagnosis _____

Powerlessness related to abrupt change in life-style.

Nursing Interventions

❑ Sit down with Miss Adams to discuss her needs and set up a routine that is agreeable to her and liveable for staff. Write the routine on her care plan so it is communicated to all caregivers. Help her identify aspects of her care/life over which she has control and those aspects which she cannot realistically change.

❑ Make sure her call light is within reach at all times. Ask her if she has anything at home that she would enjoy having at the nursing home. Plants, pictures, and other mementos may improve her morale.

❑ Deal with Miss Adams's feelings of powerlessness before the feelings progress to hopelessness. Explain to staff that without appropriate, consistent intervention, Miss Adams may develop manipulative behaviors as a way to manage her feelings of powerlessness.

❑ Encourage her to verbalize her concerns and accept her expressions of anger and frustration. Provide her with opportunities for making choices and decisions. Give her positive reinforcement for her progress.

Collaboration: Interdisciplinary Team

❑ Social Services will ask her if she would like to communicate with her brother and will arrange for her to do this if she so desires.

❑ Social Services will assist her to make contact with her banker, attorney, or other individuals she trusts to help her with her financial and legal affairs.

❑ She will be provided with assistance to go to the business office to take care of her financial concerns.

❑ Activities staff will discuss their program with Miss Adams. She may find satisfaction leading a current events discussion group, joining a reminiscing group, or actively participating in the residents' council. Ask the activities aide to visit her weekly to go over the scheduled events.

❑ Explore the possible volunteer activities available to Miss Adams and discuss with her whether or not she chooses to become involved in the activities.

❑ Miss Adams was an active church member, so Social Services will talk with her regarding attendance at the weekly services and at Bible study classes.

❑ The social worker will visit Miss Adams once or twice a week at a scheduled time to discuss her progress and plan of care. Miss Adams has agreed to have a volunteer visit her weekly to talk with her, to participate in individualized activities, or to run errands for her.

Outcome

Miss Adams will
❑ Actively participate in planning her care, making realistic choices
❑ Verbalize a sense of being in control of her life and a feeling of hope

COMMENTS

Fractured hips generally heal successfully. Postoperative complications, if they occur, are often related to cardiovascular problems or to respiratory tract or urinary tract infections.

The accident caused a sudden and overwhelming disruption in Miss Adams's life. Her recovery may be a lengthy one and her future living arrangements remain uncertain. Her feelings of powerlessness are a natural response to an unnatural situation. Explain to staff that consistent implementation of the interventions discussed earlier will prevent formation of negative behaviors.

Miss Adams needs the friendship and caring of the staff. The activities that previously provided her with fulfillment are no longer available to her. This makes it important to strive to help her find other ways and means to again make life meaningful to her.

QUESTIONS AND DISCUSSION

1. What further investigation may be needed to determine the cause of Miss Adams's falls?
2. What steps does the professional nurse need to take to assure that staff will position Miss Adams correctly?
3. What factors would need to be evaluated to determine the possibility of Miss Adams returning home?
4. What community services would she require?
5. Are there additional interventions by the interdisciplinary team that may be beneficial to Miss Adams?

REFERENCES

DaCunha, J.P. 1991. *Emergency Procedures.* Springhouse, PA: Springhouse Corporation.

Dairy Council. 1991. International Consensus Conference on Osteoporosis Held. *Nutrition Newsbreak.* April 1991.

Daleiden, S. 1990. Prevention of Falling; Rehabilitative or Compensatory Interventions? *Topics in Geriatric Rehabilitation* 5(2): 44–53.

DiDomenico, R.L. and W.Z. Ziegler. 1989. *Practical Rehabilitation Techniques for Geriatric Aides.* Rockville, MD: Aspen Publishers, Inc.

Palmieri, G.M.A. 1988. Prevention and Treatment of Osteoporosis. *Clinical Report on Aging* 2(4): 19–20, 24.

Stevens, K.A. 1990. *Rehabilitation Nursing Procedures Manual.* Rockville, MD: Aspen Publishers, Inc.

Woollacott, M.H., issue ed. 1990. *Topics in Geriatric Rehabilitation* 5(2): vii, viii.

CHAPTER 16

A Restorative Approach to Caring for the Client with Genetic Disorder of the Central Nervous System

CONTENT OUTLINE

I. Description of the disease
   A. Symptoms
II. Case study
   A. Strengths
   B. Interdisciplinary assessment
   C. Nursing diagnoses
      1. Impaired swallowing and high risk for aspiration
      2. High risk for injury
      3. Impaired physical mobility
      4. Impaired verbal communication
      5. Anticipatory grieving
      6. Decisional conflict
III. Comments

OBJECTIVES

❑ Discuss the genetic implications of Huntington's disease.
❑ Identify the characteristics of Huntington's disease.
❑ Describe the psychosocial impact of Huntington's disease on the client and the client's family.
❑ List nursing interventions that will prevent the onset of complications for the client with Huntington's disease.
❑ Identify the role of the interdisciplinary health care team in the management of the client with Huntington's disease.

DESCRIPTION OF THE DISEASE

Huntington's disease is an autosomal dominant disorder of the central nervous system characterized by choreiform movements, cognitive impairments, and psychiatric disorders. Each child of a parent with Huntington's disease has a 50 percent chance of inheriting the disease. Both males and females with the Huntington's gene can pass the disease to either sons or daughters. The disease does not "skip" a generation. If a person at risk does not have the gene, any children born to that person will be free of the disease and the chain is broken forever in that branch of the family tree. Persons who carry the gene will develop the disease if they live long enough and they may pass the gene on to the next generation (Shoulson 1981). Although the gene is present at birth, symptoms do not usually appear until ages thirty-five to forty-five. However, symptoms may begin anytime from early childhood until old age. The disease is always progressive and irreversible (Folstein 1989).

A presymptomatic (predictive) test became available in 1988. Blood samples are analyzed for the presence of DNA markers linked to the Huntington's disease gene. By tracking the inheritance of a marker, researchers can predict the probability that an at-risk person has inherited the gene. If all the markers are used and the necessary blood samples from the family are available, the test can be 99 percent accurate (Huntington's Disease Society of America 1988). The decision to be tested is a difficult one and not all persons at risk choose to be tested. Those who do are encouraged to think about what the results of the test will mean for them.

Anyone contemplating the test is required to attend classes and participate in counseling before any tests or medical exams are proposed. Individuals are made aware that the test may not even give them an informative result. It is not a yes-no type of test and in some cases is inconclusive. The test can revise the odds that the at-risk person has inherited the gene. Each child born to an HD parent has a fifty-fifty chance of inheriting the gene. After the test, they may be told, for example, that they have either a greater or lesser than 50 percent chance of inheriting the gene. The test does not identify the gene or primary gene product connected with Huntington's disease but rather patterns of inheritance linked to the gene location on the chromosome. Psychiatric and psychological screening confirm that there are no underlying problems that are beyond the person's power to deal with, given adequate support. Individuals wishing to be tested are encouraged and, at some centers, required (if possible), to have a support person share the educational and counseling sessions. This support person can serve as a sounding board in the decision to be tested. The support person can serve as a "stabilizer" if the results show increased risk or are inconclusive (McKay 1988).

Predictive testing is now available at more than twenty centers across the country. Testing is available through university-based programs and private genetics clinics, and is provided by a variety of disciplines. There are various aspects of testing that should be considered by prospective clients. Huntington's disease is a relatively rare disorder, so it is important that the program be staffed by professionals who are familiar with the genetics and characteristics of the disease. The program should provide pedigree screening, which involves the testing of family members. Blood samples, DNA, or brain tissue samples are usually needed from at least two or more people affected with Huntington's disease, or from an unaffected grandparent on the side of the family with the disease, or from an affected sibling. Samples from other at-risk unaffected relatives (or those who died at risk) may also be needed. The exact samples that are required are determined on a case-by-case basis. An essential part of the testing is an examination by a neurologist familiar with the early symptoms of Huntington's disease. Psychiatric screening, psychological assessment, counseling, and follow-up care are also included in the *Guidelines for Predictive Testing for Huntington's Disease* published by the Huntington's Disease Society of America (Quaid 1991).

Many at-risk people are ineligible for the predictive test for such reasons as inadequate family history, difficulty in obtaining the required blood samples from family members, the cost of the test, and the large areas of the country still unserved by a testing facility.

Families should know that there is a need for autopsy brain tissue, not only from people affected with HD but also from people at-risk, to assist with research. Some research has suggested that brain cell changes begin long before the symptoms of HD become apparent. By studying tissues of at-risk persons who have no symptoms, it may be possible to determine what triggers the onset of the disease.

Currently, there is no treatment that can cure, delay, or slow the course of the disease. Medications may alleviate manifestations of the disease related to involuntary movements, irritability, and depression.

Symptoms

Symptoms encompass the physical, cognitive, and emotional status of the individual. There is not a specific sequence in which the three groups of symptoms appear. The disorder of movement is the major physical clinical manifestation of Huntington's disease. There are two components: involuntary movements and abnormalities of voluntary movement. The involuntary movements are choreic and may include myoclonus (a sudden muscle spasm usually affecting the arms), dystonia (a spasm of the muscles in the shoulders, neck, and trunk), and athetosis (a writhing, involuntary movement of the hands, face, and tongue). Voluntary movements are impaired by clumsiness, bradykinesia, slowing of response time, and the inability to sustain a voluntary movement (Folstein 1989). Physical symptoms begin with fidgeting, twitching, and restlessness. The individual notes frequent falling, dropping of objects, and problems with balance. The symptoms may not yet be obvious to others. Eventually, full choreic movements are present almost constantly, except during sleep. The gait, unsteady at first, becomes broad based and slow. The rhythm is irregular and the client's knee may suddenly bend without warning. In the later stages, walking and performance of all other motor skills are impossible because of the constant involuntary movements. As a result of dysarthria, caused by weakness of the speech musculature and involuntary movements of the tongue and lips, speech becomes slurred and grunting. Speech is dysrhythmic, with bursts of words and pauses in midphrase (Folstein 1989). Because there are generally no language problems, the client can comprehend the speech of others. Dysphagia is also a problem, placing the client at risk for choking and aspiration. Voluntary control of bowel and bladder functions is lost in the later stages of Huntington's disease.

Cognitive symptoms associated with Huntington's disease are a result of a subcortical dementia. (Alzheimer's disease is a cortical dementia, so the two diseases will present differently.) Persons with Huntington's disease appear to have memory lapses, but given enough time and cues, they can generally learn new information and recall it. Judgment is impaired and the client has increasing difficulty with planning, organizing, and sequencing daily tasks (Shapira, Schlesinger, and Cummings 1986).

The initial emotional disturbances are vague. At the onset of emotional involvement, the client appears vague, listless, apathetic, and indifferent. The client may be easily irritated and quick to anger. Emotional lability and impulsive behavior are common. Some clients exhibit antisocial behavior and withdraw from the environment or misuse drugs or alcohol. Depression may be manifested by either agitation or psychomotor retardation. Bipolar depression with manic features may also occur. Some clients become overtly psychotic, experiencing hallucinations and delusions (Folstein 1989).

There are no remissions with Huntington's disease. It may however, stabilize for long periods of time. The disease may progress rapidly over a few years or slowly over fifteen to twenty years. In the early stage of Huntington's disease, the client can function independently despite the onset of signs and symptoms. There are no self-care deficits, employment can be continued, and family interactions are usually satisfactory.

The client remains independent in activities of daily living during the early intermediate stage. He/she is still employable, although usually at a lower level of capacity due to the change in functional abilities. The ability to handle daily financial affairs is retained and household management is continued, but not necessarily in the same manner as previously.

By the later intermediate stage, the client is no longer employable and is unable to manage household affairs. Considerable help is needed with financial affairs. Only minimal assistance is required with the basic activities of daily living.

The client is dependent on others for most aspects of daily life during the early advanced stage. The client may be able to function at home with a supportive family or in a long-term-care facility with minimal to moderate professional assistance.

By the advanced stage, the client requires continued professional assistance and complete support for all activities of daily living. Death usually results from an infectious process (Shoulson 1981).

CASE STUDY

Mrs. Jones, age sixty-five, was admitted to the nursing home because of problems related to Huntington's disease. She was diagnosed when she was forty-five years old at a large clinic after two years of consultation with several physicians. Mrs. Jones's father died when he was eighty-eight years old and had never exhibited symptoms. Her mother had never been ill but she died suddenly in an accident when she was thirty-five years old and Mrs. Jones was still a child. Mrs. Jones remembers the family talking in whispers about her maternal grandmother who lived the last few years of her life in a state mental hospital. Mrs. Jones feels her grandmother was the branch of the family tree carrying the defective gene.

Mrs. Jones has three adult children, ages forty, thirty-eight, and thirty-five. The two oldest are married and the thirty-eight-year-old has two children. Mr. Jones retired five years ago to care for his wife.

Strengths

- ❑ Ambulatory with assistance
- ❑ Control of bowel and bladder if toileted regularly
- ❑ Able to complete activities of daily living with assistance
- ❑ Supportive family

Interdisciplinary Assessment

Nursing and Speech Pathologist.

Mrs. Jones has a good appetite and enjoys eating. But she has a history of difficulty with swallowing, although she has never needed to have the Heimlich maneuver performed. She frequently has problems with coughing spells while eating. Her weight is satisfactory and has remained relatively stable the last five years.

Nursing Diagnosis

Impaired swallowing and high risk for aspiration related to involuntary movements of the tongue, lips, and cheeks.

Nursing Interventions

❑ Provide Mrs. Jones with a diet that she can swallow without difficulty. Try to arrange for the same people to feed her at each meal. They will become familiar with her problem and she will feel more relaxed.

❑ Instruct the caregivers to feed Mrs. Jones slowly and have her remain upright for at least thirty minutes after the meal. Be sure they know how to perform the Heimlich maneuver for obstructed airway. Have a professional nurse and suction equipment close by when she is eating to provide emergency care should it be needed. (See chapter 5.)

❑ People with Huntington's disease require twice the normal amount of calories per day because of the constant physical activity. Provide her with nourishing snacks when she is hungry. Monitor her daily intake and weigh her weekly. It may become necessary to administer tube feedings to maintain nutritional status. This procedure also poses risk because of the involuntary movements. If this becomes necessary, a gastrostomy would be less dangerous than a nasogastric tube.

Collaboration: Interdisciplinary Team

❑ If the above interventions are inadequate, arrange for the speech pathologist to complete a full swallowing evaluation.

Outcome

Mrs. Jones will
❑ Swallow without aspiration, maintaining an adequate nutritional status
❑ Maintain her present weight

Interdisciplinary Assessment

Nursing and Physical Therapist.

Impaired physical mobility places Mrs. Jones at risk for injury due to falling and accidentally harming herself by striking her moving extremities against stationary objects. The involuntary movements can also interrupt the skin integrity of her extremities. Because of poor judgment and impulsivity, Mrs. Jones places herself in dangerous situations. She has attempted to lean over while in the wheelchair, losing her balance. Her potential fall from the wheelchair was intercepted by a caregiver.

Nursing Diagnosis

High risk for injury related to involuntary movements and impaired mental status.

Nursing Interventions

❑ Use a wheelchair only for transporting Mrs. Jones. Her movements can cause the chair to tip, causing injury. When she is up, provide her with a sturdy, well-padded chair, large enough to prevent her from falling out of the chair.

The use of physical restraints increases the risk of injury for persons with Huntington's disease and are best avoided.

☐ Have Mrs. Jones use a bedside commode with padded arms instead of the toilet. Monitor her while she is up. An indwelling catheter is inappropriate for Mrs. Jones. The movements could pull on the catheter causing urethral lacerations. When she loses total control of her bowels and bladder, she will need to wear incontinent pads during the day.

☐ Pad the side rails on Mrs. Jones's bed to avoid abrasions to her extremities. When she is up, help her dress in nonrestrictive clothing that will protect the skin of her arms and legs. Jogging suits with pads for her knees and elbows may provide protection.

Outcome

Mrs. Jones will
☐ Remain free of injury
☐ Maintain skin integrity

Interdisciplinary Assessment

Nursing and Physical Therapy.

Mrs. Jones is unable to walk without assistance due to sudden and unexpected involuntary movements that throw her off balance. She had fallen several times at home prior to her nursing home admission. She has a shuffling, dancing gait and her upper body seems to advance ahead of her pelvis and legs. She also has difficulty coming to a standing position, but can walk with assistance, once she is up.

Nursing Diagnosis

Impaired physical mobility related to unsteady gait due to choreiform movements.

Nursing Interventions

☐ Teach the assistants how to ease her to the floor if she starts to fall.
☐ When Mrs. Jones transfers, again use a transfer belt and two assistants. Teach her to take her time and to make sure her feet are positioned slightly back and her trunk is flexed. Remind her to push off the bed or chair with both hands.
☐ Place Mrs. Jones on a positioning schedule and give her the help she needs to change her position.
☐ Do active assistive range-of-motion exercises twice each day on all extremities.

Collaboration: Interdisciplinary Team

☐ The physical therapist has recommended that Mrs. Jones ambulate two or three times a day with the assistance of two people and a gait belt.
☐ Be sure that anyone ambulating Mrs. Jones understands how to walk with her. The unexpected, involuntary movements can cause her to bolt away from the caregiver. There should be a person on each side of her to provide counterbal-

ance. Each person places the hand closer to the client through the gait belt. The client's hands are held at her waist level with her elbows flexed to provide better balance. Because of her unsteady movements, a cane or walker would pose additional danger.

Outcome

Mrs. Jones will
❏ Ambulate with assistance two or three times each day to the end of the hall and back

Interdisciplinary Assessment

Nursing and Speech Pathologist.
Because of the involvement of her speech musculature, Mrs. Jones's speech is slurred. The volume is low and at times almost inaudible.

Nursing Diagnosis

Impaired verbal communication (dysarthria) related to weakened speech muscles.

Nursing Interventions

❏ When Mrs. Jones prepares to speak, teach her to think of a slow start, to take her time, and to talk slowly.
❏ Place yourself at her level so you can watch her mouth for cues as to which sounds of speech she is trying to produce.
❏ Request that she speak one phrase at a time rather than attempting lengthy sentences. After she speaks a phrase, repeat it after her. This gives her opportunity for a short rest and the caregiver will know whether she was correctly understood.
❏ Give verbal or visual feedback when the client is understood. If she is not understood, ask her to repeat the phrase with different words when possible. The new words may be easier for her to produce. Assess for signs of fatigue and suggest she avoid unnecessary talking when she is tired.
❏ If these interventions are unsuccessful, an alternate means of communication needs to be established (see chapter 13).

Collaboration: Interdisciplinary Team

❏ Consult with the speech pathologist to determine the appropriateness of oral exercises (see chapter 18).

Outcome

Mrs. Jones will
❏ Be capable of communicating her needs to the staff

Interdisciplinary Assessment

Nursing and Social Services.

Mrs. Jones's symptoms and functional abilities indicate that she is in the early advanced/advanced stage of Huntington's disease. She is aware that nursing home placement is permanent and that she will eventually die here. Although her judgment is impaired and she exhibits impulsive behavior at times, Mrs. Jones is oriented. She has expressed feelings of guilt in regard to the at-risk status of her children and grandchildren and is distressed at the thought of living the rest of her life in a nursing home. She is concerned that the disease will cause her great suffering before she dies and that her family will have to witness this. Mrs. Jones needs to be allowed to grieve and resolve her feelings regarding dependence, separation from her husband, and living in the nursing home. She needs the support of the staff as well as her family to reach acceptance of her death.

Nursing Diagnosis

Anticipatory grieving related to progressive loss of health and dependence.

Nursing Interventions

❑ Actively listen to Mrs. Jones's perceptions, permitting her to express anger or fear. Be sensitive to and acknowledge her feelings. Respect her wishes if she desires not to talk.
❑ Observe her body language and monitor her patterns of eating, sleeping, and activity for signs of unexpressed emotions.
❑ Touch Mrs. Jones if it brings her comfort. Hold her hand while you are talking to her.
❑ Encourage her to recall happy memories so that she may validate the worth of her life.
❑ Avoid robbing Mrs. Jones of her abilities — do not do anything for Mrs. Jones that she is still capable of doing for herself. Encourage her to direct her care, providing her as much control as she desires.
❑ Help her maintain her current levels of mental and physical activity to avoid painful complications. Provide the assistance she needs to look attractive and well groomed every day.
❑ Avoid giving Mrs. Jones false reassurance but do not deny her hope. Assure her that you will help her deal with each problem as it arises and that you will do everything possible to maintain her comfort and dignity.
❑ Discuss with the physician, Mrs. Jones, and her family her wishes in regard to life-extending measures.
❑ Use humor therapeutically. Although Mrs. Jones's health is deteriorating, it is not natural or tolerable to constantly think of one's impending death. She will have periods of denial; this is natural. Do not force her back to reality until she is ready to be there.

Collaboration: Interdisciplinary Team

❑ The social services department has had frequent communication with Mrs. Jones and her family. They will observe interaction patterns of the client and her family and provide support to her family as appropriate.
❑ Social Services will discuss with Mrs. Jones and her family the possibility of

becoming involved with the local hospice agency. This group can provide additional assistance to everyone.

❑ Mrs. Jones needs mental stimulation within the realm of her capabilities. The activities staff will be challenged to provide her with activities appropriate to her changing needs.

Outcome

Mrs. Jones will
❑ Feel comfortable expressing her feelings honestly
❑ Maintain control of her care as long as she desires
❑ Maintain hope, take one day at a time, and look forward to tomorrow

Interdisciplinary Assessment

Nursing and Social Services.

The Jones children were ages twenty, eighteen, and fifteen when their mother was diagnosed with HD twenty years ago. At that time, they were counseled and advised of their at-risk status. The eldest and his wife have made the choice not to have children. The middle child and her husband have a son and daughter ages ten and twelve who have not been told about HD. The youngest daughter is not married at this time. The children have been unable to make a decision regarding testing.

Throughout the years of their mother's illness, the family has generally coped adaptively. Family members fluctuate at times between feelings of despair and optimism, but for the most part are satisfied with their lives. Mrs. Jones denied her illness for a lengthy time after diagnosis, but eventually came to accept the implications of the disease. For many years, she has periodically wrestled with overwhelming feelings of guilt when she blames herself for "inflicting" this on her family.

The decision to be tested is a difficult one and a large percentage of at-risk individuals have not availed themselves of the test. When the Jones's grandchildren should be told about HD is a decision that will have to be made by the parents. Regardless of when they are told, they will be devastated. Support and counseling may provide them with the strength to pick up the pieces and live productive lives. Children are very perceptive and it is possible they are already aware of something happening in their lives. For better or worse, children have the right to know about major facts that affect their lives so they can make sound decisions regarding their present and future. It is the parents' role to provide the children with this information which can be reinforced, if necessary, by the physician, genetic counselor, or relative. Whether the grandchildren participate in predictive testing is a decision they must make when they reach the age of consent. By that time, the specific gene may be identified, making testing more conclusive.

Nursing Diagnosis

Decisional conflict related to family members' inability to make a decision regarding predictive testing.

Nursing Interventions

❏ The physician has referred the family to a testing center and genetic counselor for further information on predictive testing. It is not the responsibility of the nursing home staff to counsel the family in regard to testing. However, the staff should be well informed on the subject so they understand the stress of the family at this time.

❏ At risk family members require your care and understanding. They are witnessing the deterioration of a loved one, realizing they may be the person in bed at some point in time.

❏ Remember that the state of being at risk is very different from knowing definitely that one is sick or one is healthy. A 50 percent chance of developing the disease is 50 percent yes and 50 percent no. In the minds of at-risk persons, the certainty changes for the individual from moment to moment. This fluctuation is a normal means of coping.

❏ Avoid smothering the family with sympathy, but do be empathetic, listen to them, and allow them to verbalize their feelings. Remember that it is not the role of staff to give advice regarding predictive testing.

❏ Avoid minimizing the family's concerns but give realistic hope. Spouses and friends of at-risk persons often encourage denial. While denial is necessary at times as a coping mechanism, being told "Don't worry, it won't happen" implies to the at-risk person that "This is so horrible, I can't talk about it."

❏ At-risk persons are "symptom searching" — being on the alert for any indication of HD symptoms. Stumbling, falling, forgetting, or personal life changes may be interpreted as the onset of the disease. This too is a normal reaction to an abnormal situation. If this response interferes with their lives, intervention is needed.

❏ The Jones children may feel guilty at times. This may stem from feelings of anger toward their mother for "giving" them the disease. The middle daughter may experience guilt because of her decision to have children and placing them at risk. These too are expected reactions that must be worked through.

❏ Do not forget Mr. Jones and the children's spouses. Although they are not at risk, they too may feel overwhelmed at times with the unpredictability of their futures. Their concern and love for the family may cause them to overextend themselves.

❏ Mr. Jones has been in limbo for the last few years, putting aside his own interests and hobbies in order to care for his wife. He has been criticized by some of their friends and relatives for placing Mrs. Jones in the nursing home. Mr. Jones and other family members may benefit from joining a support group. If there is not a group in the area for Huntington's disease, an Alzheimer's support group may be helpful.

Collaboration: Interdisciplinary Team

❏ The social worker is an integral member of the team. With HD, it is sometimes difficult to sort out who needs the care — client or family? Referrals may need to be made for family members for additional counseling. Mrs. Jones may require psychiatric intervention for treatment of depression.

Outcome_____

The Jones family will
☐ Verbalize their feelings to the nurse, social worker, physician, and/or genetic counselor
☐ Continue to support each other
☐ Arrive at a decision that is compatible with the family's desires

COMMENTS

Persons with Huntington's disease usually die from an infectious process. Maintain preventive measures, especially for respiratory and urinary tract infections. Depression is an inevitable component of HD. This can generally be treated with medication and intervention by a mental health therapist or psychiatrist. Staff need to be aware that individuals with subcortical dementias are at high risk for suicide. Tell them to report immediately any comments or behaviors of Mrs. Jones that may indicate suicidal thoughts. Some clients with HD experience a loss of sexual inhibitions. Limits need to be placed on inappropriate behavior and rules established. Always strive to maintain the client's dignity and avoid being judgmental.Clients with HD seek structure in their lives. Establish a routine with Mrs. Jones both in terms of her schedule and the way in which procedures and care are completed. Consistent caregivers will add to her sense of security, facilitating adaptation.

When the diagnosis is Huntington's disease, it is given to the entire family. Research is being conducted around the country on potential therapies and to locate the responsible gene thereby improving predictive testing results. Persons at risk have much to be hopeful for. In the meantime, health care professionals must continue to be advocates, educators, and responsible caregivers.

Arrange to do an in-service for the staff on Huntington's disease and Mrs. Jones's care. Most larger nursing homes have at least one client with HD at any given time. However, it is not a common disease and it is likely that many staff, including professionals, have a limited knowledge of HD. Health care professionals who have experience in caring for clients with Huntington's disease are frequently called upon to educate emergency staff, paramedics, and fire department personnel about the disease. It is frequently confused with substance abuse, mental retardation, or other central nervous system disorders.

QUESTIONS AND DISCUSSION

1. What social services and community resources are available in your area for clients with Huntington's disease and their families?
2. If you have ever provided nursing care for a client with HD, which client problems required the most intricate planning? Were the problems resolved and if so, which interventions were successful?
3. Discuss the psychosocial implications of genetic testing. What possible effects would either result have on the individual and the family?
4. What can the nurse do to facilitate the client's acceptance of the prognosis?
5. What can the nurse do to provide psychosocial support to the family?
6. What additional interventions can be implemented by members of the interdisciplinary health care team?

REFERENCES

Folstein, S.E. 1989. *Huntington's Disease, A Disorder of Families*. Baltimore: The Johns Hopkins University Press.
Huntington's Disease Society of America. 1988. Integrated Genetics Announces Availability of Predictive Test. *The Marker* 2(3): 3.
McKay, C. 1988. Health Professionals Attend HDSA-NIH Testing Workshop. *The Marker* 2(1): 1, 3.

Quaid, K.M. 1991. What to Look for in a Presymptomatic Testing Program. *The Marker* 4(2): 4, 6–7.

Shapira, J., R. Schlesinger, and J.L. Cummings. 1986. Distinguishing Dementias. *American Journal of Nursing* 86(6): 699–702.

Shoulson, I. 1981. *Clinical Care of the Patient and Family with Huntington's Disease.* New York: Committee to Combat Huntington's Disease, Inc.

CHAPTER 17

A Restorative Approach to Caring for the Client with Multiple Neurological Deficits Related to Demyelinating Disease

OBJECTIVES

- List the possible courses of multiple sclerosis.
- Describe the diagnostic process.
- Identify the neurological deficits common in multiple sclerosis.
- Describe appropriate nursing interventions for these deficits.
- Describe the mobility problems associated with multiple sclerosis.
- Outline a program of physical activity for a client with multiple sclerosis.
- Recognize the implications for the family of the client with multiple sclerosis.
- Identify the role of the interdisciplinary team in the management of a client with multiple sclerosis.

DESCRIPTION OF THE DISEASE

Multiple sclerosis (MS) is a neurological disorder that attacks the myelin sheath, resulting in widely distributed neurological deficits. The myelin sheath is a white, fatty tissue that covers axons and assists in the conduction of nerve impulses. In multiple sclerosis, the ones affected are those that connect neurons in the brain and spinal cord.

The cause is unknown, but several theories are under investigation. One theory is that a slow, progressive viral infection is the causative factor. Other theories suggest that it is an autoimmune reaction or that there is a deficit in the person's immune system (Chipps, Clanin, and Campbell 1992).

The incidence of multiple sclerosis in the United States and Canada is forty to sixty cases per 10,000 people. Women are affected slightly more often than men. Symptoms usually first appear in young adulthood, between twenty and forty years of age, but MS has also been diagnosed in the fourth and fifth decades. The survival rate for individuals with multiple sclerosis is approximately 85 percent of that for the general population (Chipps, et al. 1992). For this reason, many individuals with a progressive form of the disease will eventually seek admission to long-term-care facilities. The disease is not fatal and death usually results from complications associated with an infectious process or other medical problems. While MS is generally considered a young person's disease, there are large numbers of elderly people dealing with the effects of the disease.

Medical Diagnosis

There are no specific tests for the diagnosis of multiple sclerosis. The diagnosis is based on the clinical history, neurological examination, and the ruling out of other central nervous system disorders. Magnetic resonance imaging (MRI) is the most important diagnostic advance in the last several years. It detects and measures the number, severity, and extent of lesions resulting from multiple sclerosis (McCann 1991). Approximately nine out of ten persons who have a definite diagnosis of MS based on clinical criteria also have multiple lesions visible on the MRI scan. The physician may perform a lumbar puncture for the withdrawal of cerebrospinal fluid. Electrophoresis is done on the fluid to detect a pattern called oligoclonal banding. Positive oligoclonal banding is found in more than 90 percent of persons diagnosed with MS. Positive findings may be an indication of a number of other neurological conditions. Evoked potentials (EP) is a test that records the brain's response to sensory stimuli. A slowing of nerve conduction is a sign of demyelination. Myelography may be used to differentiate multiple sclerosis from conditions such as nerve compression syndromes. This procedure is rarely used because of the availability of noninvasive tests (Calvano 1987).

Course of the Disease

Unpredictability is the key feature of MS. After diagnosis, the client learns the disease may improve, remain mild, or progressively worsen. There is little known about what the client might do to change the course of events. There are four possible courses the disease may follow. Twenty percent of cases are the benign form, characterized by mild attacks occurring intermittently with long symptom-free periods. This form has minimal or no disability. The person with the exacerbating-remitting type has periods of illness that occur with acute onset and may be severe. This is followed with partial or complete recovery and a plateau of stable disability. Residual weakness may continue through the remissions. The exacerbations can occur in rapid succession or there may be years in between. About 25 percent of persons with multiple sclerosis have the exacerbating-remitting type. Chronic-progressive multiple sclerosis affects 15 percent of cases. It has no clear cut exacerbations or remissions but follows a slow, steady course of deterioration with increasing levels of disability. Chronic-relapsing multiple sclerosis, affecting 40 percent of diagnosed individuals, is disabling and is characterized by a continual deterioration with fewer remissions over a period of months or years (Chipps et al. 1992).

There is a wide spectrum of presenting symptoms due to the variability of sclerotic patch formation in the central nervous system. Some symptoms may be transient and others permanent. Initially, the client may complain of visual disorders, muscle weakness and poor coordination, slurred speech, numbness, and tingling sensations. The client often does not seek diagnosis for a period of time due to the erratic, mild, subjective, and sometimes temporary nature of the symptoms. The client appears healthy and capable.

Optic neuritis is often a first symptom of multiple sclerosis. It begins with a loss of vision in one eye and can produce blind spots in the field of vision, blurriness, and color blindness. Total blindness occasionally results. Recovery may be accelerated with treatment of ACTH or oral steroids, but recurrence is common. Diplopia (double vision) occurs because of muscle imbalance between the two eyes. The eyes do not move together in a coordinated manner and do not see the same thing at the same time. This occurs because demyelination of the nerve fibers disrupts the mechanism that coordinates movement of both eyes. This usually improves after a few months. Nystagmus is another visual impairment characterized by jerky, involuntary eye movements. The eyeball may move in a horizontal, vertical, or rotational direction. The client experiences blurring of vision, dizziness, and sensation of movement. Nystagmus is usually temporary (Frames 1987). Lhermitte's sign is frequently noted in multiple sclerosis. This is described as a tingling, shocklike sensation that radiates down the trunk and limbs after neck flexion (Chipps et al. 1992). Fatigue is an outstanding and disabling feature of multiple sclerosis, affecting 80–90 percent of individuals with the disease. This is a physical phenomenon rather than an emotional or intellectual one. It is characterized by a generalized low-energy feeling and is not related to depression. It is worse on hot, humid days and tends to make other symptoms worse (Shaw 1989). It can be most distressing to the client and is poorly understood by family, friends, and sometimes even health care professionals. Tremor can be another disabling symptom of multiple sclerosis and seems to defy intervention. It is called "intention tremor" because it occurs when the individual intends or attempts to do a specific task, such as reaching for an object, writing, or eating. Anxiety and stress tend to increase the tremor (Frames 1987). As the disease progresses, muscle spasticity, pain, and paralysis, dysphagia, speech impairment, emotional lability, mild depression, irritability, and alterations in bowel and bladder functions eventually occur.

Clients with MS are seen in all health care settings. The nurse in long-term care, whether in a nursing home or the community, is generally involved with clients who were diagnosed several years earlier. Complications and varying levels of disability often present challenges to the nursing staff. Evaluating the client in terms of existing abilities rather than disabilities and emphasizing function rather than dysfunction are important. An interdisciplinary team approach provides comprehensive care with an holistic view of the client, enabling the client to function at an optimal level.

CASE STUDY

Mr. Nelson, sixty-five years old, was diagnosed with multiple sclerosis twenty-five years ago. He was a self-employed accountant and continued with his work for several years. Mrs. Nelson is a school teacher and plans to retire in two years. The Nelsons have three adult children and several grandchildren, all of whom live within fifty miles. After Mr. Nelson was diagnosed with MS, the couple sold their large, two-story home and moved to a smaller house with minimal upkeep.

Mr. Nelson has a chronic-progressive form of the disease, but has managed for several years to remain independent with minimal assistance from his family. Mrs. Nelson helps her husband with morning care and breakfast before she goes to work. Mr. Nelson has just returned home after a week in the hospital for treatment of a urinary tract infection. Reassessment by his case manager (a registered nurse) is indicated at this time so that an appropriate plan of care can be reestablished.

Strengths

□ Until the recent urinary tract infection, Mr. Nelson was in basically good health. With recuperation, he should return to his previous state of health.
□ Appetite is good.
□ Absence of cognitive impairments
□ Lives in safe neighborhood
□ Knowledgeable about his physical condition.
□ Strong family support system

Interdisciplinary Assessment

Nursing and Physical Therapy.

Persons with MS report a number of problems affecting gait. These include weakness, ataxia, and sensory problems such as numbness, tingling, and spasticity (Frames 1989). Because of the acute and debilitating results of the urinary tract infection, Mr. Nelson has residual weakness of both lower extremities, which may or may not be permanent. Sclerotic lesions in the central nervous system cause exaggerated responses to stimuli, resulting in spasticity. This increased muscle tone is experienced by Mr. Nelson as tight, stiff sensations and painful spasms in the calf and thigh muscles. This causes Mr. Nelson to walk stiffly. Foot drop and toe drag are noted during the swing phase of ambulation. Mr. Nelson appears to weave from side to side, which is characteristic of ataxia. He reports numbness and tingling in both legs. Regular exercise can improve Mr. Nelson's endurance, strength, flexibility, and general well-being. Mr. Nelson reports that he is occasionally experiencing tremors in his upper extremities. The tremors tend to interfere with his ability to complete his activities of daily living.

Nursing Diagnosis

Impaired physical mobility related to spasticity, weakness, and ataxia.

Nursing Interventions

□ Exercises
—If medication for spasticity is given, exercise should begin about one hour afterward. Do passive range-of-motion exercises slowly to allow joints and muscles to respond to the stretch by relaxing.
—If spasticity is present in the back muscles, help Mr. Nelson stretch by having him sit on the bed or floor with his legs straight out in front. Then gently push forward until his arms reach toward his feet. *Do not do this exercise unless there is tightness present* (Kimberg 1985). Remember that moving a spastic muscle passively or actively can increase the spasticity. Use gentle, slow movements.
—Teach Mr. Nelson to do active range-of-motion exercises on all extremities, his head, and his neck as he gets stronger. If Mr. Nelson experiences the sensation associated with Lhermitte's sign, he should discontinue the exercise until he checks with his physician (Kimberg 1985).

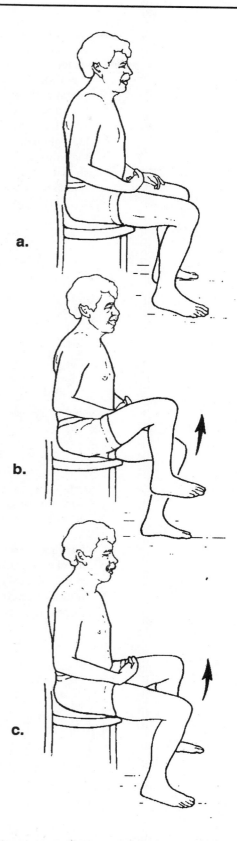

Figure 17–1 *(Reprinted from Iris Kimberg, MS, OTR, RPT, Moving with Multiple Sclerosis. © 1985 by National Multiple Sclerosis Society.)*

—Coordination and balance exercises are helpful for persons with ataxia. These involve repetitive movements of the extremities while lying, sitting, standing, or walking.

—Have Mr. Nelson sit unsupported. Have him try to maintain his balance keeping his arms in his lap, Figure 17–1a. If he is able to do it, have him lift up one leg, then the other, Figure 17–1b and Figure 17–1c.

—With his arms at his side and elbows bent to ninety degrees, have him turn his right hand so that his palm faces up. Have him turn his left hand so that the palm faces down, Figure 17–2a. Then tell him to simultaneously switch so that the right palm is down and left palm is up, Figure 17–2b. Repeat in rapid succession.

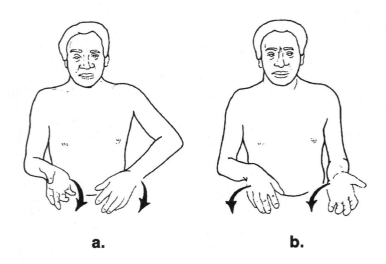

a.　　**b.**

Figure 17–2 *(Reprinted from Iris Kimberg,* MS, OTR, RPT, *Moving with Multiple Sclerosis. © 1985 by National Multiple Sclerosis Society.)*

—For this exercise, have Mr. Nelson start with both hands in the middle of his chest, Figure 17–3a. Then have him bring one arm up and forward while simultaneously stretching his other arm back, Figure 17–3b. Then have him return to original position and repeat in opposite direction, Figure 17–3c. Repeat this sequence five times.

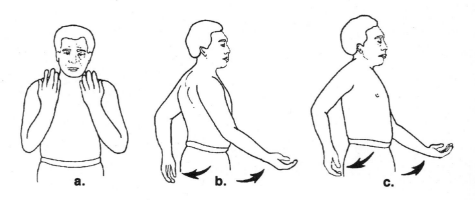

a.　　**b.**　　**c.**

Figure 17–3 *(Reprinted from Iris Kimberg,* MS, OTR, RPT, *Moving with Multiple Sclerosis. © 1985 by National Multiple Sclerosis Society.)*

—The next set of exercises is for ambulatory persons. Evaluate Mr. Nelson's ability to complete these. These are all done by assuming a hands-and-knees position to start, Figure 17–4a. First, tell him to reach forward with his right arm, shift his weight forward toward his right arm, hold for a count of five, and then return to original position, Figure 17–4b.

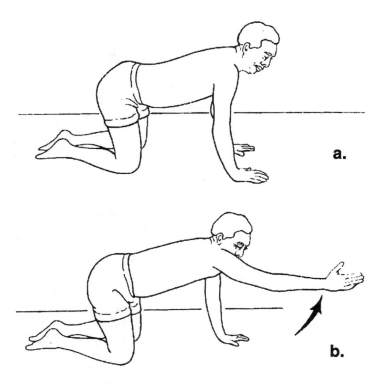

Figure 17–4 *(Reprinted from Iris Kimberg, MS, OTR, RPT, Moving with Multiple Sclerosis. © 1985 by National Multiple Sclerosis Society.)*

Now tell Mr. Nelson to reach forward with his left arm, shifting his weight toward his left arm, hold for a count of five, and return to original position.
—For the next exercise, still on hands and knees, tell him to point backward and straighten his right leg, shifting his weight back toward his leg, hold right leg extended for a count of five and then return to original position, Figure 17–5.

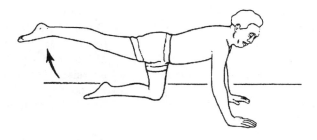

Figure 17–5 *(Reprinted from Iris Kimberg, MS, OTR, RPT, Moving with Multiple Sclerosis. © 1985 by National Multiple Sclerosis Society.)*

Now have him point backward and straighten his left leg, hold left leg extended for a count of five, then return to original position.

— If Mr. Nelson was able to do those without difficulty, have him try these. Tell him to simultaneously reach forward with his right arm and straighten his left leg in a backward direction, hold for a count of five, and return to original position, Figure 17–6.

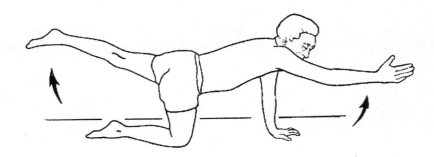

Figure 17–6 *(Reprinted from Iris Kimberg, MS, OTR, RPT, Moving with Multiple Sclerosis. © 1985 by National Multiple Sclerosis Society.)*

This is the last exercise on the hands and knees. Tell Mr. Nelson to simultaneously reach forward with his left arm while straightening out his right leg in a backward direction, hold for a count of five, then return to original position.

— For this exercise, Mr. Nelson will need to assume a kneeling position. With his arms at his side, have him rise to a half-kneeling position (right leg first), Figure 17–7, and then stand. Tell him to use his arms to balance himself, then try coming down to a kneeling position, leading with his right knee. Now have him try to repeat the sequence with his left leg.

— The next two exercises are done by standing and holding the back of a chair. Tell Mr. Nelson to lift his right foot and leg at least three inches from the floor and attempt to maintain balance on his left foot, Figure 17–8. Hold for a count of ten if possible, then return right foot to floor and try lifting up the left foot and maintaining balance.

Now have him alternate rising up on his toes and back on his heels ten times in succession, Figure 17–9.

— For this exercise (braid walking), tell Mr. Nelson to stand with his feet two feet apart. Have him sidestep, bringing his left foot behind his right foot, then have him move the right foot over two feet past his left foot, Figure 17–10. Tell him to repeat the sequence five times, then reverse direction.

— Have Mr. Nelson try walking forward and backward in a straight line, Figure 17–11.

❑ Positioning

— Teach Mr. Nelson how to position pillows when he is lying on his side (chapter 3). Persons with spasticity usually demonstrate synergy patterns of flexor or extensor spasticity. Instruct Mr. Nelson to avoid positions and exercises that increase these patterns (see chapter 21).

— Encourage Mr. Nelson to try the prone position several times when he is in bed. This position is especially effective for flexor spasticity of the lower extremities.

— The use of forearm crutches and a four-point gait or two canes effectively provide this support. (See chapter 3).

— Heat is poorly tolerated by many persons with MS and can accentuate the

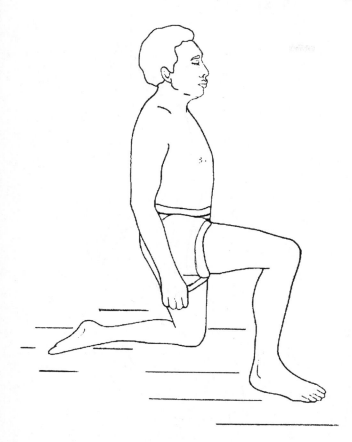

Figure 17-7 *(Reprinted from Iris Kimberg, MS, OTR, RPT, Moving with Multiple Sclerosis. © 1985 by National Multiple Sclerosis Society.)*

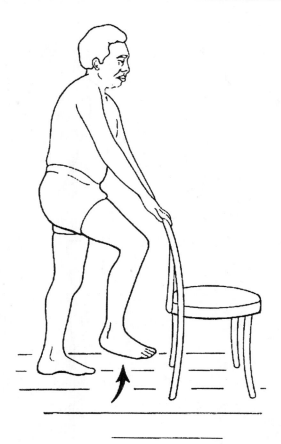

Figure 17-8 *(Reprinted from Iris Kimberg, MS, OTR, RPT, Moving with Multiple Sclerosis. © 1985 by National Multiple Sclerosis Society.)*

symptoms of the disease. Exercise, especially those with highly resistive techniques, may increase body temperature, so instruct Mr. Nelson to pace himself and avoid overexertion.

❑ Suggest that Mr. Nelson implement these interventions for tremor:
— Stabilize the arm and elbow against the table for such activities as eating.
— Stabilize the arm against his body.
— Try relaxation exercises.
— If one hand is not affected, use that hand for completing tasks.

Collaboration: Interdisciplinary Team

❑ Consult with a physical therapist if Mr. Nelson continues to have problems with spasticity. He may benefit by specific gait exercises and walking exercises in a therapeutic pool.

❑ The physician may order medication for the spasticity. Drugs commonly prescribed include baclofen (Lioresal®), diazepam (Valium®), and dantrolene sodium (Dantrium®). Some physicians feel that spasticity is not all bad and that it may be beneficial if the alternative is weak and rubbery legs. Spasticity can be an isometric exercise, maximizing the client's ability to walk and stand (Frames 1989). Cortisone therapy is used by some physicians to combat

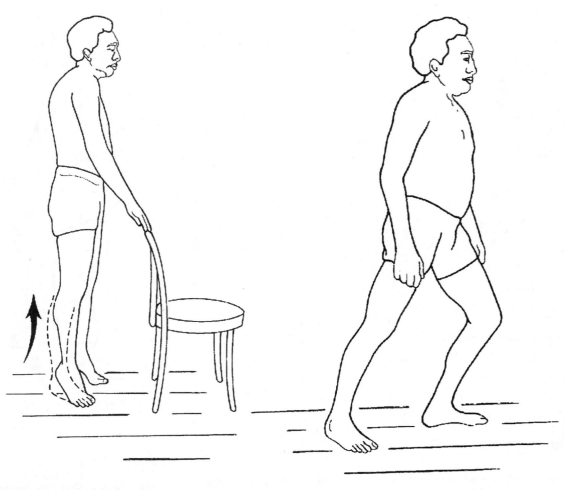

Figure 17–9 *(Reprinted from Iris Kimberg, MS, OTR, RPT, Moving with Multiple Sclerosis. © 1985 by National Multiple Sclerosis Society.)*

Figure 17–10 *(Reprinted from Iris Kimberg, MS, OTR, RPT, Moving with Multiple Sclerosis. © 1985 by National Multiple Sclerosis Society.)*

weakness. This reduces spinal cord inflammation, facilitating nerve conduction. Amantadine is prescribed by some physicians for fatigue.
□ An ankle-foot orthoses (AFO) may be prescribed by the physician and fitted by the orthotist to correct the foot drop and toe drag. A wider base of support compensates for disturbances in balance and coordination.

Outcome

Mr. Nelson will
□ Maintain current levels of range of motion
□ Increase his endurance
□ Experience less spasticity
□ Improve his balance and coordination
□ Experience a sense of well-being

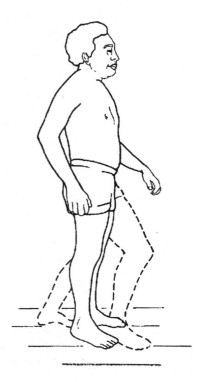

Figure 17–11 *(Reprinted from Iris Kimberg, MS, OTR, RPT, Moving with Multiple Sclerosis. © 1985 by National Multiple Sclerosis Society.)*

Interdisciplinary Assessment

Nursing and Occupational Therapist.

Mr. Nelson states that he frequently has no energy. He feels completely weak and drained at these times. He reports that the fatigue interferes with activities he has planned, even though he tries to force himself to complete the activities.

Nursing Diagnosis

Fatigue related to disease process.

Nursing Interventions

❑ Teach Mr. Nelson and his family that fatigue is due to the disease, not to him. The fatigue bears no relationship to depression, but fatigue can induce depression. If this occurs, the physician may order medication to relieve the depression. This will not relieve the fatigue.

❑ Advise Mr. Nelson to accept the fatigue and not try to fight or deny it. If a particular time of the day seems worse, he should schedule activities so he can rest during that time. For most people with multiple sclerosis, afternoon is worse.

❑ Encourage Mr. Nelson to set priorities to allow him to enjoy the activities that are important to him. For example, if he and his wife wish to go out in the evening, he should plan for a quiet day with rest periods.

❏ Encourage Mr. Nelson to parcel his energies. He should have a wheelchair or electric scooter available to use for those times when he needs his energy for activities other than walking.

❏ Suggest to Mr. Nelson that he remain indoors on hot, humid days and to avoid places that are not air-conditioned, since heat affects fatigue. Hot baths also increase fatigue.

❏ Stress is another factor that increases fatigue. If his usual coping mechanisms are ineffective in dealing with stressful events in his life, Mr. Nelson may need additional help.

Collaboration: Interdisciplinary Team

❏ An occupational therapist can devise energy-saving adaptations for Mr. Nelson that may alleviate some of the fatigue he is experiencing.

Outcome

Mr. Nelson will
❏ Effectively manage his fatigue, enabling him to have energy to participate in those activities that are most important and enjoyable to him.

Interdisciplinary Assessment

Nursing.

Spasticity and reduced activity increase the risk of pressure-ulcer development. Mr. Nelson spends a large part of his day sitting in a chair. The coccyx and sacral areas are especially at risk for skin breakdown. Mr. Nelson lacks sensation due to the central nervous system involvement.

Nursing Diagnosis

High risk for impaired skin integrity related to spasticity and reduced activity.

Nursing Interventions

❏ In addition to the exercise regime described above, suggest to Mr. Nelson that he shift his position frequently to alleviate the pressure on his buttocks. Teach him to do chair push-ups ten to thirty times at frequent intervals.

❏ Teach Mr. Nelson to do a skin inspection at least once every day, using a mirror so he is able to see any signs of redness or breaks in the skin. Tell him to report these signs immediately. Ask his wife to give him a lotion massage every evening.

❏ Suggest placing a foam overlay on his mattress. Instruct him to change his position at least every one to two hours when he is in bed.

Outcome

Mr. Nelson will
❏ Remain free of skin irritations and breakdown

Interdisciplinary Assessment

Nursing.

Alterations in bladder elimination are a frequent occurrence in MS. Problems are related to storage dysfunction, emptying dysfunction, or a combination of both (Holland and Francabandera 1987). Mr. Nelson's problem is one of emptying dysfunction or failure to empty. This is due to weakness of the detrusor. The detrusor is the external layer of the muscular coat of the bladder. It is innervated by fibers from the 3rd and 4th sacral nerves. The sphincter is spastic and tightens instead of relaxing when the bladder muscle provides an expulsive force to evacuate urine (Holland and Francabandera 1987).

In the hospital, postvoid residuals (PVR) were 100–150 ml. PVR greater than 100 ml or 20 percent of the voided volume are considered significant. Bacteria multiply rapidly in the residual urine, causing urinary tract infection. Over time, the retained urine may stretch the bladder muscle beyond recovery, resulting in reflux of urine to the kidneys. Substantial kidney damage may occur before this is detected. In addition to the PVR, Mr. Nelson has symptoms of urinary hesitancy and a sensation of incomplete bladder emptying after voiding. Overflow incontinence may occur if the emptying dysfunction is neglected. A major goal of bladder management is to resolve the problem of PVR in order to prevent the recurrence of urinary tract infection.

Nursing Diagnosis

Alterations in bladder elimination related to failure to empty.

Nursing Interventions

❑ Instruct Mr. Nelson to establish a regular voiding schedule. Teach him to trigger detrusor contractions to ensure bladder emptying. To do this, tell him to tap the suprapubic area, to stroke the glans penis, rub his thighs, or gently pull the pubic hair. Gently touching the urinary meatus with toilet tissue may also help in releasing more urine.

❑ Encourage Mr. Nelson to drink three or four glasses of cranberry juice a day to decrease the urinary pH. Citrus juices tend to increase urinary pH. Tell Mr. Nelson to maintain a minimum daily fluid intake of 2500 ml. The physician has ordered Vitamin C, 1 gm four times a day to acidify the urine, reducing the risk of another urinary tract infection.

❑ The physician has ordered regular postvoid catheterization to evaluate the effectiveness of this regime. As you do these, observe the urine for symptoms of infection.

❑ If the PVR remain consistently high, the physician may order intermittent catheterization. The goals of intermittent catheterization are to eliminate residual urine, prevent bladder distention, and prevent kidney damage caused by reflux (Holland and Francabandera 1987). You will then need to teach Mr. Nelson this procedure (see chapter 7). He can plan to fit this into his daily routine. Explain that he may meet resistance when he tries to insert the catheter. This is from a spastic sphincter. Tell him to wait a few seconds, relax, and then try again. Spasms of the legs may occur as the catheter is passed. This too will pass if Mr. Nelson pauses until the spasms stop before continuing with the catheter insertion. Mr. Nelson has a mild intention tremor in his right (dominant) hand. By bracing his arm against his body he should be able to use his hand to insert the catheter. If this does not work, he may learn to use his left hand. A plastic catheter is more rigid than rubber and therefore easier to insert (Holland and Francabandera 1987). Should Mr. Nelson lose the ability to do this procedure, his wife may be taught to perform the procedure for him. Remember that for some individuals, it is difficult to be responsible for such procedures and to continue to view the spouse as a sexual person. If it becomes necessary, speak with Mrs. Nelson about her feelings regarding this procedure. Depending on her feelings, it may be preferable to have a home health nurse perform this function. An indwelling catheter is a last resort but may be necessary at some point in time.

Outcome

Mr. Nelson will
❑ Have reduced postvoid residuals and remain free of urinary tract infections.

Interdisciplinary Assessment

Nursing and Social Services.

When Mr. Nelson was diagnosed with MS twenty-five years ago, he and his family were given little information on the physical aspects of the disease. They knew nothing about the possible course of the illness or actions that could be implemented to assist Mr. Nelson optimize his potential. His physician's recommendation at that time was "go home and live with it."

Had they been given more information, they may have experienced shock, anger, and resentment. However, they would have had the opportunity to work through these feelings and get on with the business of living. Because of a lack of understanding of the disease and how to deal with it, the family's expectations of Mr. Nelson were incorrectly perceived and he was placed in a dependent role prematurely. Although Mr. Nelson worked for ten years after the diagnosis was established, he accepted the dependent role in all other aspects of his life. He gave up most leisure time activities and household responsibilities. Since retiring, he spends most of the day watching television or reading. Although he feels guilty because his wife has to work, he is frequently critical of her efforts to maintain the yard and do household repairs.

After Mr. Nelson was diagnosed with MS, his wife took over all the household responsibilities that her husband had previously assumed. She frequently feels tired and edgy and has become increasingly resentful of the burden she has carried for so many years. As a school teacher, Mrs. Nelson spent her summers golfing and doing volunteer work. For the last several years, she has had to work as a tutor to earn extra money for household expenses.

Mr. and Mrs. Nelson love and respect one another. They have shared many enjoyable and satisfying moments during their years of marriage. They are proud of their children and grandchildren and look forward to their visits. On the whole, they are grateful for the many blessings that they have. However, the lack of communication and the escalation of negative emotions are eroding their marriage. The unspoken feelings of both partners have diminished their affection and demonstrativeness, causing frustration with their sexual relationship. At times, they are both overwhelmed by feelings of isolation and loneliness. Sexuality plays a major role in determining how individuals feel about themselves. Individuals coping with multiple sclerosis frequently experience changes in their feelings about themselves and their bodies. These changes may affect one's sex life. Difficulties in sexual function of persons with MS may be influenced by the physical and emotional effects of the disease (Kalb, LaRocca, and Kaplan 1987).

Nursing Diagnosis

Altered family processes related to the long-term illness of Mr. Nelson and the role changes experienced by both Mr. and Mrs. Nelson.

Nursing Interventions

- ❑ None of the problems faced by the Nelsons will be resolved until the channels of communication are open. They need to acknowledge and face their feelings before they can effectively solve the other problems.
- ❑ Provide Mr. and Mrs. Nelson with educational materials from the National Multiple Sclerosis Society and suggest they attend the meetings of the local chapter. This group can help them learn more about the disease and how to cope with the associated problems.
- ❑ Encourage Mr. Nelson to carry out the exercise regime described earlier so he will feel better physically and mentally. In addition to this, he needs activity commensurate with his abilities that will give him a feeling of accomplishment and contribution. In the early years of their marriage, Mr. Nelson enjoyed cooking. Suggest that he take over preparation of the evening meal. Advise him to do this early in the day when his energy is higher. It can be warmed in the microwave later. This will give his wife a welcome respite and allow her time to relax after arriving home. If he is able to complete this activity on a consistent basis, he may undertake other household tasks within his capabilities.
- ❑ Encourage the Nelsons to reestablish a social life that can add zest and stimulation to their routine. Spending time with old friends or going out to dinner or to a movie are pleasant ways to spend an evening.

TABLE 17–1	Sexual Considerations of Multiple Sclerosis
Sexuality	is a part of lifelong being. For each person it defines maleness or femaleness, identity as a sexual being, and interactions with other people. Regardless of age or disability, sexuality is a part of one's total self.
Sexual function	or sexual physical activity may or may not be a component of sexuality. Sexual satisfaction through sexual response may be alone or with a partner. The physical and emotional aspects of sexual functioning are interwoven.
Sexual dysfunction	is an alteration in sexual patterns that is viewed as inadequate, unsatisfying, or unrewarding to the person(s) involved.
Sexual response	involves functioning of the somatic and autonomic nervous system. Demyelination can interfere with different aspects of sexual response.
Problems/Interventions	❑ Fatigue can be helped with medication. Morning may be a better time for sexual activity when energy is greater. ❑ Diminished genital sensation may be aided by use of a vibrator or oral stimulation. Painful sensations can be controlled with medication. ❑ Inadequate vaginal lubrication can be corrected with water-soluble lubricants.

Continues

❑ Alterations in bladder function may be remedied by reducing fluid intake and emptying the bladder before sexual activity. Males with indwelling catheters can apply a condom over the penis and catheter, folding the catheter up along the penis. Females with catheters can remove them during sexual activity or bring it over to the side and tape it to the lower abdomen.

❑ Spasms can sometimes be controlled with medication.

❑ Impotence should be evaluated by a physician to determine proper therapy.

Collaboration: Interdisciplinary Team

❑ Referral to a mental health clinic is appropriate at this time. The counselor can assist them to regain a sense of control over their lives and provide them with direction in planning their future. Mrs. Nelson hopes to retire in two years and this will require additional adjustment from both of them.

❑ Because Mr. Nelson has never been thoroughly evaluated, he may benefit from undergoing an evaluation at a multiple sclerosis clinic associated with a medical center or rehabilitation hospital. Multiple sclerosis involves many emotional and mental health issues, as well as having physiological implications. An interdisciplinary assessment team may provide many helpful suggestions to improve Mr. Nelson's quality of life.

Outcome

Mr. and Mrs. Nelson will
❑ Express their feelings openly and constructively
❑ Establish a household routine that is agreeable to them both
❑ Utilize effective problem-solving skills
❑ Express understanding of MS and its effects
❑ Enjoy a relationship that is satisfying to them both

COMMENTS

Mr. Nelson has many strengths upon which to draw. Utilization of his abilities and adaptation to his disabilities will optimize his potential and increase the quality of his life. Multiple sclerosis requires continual adjustment and adaptation, not only for the client, but for everyone connected with the client. The Nelsons would be wise to return for counseling during periods of crisis in their lives. The Nelson children have a stable relationship with their parents. The lack of communication between the Nelsons concerning Mr. Nelson's illness also extended to the children. It will be beneficial to everyone if they understand the ramifications of the disease and the impact it has on families.

If Mr. Nelson's condition deteriorates, he will need more comprehensive health care. Dysphagia and speech impairments are common in advanced cases of MS. If Mr. Nelson experiences these situations, the speech pathologist can complete an assessment and directions for working with these problems. The disease has progressed slowly to this point, so it is possible that Mr. Nelson may never experience the extreme disability associated with some cases of multiple sclerosis. If Mr. and Mrs. Nelson are willing to put forth time and effort to repair and revitalize their marriage, they can enjoy many years together as friends, as lovers, as sources of strength and support for each other — the best possible combination.

QUESTIONS AND DISCUSSION

1. Visit a multiple sclerosis support group in your community to learn more about this disease.
2. What benefits do you think this group can provide for the Nelsons?
3. Can you instruct a client in the use of forearm crutches and a four-point gait?
4. What adaptations can you suggest to Mr. Nelson for preparing meals? How can he avoid unnecessary efforts?
5. Can you provide Mr. and Mrs. Nelson with information to assist them in enhancing their relationship?
6. Many long-term-care facilities admit younger individuals with multiple sclerosis. What suggestions do you have for facilitating psychosocial adjustment for these young people?
7. Discuss additional interventions from the interdisciplinary team for management of the client with multiple sclerosis.

REFERENCES

Calvano, M. 1987. The ABCs of Diagnosing MS. *MS Facts and Issues* II(2): 2.

Chipps, E., N. Clanin, and V. Campbell. 1992. *Neurologic Disorders*. St. Louis: Mosby-Year Book, Inc.

Frames, R. 1987. Insight into Eyesight. *MS Facts and Issues* II(3): 1, 2.

Frames, R. 1987. Tremor, Can We Manage It? *Inside MS* 5(1): 27–29.

Frames, R. 1989. Getting a Grip on Gait. *Inside MS* 7(1): 27–29.

Frames, R. 1989. Sexual Dysfunction, Dare We Discuss It? *Inside MS* 7(4): 24–27, 29, 31.

Holland, N.J. and F. Francabandera. 1987. In L. Scheinberg and N.J. Holland, eds. *Multiple Sclerosis: A Guide for Patients and Their Families*. New York: Raven Press.

Kalb, R.C., N.G. LaRocca, and S.R. Kaplan. 1987. In L. Scheinberg and N.J. Holland, eds. *Multiple Sclerosis: A Guide for Patients and Their Families*. New York: Raven Press.

Kimberg, I. 1985. *Moving with Multiple Sclerosis*. New York: National Multiple Sclerosis Society.

McCann, J.A.S. 1991. *Diagnostic Test Implications*. Springhouse, PA: Springhouse Corporation.

Shaw, P. 1989. Digging for Clues to Fatigue. *Inside MS* 7(4): 16–17.

SUGGESTED READINGS

Davis, F.A., M.M. Pavlous, and M.F. Hartings. 1986. *Emotional Aspects of Multiple Sclerosis*. New York: National Multiple Sclerosis Society.

Francabandera, F.L., J. Holland, P. Wiesel-Levison, and L.S. Scheinberg. 1988. Multiple Sclerosis Rehabilitation: Inpatient vs. Outpatient. *Rehabilitation Nursing* 13(5): 251–53.

Halper, J. 1990. The Functional Model in MS. *Rehabilitation Nursing* 15(2): 77–79.

Kelley, B. and S.M. Mahon. 1988. Nursing Care of the Patient with Multiple Sclerosis. *Rehabilitation Nursing* 13(5): 238–43.

LaRocca, N.G. 1990. The Mind and MS. *Inside MS* 8(1): 16–19.

Larsen, P.D. 1990. Psychosocial Adjustment in Multiple Sclerosis. *Rehabilitation Nursing* 15(5): 242–47.

Marks, S.F. and R.W. Millard. 1990. Nursing Assessment of Positive Adjustment for Individuals with Multiple Sclerosis. *Rehabilitation Nursing* 15(3): 147–51.

McBride, E.V. and K. Distefano. 1988. Explaining Diagnostic Tests for Multiple Sclerosis. *Nursing 88* 18(2): 68–71, 72.

Scheinberg, L. and C.R. Smith. 1989. *Rehabilitation of Patients with Multiple Sclerosis*. New York: National Multiple Sclerosis Society.

CHAPTER 18

A Restorative Approach to Caring for the Client with Progressive Disorder of the Extrapyramidal System

---

CONTENT OUTLINE

I. Description of the disease
II. Case study
   A. Strengths
   B. Interdisciplinary assessment
   C. Nursing diagnoses
      1. Impaired physical mobility
      2. Self-care deficit (dressing)
      3. Altered nutrition, less than body requirements
      4. Impaired verbal communication
      5. High risk for respiratory tract infection
      6. Body image disturbance
      7. Altered patterns of sexuality
III. Comments

OBJECTIVES

❑ Describe the pathophysiology related to the symptoms of extrapyramidal damage.
❑ Distinguish between parkinsonism and Parkinson's disease.
❑ Identify the expected functional deficits related to extrapyramidal damage.
❑ Plan effective nursing interventions for the functional deficits.
❑ Develop an exercise program to prevent or delay the progression of the disease.
❑ Identify the drugs used for Parkinson's disease and recognize the side effects specific to each drug.
❑ Identify the role of the interdisciplinary health care team in the management of the client with Parkinson's disease.

DESCRIPTION OF THE DISEASE

Parkinson's disease is a chronic, progressive disorder of the brain, resulting from damage to the extrapyramidal system. The substantia nigra in the cerebrum consists of pigmented cells containing neuromelanin, which produces and stores the neurotransmitter dopamine, which has an inhibitory effect on movement. These cells synapse with the cells in the striatum that control movement, balance, and walking. Messages pass between cells in the substantia nigra and the striatum through dopamine. In Parkinson's disease, the cells in these two areas are damaged, causing a deficiency in dopamine production. Acetyl choline, which has an excitatory effect on movement, is produced in the striatum and is normal in Parkinson's disease. But for the striatum to function, a balance between dopamine and acetyl choline is necessary. The dopamine deficiency disturbs this balance (Chipps, Clanin, and Campbell 1992). Parkinsonism describes syndromes that mimic the characteristics of Parkinson's disease but do not have the identifying neurological features. Psychotropic drugs and medications containing reserpine may have side effects that involve extrapyramidal symptoms.

The outstanding symptoms of Parkinson's disease are resting tremor, rigidity (cogwheeling), and bradykinesia. This disorder usually begins in one side of the body, gradually involving both sides. Tremor is the most obvious symptom, but is not as disabling as the bradykinesia. Tremor (often a thumb-to-finger movement called pill-rolling) worsens when the client is anxious, angry, or frightened. The tremor is noted at rest, diminishes with action, and disappears during sleep. The tremor begins unilaterally, but soon spreads to the other upper extremity. Persons with advancing Parkinson's disease have problems with posture, all aspects of mobility, speech, chewing, swallowing, and respiration. As the disease progresses, symptoms of depression may be evident because of the increasing dependency. A few persons experience intellectual decline, exhibiting symptoms of dementia. Symptoms may appear at any age, but are uncommon before thirty and most prevalent after sixty years of age (DeLaney 1988). Some cases progress steadily while others remain mild. There is no cure for Parkinson's disease. However, judicious use of medications and restorative care can improve symptoms and delay progression of the disease and associated complications.

CASE STUDY

Mr. Jenkins, seventy-eight years old, was admitted to Park Manor Nursing Home from the local hospital where he was treated for viral pneumonia. He was diagnosed with Parkinson's disease three years ago and is experiencing slow progression of symptoms. Upon questioning, it became evident that neither Mr. nor Mrs. Jenkins had much information about the disease. Before the onset of acute illness, he was able to manage at home with the assistance of his wife. Increased functional deficits were noted during the hospitalization. This is a result of the enforced inactivity and fatigue related to the acute illness, rather than to the disease process. Convalescence will continue at the nursing home with emphasis on increasing Mr. Jenkins's strength and endurance. Discharge planning will begin immediately so Mr. Jenkins can return home as soon as his condition permits. Both Mr. and Mrs. Jenkins will participate in the client teaching process so that after returning home, complications will be prevented and further deterioration may possibly be avoided. Community resources will be investigated in an attempt to ease the responsibilities of Mrs. Jenkins in an effort to maintain her strength and health status.

Strengths

- ❏ Supportive, capable wife and two adult children who are willing to provide assistance
- ❏ Comfortable home and sufficient financial resources to cover nursing home charges for several weeks
- ❏ Community resources are available.
- ❏ Ties with community and church
- ❏ Positive health history and life-style habits
- ❏ Readiness for learning about Parkinson's disease

Interdisciplinary Assessment

Nursing and Physical Therapy.

Mr. Jenkins walks on the balls of his feet with his heels raised and uses a shuffling, accelerating gait, with a tendency to stoop forward. A lack of arm swing during ambulation tends to affect his balance. During the assessment, Mr. Jenkins had several freezing episodes, unable to raise either foot from the floor. He stated that this happens frequently, causing him to avoid walking in public. In addition, Mr. Jenkins has difficulty getting out of bed, sitting down, and arising from chairs. His strength and endurance are limited since his recovery from pneumonia.

Nursing Diagnosis

Impaired physical mobility related to bradykinesia, stooped posture, and incoordination.

Nursing Interventions

- ❑ Teach Mr. Jenkins to wear shoes with a nonstick sole to facilitate walking.
- ❑ Teach him to use a wide-based gait, keeping his feet about eight inches apart, and to think about moving his arms in a normal swing. He needs to concentrate on what he is doing. Suggest that he avoid talking or other activities while walking.
- ❑ When turning corners, teach him to keep his feet apart, head up, and to walk into the turn by making a semicircle.
- ❑ When freezing occurs, have Mr. Jenkins raise his head and relax back on his heels without trying to take any more steps. Then tell him to straighten his knees, hips, and trunk. The next step is to rock from side to side and then take some marching steps in place. Begin walking by placing heels down first. Keep obstacles out of the way and advise Mr. Jenkins to avoid crowded places, and narrow doors and hallways if possible (Talotta and Lisanti 1989). He does not need any assistive devices at this time but may require a walking aid in the future. A cane may be difficult to use for someone with Parkinson's disease because of the lack of normal arm swing. A walker with wheels on the front legs eases movement and provides maximum security because the wheels lock when weight is applied.
- ❑ To get out of bed, teach Mr. Jenkins to clasp his hands either behind his head or in front, rolling his body back and forth to gain momentum. Have him roll onto his side and slide his feet to the edge of the bed. Instruct him to use his hands to push to a sitting position and his feet will swing to the floor (Lieberman, Gopinathan, Neophytides, and Goldstein).
- ❑ Sitting down and getting up from a chair is easier if a straight chair with armrests is used. Movement in and out of the chair is facilitated by placing 2" x 4" blocks under the back legs (Schwab and Doshay 1986). Teach Mr. Jenkins to get out of the chair by sliding to the edge, with his feet about eight inches apart, placing one foot further forward. Have him put his weight on the ball of the foot in back and then teach him to rock forward and back to gain momentum. On the count of three, tell him to push down with his hands on the armrests and stand up. To sit down, teach Mr. Jenkins to back up so the chair touches the back of his legs. Then have him bend his knees, lean slightly forward, grasp the armrests, and slowly lower himself into the chair (Côté and Riedel).

❑ Place Mr. Jenkins in an exercise program and ask his wife to accompany him so she can help him continue with the exercises after he returns home.
— Place a number of strips of tape twelve inches apart on the floor and have Mr. Jenkins practice stepping over the tape.
— In an area with sufficient space, practice marching and walking sideways, backward, and in circles.
— Do range-of-motion exercises twice a day. Teach Mr. Jenkins to do active range of motion with his head and neck and active assistive range of motion with his other joints. Stretching exercises can be carried out with these. (See chapter 3, "Exercise and Activity.")
— Pulley exercises for the shoulders can be carried out at home by installing a rope and pulley in a doorway. Instruct Mr. Jenkins to sit in a chair underneath and hold one end of the rope in each hand, pulling first with one hand and then with the other, fully elevating each hand. By moving the chair, a full range of exercises for the shoulder can be carried out (Côté and Riedel).

Collaboration: Interdisciplinary Team

❑ Ask the physical therapist to suggest additional exercises to increase or maintain strength, endurance, and range of motion.

Outcome

Mr. Jenkins will
❑ Maintain current range of motion in all extremities
❑ Walk to and from the bathroom independently
❑ Gradually increase his ambulation by walking to and from the dining room for each meal as his strength and endurance increase
❑ Experience fewer freezing episodes and will know what to do when one occurs
❑ Get out of bed independently
❑ Sit down and arise from the chair independently

Interdisciplinary Assessment

Nursing and Occupational Therapy.
Mr. Jenkins has difficulty manipulating buttons, putting on a necktie, and tying his shoes. He can eventually manage these tasks but becomes very fatigued and frustrated because of the length of time it takes to complete getting dressed. As a result, he has less energy available for eating, exercises, and other activities of his choice. Mr. Jenkins resists offers of assistance.

Nursing Diagnosis

Self-care deficit (dressing) related to rigidity of hand and tendency to fatigue.

Nursing Interventions

❑ Ask Mrs. Jenkins to bring in polo shirts that are loose fitting and stretchy. Buttons on cardigan style clothing can be resewn with elastic thread, allowing the garment to remain buttoned during dressing. It is often easier to slip the garment over the head than to manipulate buttons. Teach Mr. Jenkins to put the shirt in front of him, put his hands into the sleeves, raise his arms over his head, and duck his head under the tail of the shirt (Côté and Riedel). Replace neckties with clip-on ties. Shoes with elastic shoelaces or velcro closures or well-fitting slip-ons are easier to get into.

□ Teach Mr. Jenkins to dress while sitting in the chair, putting on upper body clothing first, then socks to prevent his toes from catching in the clothes. Then have him put his pants on, pulling them up as far as he can while seated, then his shoes. A long-handled shoehorn prevents the need to lean forward, which might cause him to loose his balance. After he stands, he can pull his pants up over his hips, buckling the belt first and then closing the zipper. It is easier to wear beltless pants, or to put the belt in the pants before putting them on.

□ Talk with Mr. Jenkins, assuring him that accepting help when he needs it will allow him to have more energy for the activities of his choice later in the day.

□ Instruct the staff to monitor his dressing, providing him privacy and offering assistance when he appears to be getting tired or frustrated.

Collaboration: Interdisciplinary Team

□ The occupational therapist has suggested the following exercises to help Mr. Jenkins maintain dexterity and strength in his hands and fingers. He can continue to do these at home. The exercises will help him maintain his functional skills.

— Physical therapy putty is available in different consistencies. Have him squeeze and mold it with each hand and use his thumbs and index fingers to pinch off small bits.

— Instruct Mr. Jenkins to use a hand gripper several times with each hand.

— Place various-sized coins over a table top and have Mr. Jenkins use his thumb and index finger to pick them up.

— Activities such as marbles, checkers, and puzzles provide exercise as well as socialization.

Outcome

Mr. Jenkins will

□ Maintain current levels of hand and finger dexterity by carrying out exercises as instructed

□ Dress and undress himself independently, allowing staff/wife to help him if necessary, preventing fatigue and frustration

Interdisciplinary Assessment

Nursing and Dietary.

Mr. Jenkins lost four pounds over a two-month period prior to being ill with pneumonia. During hospitalization, his weight dropped by two more pounds. His wife indicates that he often becomes too tired to complete a full meal. Mr. Jenkins frequently complains of food getting stuck in his throat.

Nursing Diagnosis

Altered nutrition, less than body requirements, related to difficulty chewing and swallowing and fatigue due to the length of time required for eating.

Nursing Interventions

- Use a thermal plate to keep foods hot, making them more appetizing. Place a nonslip mat under the plate and use a plate guard and a stationary flexible straw to facilitate self-feeding. Utensils with built-up handles may be easier to grasp.
- Teach Mr. Jenkins to sit upright while eating and to remain upright for thirty minutes after finishing. Tell him to take small bites and after chewing, move the food to the back of his mouth. Then instruct him to tilt his head slightly forward before swallowing.
- Weigh Mr. Jenkins weekly.
- Before his discharge from the nursing home, teach Mrs. Jenkins how to do the Heimlich maneuver, to prepare her if her husband experiences choking.

Collaboration: Interdisciplinary Team

- Mr. Jenkins needs foods that are easy to chew and swallow but attractive and appetizing. Rather than serving pureed foods, the dietician will offer a choice of regular foods that are manageable for Mr. Jenkins and high in fiber.
- The dietician has suggested the use of commercial thickeners to make liquids more manageable. These do not affect the taste and foods can be prepared to the desired consistency.
- Protein affects the action of levodopa, so persons taking this medication are advised to maintain an adequate level of protein intake without increasing it.
- Dietary will serve Mr. Jenkins six small meals per day instead of three larger ones. This will conserve his energy.
- Consult with the speech pathologist for a swallowing evaluation.

Outcome

Mr. Jenkins will
- Consume 80–90 percent of his meals without becoming fatigued
- Have fewer complaints of food getting stuck in his throat
- Gain one-half pound per week until his usual body weight is attained

Interdisciplinary Assessment

Nursing and Speech Pathologist.

Mr. Jenkins's speech is indistinct and accelerates at the end of sentences. His voice is breathy and tremulous with decreased volume. It is becoming more difficult for others to understand him.

Nursing Diagnosis

Impaired verbal communication (dysarthria) related to rigid vocal muscles and stiff mouth and facial muscles.

Nursing Interventions

- Limit distractions when Mr. Jenkins wishes to converse. Turn off the television or radio and provide a quiet, private environment without interruptions. Have him face the person with whom he is speaking.

❑ Monitor his fatigue level and avoid conversation when he is tired, asking only yes and no questions, if necessary.

❑ Instruct him to take in air before speaking, and then to speak as he exhales. Teach Mr. Jenkins to think of his lips, tongue, and jaws as he concentrates on forming one word at a time.

❑ Reading aloud and singing will further facilitate verbal communication skills.

Collaboration: Interdisciplinary Team

❑ The speech pathologist has suggested the following exercises.

TABLE 18–1	Oral Exercises for Clients with Parkinson's Disease
	Use a mirror to help you do these exercises. Practice two to three times a day for five to ten minutes. Try them all.

❑ Open and close your mouth slowly several times. Be sure lips are all the way closed. Pucker your lips as for a kiss, hold, then relax. Repeat several times.

❑ Spread lips into a big smile, hold, then relax. Repeat several times.

❑ Pucker, hold, smile, hold. Repeat this alternative movement several times. Open your mouth, then try to pucker with your mouth wide open.

❑ Close your lips tightly and press together. Relax and repeat.

❑ Close your lips firmly. Slurp all the saliva onto the top of your tongue.

❑ Open your mouth and stick out your tongue. Be sure your tongue comes straight out of your mouth and doesn't go off to the side. Hold tongue out and then relax and repeat several times. Work toward sticking your tongue out farther each day.

❑ Stick your tongue out and move it slowly from corner to corner of your lips. Hold in each corner. Relax and repeat several times. Be sure your tongue actually touches the corner each time.

❑ Stick out your tongue and try to reach your chin with the tongue tip. Hold it out at the farthest point. Relax, repeat.

❑ Stick out your tongue and try to reach your nose with tongue tip. Pretend you are licking a popsicle from your top lip. Hold tongue up as far as possible. Relax, repeat.

❑ Stick out your tongue. Hold spoon against tip of your tongue and try to push the spoon even farther away with your tongue while your hand is holding the spoon readily in place. Hold spoon upright. Repeat.

(Coddington)

Outcome

Mr. Jenkins will

❑ Attempt to prevent further deterioration of verbal communication by carrying out oral exercises regularly

❑ Communicate verbally so that he is understood by others

❏ Indicate to staff and visitors when he is too tired to converse

Interdisciplinary Assessment _____

Nursing.

Mr. Jenkins's recent bout of pneumonia and his problems with speech indicate a predisposition for respiratory infections.

Nursing Diagnosis _____

High risk for respiratory tract infection related to impaired throat and chest movements and recent pneumonia.

Nursing Interventions _____

❏ Teach Mr. Jenkins breathing exercises to increase his chest expansion and lung ventilation. (See chapter 19.)
❏ Advise him to get an influenza immunization each fall and to get pneumococcal vaccine if he has not previously been vaccinated.
❏ Suggest he prevent exposure to respiratory infection by avoiding crowds during peak infection times.

Outcome _____

Mr. Jenkins will
❏ Reduce his risk for respiratory tract infections

Interdisciplinary Assessment _____

Nursing and Social Services.

An individual's body image is related not only to physical appearance, but also to how one views oneself in terms of abilities. Mrs. Jenkins states her husband has always been a very independent person who took pride in maintaining their yard and garden. He retired five years ago but continued an active schedule by increasing his community and family involvement until his diminishing abilities forced him to relinquish many responsibilities. Being well groomed and dressed is important to him. Mr. Jenkins states he is ashamed of his inability to carry out his chores as the "man of the house." He is fearful that his decreased facial expressions cause him to appear disinterested. Because of this, Mr. Jenkins is reluctant to socialize with friends. He is hesitant about going out in public, due to his fear of falling.

Nursing Diagnosis _____

Body image disturbance related to the visible evidence of his disease process and the inability to carry out household and community activities.

Nursing Interventions _____

❏ Encourage Mr. Jenkins to direct his care by giving choices in clothing selection, activities, and scheduling his day. Instruct staff to give him the opportunity to do as much as possible for himself and to intervene with help only when necessary.

□ Advise the family to avoid treating him as an invalid by including him in all activities and all decisions. After he regains some strength and endurance, encourage his family to take him out to church or for lunch to assist him in regaining his self-confidence. Plan outings for early arrival or less-busy times to avoid crowds, thus alleviating the stress associated with being in public.

Collaboration: Interdisciplinary Team

□ Ask the social worker to consider counseling Mr. and Mrs. Jenkins. This will provide Mr. Jenkins opportunity to ventilate his fears without feelings of shame. Discuss his remaining strengths and abilities. With Mrs. Jenkins, he can find ways in which he can use these to maintain activities that are most important to him.

□ Arrange with a community services agency to schedule a homemaker for weekly visits to assist Mrs. Jenkins with household chores.

□ Suggest to Mr. Jenkins that he use his leadership abilities by participating in the residents' council of the nursing home. Have Activities staff review his admission assessment and invite him to activities of his choice.

□ Drugs play a major role in the treatment of Parkinson's disease by improving the symptoms that are related to disturbances in body image. Consult with the pharmacist for additional information on these drugs, their actions, and side effects.

Outcome

Mr. Jenkins will
□ Verbalize positive statements about himself and his abilities
□ Make decisions regarding his personal care and activities
□ Maintain his role in the family by participating in discussions with wife and family
□ Participate in activities of his choice

Interdisciplinary Assessment

Nursing and Social Services.

Mr. and Mrs. Jenkins have enjoyed a close, intimate relationship throughout their forty-five years of marriage. Until his illness, they had regular sexual activity. Mrs. Jenkins revealed that with her husband's disability, she is fearful that continuing this activity is dangerous and inappropriate. Mr. Jenkins is hesitant to initiate sexual activity because of his fear of failure. He frequently has difficulty in getting and maintaining a firm erection for a long enough period of time to allow for penetration.

Nursing Diagnosis

Altered patterns of sexuality related to physical deficits and disturbance in body image.

Nursing Interventions

❑ Sexuality is a quality-of-life issue. Advise Mr. and Mrs. Jenkins to continue with expressions of sexuality that provide satisfaction and gratification to them both. Teach Mrs. Jenkins that continuing sexual activity is not dangerous or inappropriate. Suggest they plan sexual activity for times when they are rested. Encourage them to experiment using positions that are most comfortable. Remind them to enjoy these times for what is possible at the moment.

❑ Advise them that masturbation or oral sex can be a physically and psychologically appropriate alternative means of sexual expression, if this is acceptable to both of them.

❑ Whether or not Mr. and Mrs. Jenkins choose to continue with sexual intercourse, it can be therapeutic to them both to participate in other forms of intimacy, such as kissing, holding each other, and caressing. Because of their long-standing, loving relationship, they may discover aspects of sexuality that extend beyond physical expression.

Collaboration: Interdisciplinary Team

❑ Should problems related to sexual activity continue or increase, it may be necessary to undergo further investigation to uncover the precise cause. Numerous factors may have to be considered.
— Medications: antihypertensives, tranquilizers, antidepressants, and hypnotics can all influence sexual activity.
— Urologic problems
— Depression
— Symptoms related to the functioning of the autonomic nervous system: alterations in bowel or bladder function, heart and blood pressure, sweating, and body temperature

❑ Resolving these problems would require the intervention of several members of the interdisciplinary team.

Outcome

Mr. and Mrs. Jenkins will
❑ Continue with a relationship and expressions of sexuality that are gratifying to both of them

COMMENTS

The Jenkins family should all be prepared for Mr. Jenkins's eventual discharge. Invite the Jenkins children to the care plan conference after consulting with both Mr. and Mrs. Jenkins. Discuss plans for discharge at the care plan conference with both Mr. and Mrs. Jenkins present. Make a home visit before discharge to evaluate the environment for safety and advise changes that may be needed.

TABLE 18–2	Preparing for Discharge to Home
Preventing Falls	❑ Remove loose rugs and doorsills. ❑ Arrange space for ambulating around rooms and halls. ❑ Place lamps and other objects in areas where they are not accidentally toppled. ❑ If climbing stairs cannot be avoided, install secure rails on both sides. If disease progresses, an electric chair lift will increase safety and reduce fatigue. ❑ Install metal or wooden handles on walls adjacent to doorknobs so client can hold handle on wall with one hand while pulling doorknob with the other hand.
Bathroom Adaptations	❑ Install elevated toilet seat and bar for support at side of toilet. ❑ If there is no shower, install hand-held shower device for use in tub. Place nonslip mats on tub floor. Use tub chair. ❑ Place grab rail on wall next to tub.
Chairs and Bed	❑ Designate a special chair for client and attach 2" x 4" blocks under back legs or lengthen back legs by two inches. ❑ Tie a sheet to the bedpost and a make a knot in the other end to facilitate getting out of bed.
Room Temperature	❑ Maintain temperature warm enough so client can wear fewer items of clothing. This makes dressing easier.

TABLE 18–3		Antiparkinson Drug Summary		
Drug	**Stage**	**Action**	**Effectiveness**	**Side Effects**
Amantadine (Symmetrel®)	Mild–moderate	Releases dopamine. May block acetyl choline	Improves all symptoms	Mottling of skin, swelling of feet, confusion, hallucinations
Anticholinergics Artane®, Akineton®, Cogentin®, Kemadrin®	Mild–moderate	Block acetylcholine	Improves rigidity, tremor and drooling	Dry mouth, blurred vision, mental changes, difficulty in voiding, constipation
Antidepressants with anticholinergic activity Elavil®, Pamelor®, Tofranil®	Patients with depression All stages of PD	Block the re-uptake (inactivation) of dopamine, norad-renalin, serotonin	Improves depression and sleep. May improve anxiety	Same as anticholinergics

Continues

Antidepressants without anticholinergic activity Desyrel®, Prozac®, Well butrin®	Patients with depression All stages of PD	Block the re-uptake of dopamine, norepinephrine, serotonin	Improves depression. May improve sleep, may improve anxiety	Mental changes
Antipsychotomimetics Mellaril®, Mobane®, Clozaril® (special precautions may be needed)	Patients with delusions, hallucinations, on antiparkinson medcation	Block the activity of dopamine on nerve cells outside the basal ganglia	May lessen the hallucinations and delusions	Mental changes
Dopa decarboxylase inhibitor combined with levodopa (Sinemet®) (Sinemet controlled release)	Mild Moderate Advanced	Blocks conversion of levodopa to dopamine outside brain while allowing conversion inside brain	Improves all symptoms	Involuntary movements, mental changes, dizziness
Dopamine agonists (Parlodel®) (Permax®)	Mild Moderate Advanced	Stimulate dopamine receptors directly	Improves all symptoms	Nausea, dizziness on standing, mental changes
Selegeline (Eldepryl® Jumex)	Mild Moderate Advanced	Blocks monoamine oxidase "B" activity in brain	May slow the progression of PD. Increases effectiveness of levodopa	Dizziness, nausea, insomnia

Courtesy American Parkinson Disease Association, *Parkinson's Disease Handbook*

Provide Mr. and Mrs. Jenkins with information concerning his medication regime. (See Table 18–3.) Tell them the signs of respiratory tract infection and advise them to report these promptly to the physician. Mr. Jenkins may need to irrigate his eyes with artificial tears if reduced frequency of spontaneous eye blink leads to irritation. The family needs to be aware of signs of depression — sleep disturbances, anorexia, or apathy. Instruct them to relay these to the physician for further evaluation.

Attention to personal hygiene is important because of increased skin oiliness and perspiration associated with Parkinson's disease. Encourage Mr. Jenkins to continue to do as much as he is able without becoming fatigued. If further deficits are noted, consider adaptations in environment or use of devices to prolong his independence. The person with Parkinson's cannot perform more than one motor act at a time. Instruct Mr. Jenkins to concentrate on doing tasks consecutively rather than concurrently. Remind him and the family that additional time is needed for all activities and that feeling pressured or hurried is counterproductive. Constipation is frequently a problem, so advise Mr. Jenkins on techniques to maintain normal bowel function (see chapter 6).

Encourage the family and Mr. Jenkins to discuss the future and to make tentative plans if the disease progresses. Mr. Jenkins is blessed with an understanding, adaptive wife and supportive family, the most important assets for coping with chronic illness.

QUESTIONS AND DISCUSSION

1. Which medications are prescribed most frequently for Parkinson's disease?
2. What side effects would you look for with these medications and what interventions would you implement?
3. Do you have further suggestions for Mrs. Jenkins so that her physical and emotional energies can be preserved?
4. How can you assist the Jenkins children to cope with the stress associated with a father with a chronic illness, a mother who needs emotional support, and at the same time, fulfill their own responsibilities and needs?
5. Are there restaurants and other public socialization facilities in your community that are accessible to persons with impaired mobility?
6. Are there other aspects of Mr. Jenkins's care that would benefit from additional interventions by the interdisciplinary team?

REFERENCES

Chipps, E., N. Clanin, and V. Campbell. 1992. *Neurologic Disorders*. St. Louis: Mosby-Year Book, Inc.

Coddington, J. In L. Côté and G. Riedel. (no date). *Exercises for the Parkinson Patient with Hints for Daily Living*. New York: Parkinson's Disease Foundation.

Côté, L. and G. Riedel. (no date). *Exercises for the Parkinson Patient with Hints for Daily Living*. New York: Parkinson's Disease Foundation.

DeLaney, J. 1988. Parkinson's/Alzheimer's Disease. *Extended Care Facilities Special Clinical Topics*. Kansas City: Marion Laboratories, Inc.

Lieberman, A.N., G. Gopinathan, A. Neophytides, and M. Goldstein. (no date). *Parkinson's Disease Handbook*. New York: The American Parkinson Disease Association.

Schwab, R.S. and L.J. Doshay. 1986. *The Parkinson Patient at Home*. New York: Parkinson's Disease Foundation.

Talotta, D. and P. Lisanti. 1989. Countering Parkinson's Assault on Your Patient's Will. *RN* (November): 34–39.

SUGGESTED READINGS

Duvoisin, R.C. 1990. *Parkinson's Disease. A Guide for Patient and Family*. 3d ed. New York: Raven Press.

Freed, C.R. 1990. Transplantation of Human Fetal Dopamine Cells for Parkinson's Disease. *Parkinson Report* 11(3): 8.

Gasser, T., M.S. Seiler, B. Perleth, H. Ellgring, P.T. Liebenstand, and W.H. Oertel. 1990–1991. Non-Medical Treatment of Parkinson's Disease—Part I. *The American Parkinson Disease Association*. pp 1, 5.

Levin, B.E. and W.J. Weiner. 1990. Psychological Aspects of Parkinson's Disease. *Parkinson's Report* 11(3): 5–7.

Robinson, M.B. 1989. *Equipment and Suggestions to Help the Patient with Parkinson's Disease in the Activities of Daily Living*. New York: The American Parkinson Disease Association.

Singer, C. 1990. Sexual Dysfunction in Parkinson's Disease. *Parkinson Report* 11(3): 3–5.

Weiner, W.J. 1990. Parkinson's Disease and Walking. *Parkinson Report* 11(3): 1–3.

Wichmann, R. 1990. *Be Active!* Staten Island, NY: American Parkinson Disease Association.

CHAPTER ■19■ A Restorative Approach to Caring for the Client with Chronic Airflow Limitation

OBJECTIVES

❏ Identify the signs and symptoms associated with chronic airflow limitation.
❏ Describe the pathophysiology related to chronic airflow limitation due to obstructive pulmonary disease.
❏ Demonstrate breathing self-help techniques.
❏ Demonstrate techniques for chest physical therapy, including postural drainage, percussion, and vibration.
❏ Describe measures to prevent respiratory infection for the client with chronic pulmonary disease.
❏ List the signs and symptoms indicative of respiratory infection.
❏ Demonstrate effective relaxation techniques.
❏ Identify the role of the interdisciplinary health care team in the management of the client with chronic airflow limitation.

DESCRIPTION OF THE DISEASE

Age-related changes by themselves should not impair the respiratory process. However, these changes in combination with lung pathology can result in severe disability. Chronic airflow limitation results from chronic pulmonary disease. While one disease may predominate, chronic obstructive pulmonary disease (COPD) is a combination of three closely related conditions: emphysema, chronic bronchitis, and asthma. The condition is characterized by airway obstruction, air trapping, and hypoxemia. It is progressive, irreversible, and degenerative, causing only minimal disability in some people, but overwhelming respiratory distress in others. COPD is a serious health problem, affecting 17 million Americans. Of all the risk factors, smoking is the most significant (Dennison 1991).

In emphysema, the bronchioles and alveolar walls are destroyed as a result of an imbalance between a lung protease called elastase, which breaks down elastin, and alpha-1-protease inhibitor, the substance that inhibits elastase. Elastase is produced by neutrophils. Normally, these antiproteases form a protective screen for the lung. The abnormalities of elastin result in collapse or narrowing of the bronchioles and enlargement of the alveolar sacs and loss of elastic recoil. The respiratory flow is obstructed because the lungs can no longer empty efficiently. In the majority of cases, this imbalance is due to cigarette smoking. Inhaled tobacco smoke stimulates excessive release of protease from the lung cells (National Institutes of Health 1986).

Chronic bronchitis is defined as a cough and expectoration that lasts at least three months out of the year for two consecutive years or for six months during one year. Inflammation of the mucosal lining causes thickening of the bronchi walls and hypertrophy of the bronchial mucous glands. The excessive mucous secretion leads to persistent, productive cough. Smoking and inhaling environmental irritants are the major causes of chronic bronchitis. Lung damage caused by severe, recurrent infections may also lead to chronic bronchitis (National Institutes of Health 1986).

Asthma is characterized by contraction of the smooth muscles in the bronchioles resulting in bronchospasm. Sticky, tenacious mucous is produced. The asthma of COPD is usually adult-onset and not related to allergies.

Varying degrees of chronic cough and shortness of breath are present in all persons with COPD. Decreasing ability to carry out physical activities gradually results in dyspnea with even minimal exertion. Through the course of the disease, respiratory tract infections occur more frequently, are more severe, and require lengthier recovery periods. During infections, dyspnea and coughing are more noticeable, wheezing is more likely to occur, and the sputum may be yellow or greenish. In advanced stages, it is usually possible to sleep only in a semisitting position and the client may awaken at night complaining of a choking feeling (Gyetvan and McCann 1988). Cor pulmonale, congestive heart failure, myocardial infarction, pulmonary embolism, stroke or cardiac arrhythmias may cause death from cardiorespiratory failure.

Diagnostic Procedures

The onset of COPD is so gradual that the disease is usually present for several years before medical attention is sought. Tests measuring lung capacity and lung volume differentiate between restrictive and obstructive forms of lung disease. They evaluate the ventilatory function of the lungs and chest wall and evaluate the severity of the disease process. The tests can also evaluate the client's response to bronchodilator therapy (McCann 1991). Radiographic tests assess structure, function, and vascular status. Blood tests indicating deficient or absent serum levels of Alpha 1-Antitrypsin can detect clients at risk for emphysema or in early stages of the disease.

Arterial blood gases (ABGs) evaluate the client's ability to exchange carbon dioxide for oxygen. ABGs measure the partial pressure that each gas exerts in the blood. The partial pressure increases as the concentration of the gas rises.

Analysis of the client's ABG results provide an evaluation of the acid-base balance and oxygenation (DaCunha 1991).

CASE STUDY

Mr. Swenson, a seventy-eight-year-old man, was admitted to a long-term-care facility from his home. The niece who had been caring for him had managed his household since the death of his wife several months ago. She is now unable to continue to do this and Mr. Swenson is agreeable to nursing home placement. His primary medical diagnosis is emphysema with secondary diagnoses of chronic bronchitis and generalized osteoarthritis. The general long-term goal is to improve Mr. Swenson's breathing patterns to maximize respiratory function. If he is willing to work at learning, it is possible he can be discharged to a less restrictive environment. It is unlikely he will return home because of a scarcity of services in the small community where he lives.

Strengths

- ❏ Skin condition is good
- ❏ Continent of bladder and bowels, if he stays close to a bathroom
- ❏ Able to walk short distances
- ❏ Oriented to person, place, and time
- ❏ Requires only partial assistance with activities of daily living
- ❏ Stopped smoking two years ago, resumed smoking after his wife's death, but quit again three months ago
- ❏ Enjoys listening to the radio
- ❏ Enjoys visiting, but becomes short of breath with extensive conversation

Interdisciplinary Assessment

Nursing.

Mr. Swenson becomes short of breath when he walks more than five to ten steps, during activities of daily living, and during lengthy conversations. His shortness of breath is identified by increases in respiratory rate with a prolonged expiratory rate. This causes Mr. Swenson to become anxious, thereby increasing the respiratory distress. Observation of breathing in the supine position indicates he uses the accessory muscles of the upper chest and neck for breathing. Blood gases are within normal limits.

Nursing Diagnosis

Ineffective breathing patterns related to obstruction of airflow during exhalation.

Nursing Interventions

- ❏ The nursing care of Mr. Swenson is directed toward teaching self-help techniques to make breathing easier. Elevate the head of the bed to a position of comfort to allow his lungs to expand more easily. Tell him to let his shoulders relax and place pillows under his elbows to prevent strain on the shoulders.
- ❏ Pursed Lip Breathing
    — Teach Mr. Swenson to practice pursed lip breathing several times a day and to use this technique whenever he is short of breath. Pursed lip breathing allows more oxygenated air to be inhaled and maintains the patency of the

airway during expiration, which helps him empty his lungs. This process will also slow his respiratory rate.

— Help Mr. Swenson to sit upright with his hands on his thighs, to lean forward with his elbows propped on a table. Instruct him to breathe in slowly through his nose with his mouth closed. Now have him purse his lips as though whistling and breathe the air out through his mouth slowly and evenly, without forcing it. Have him contract his abdominal muscles while breathing out. Exhalation should take at least twice as long as inhalation (Schull 1992).

❑ Diaphragmatic Breathing

— After Mr. Swenson feels comfortable with pursed lip breathing, teach him diaphragmatic breathing exercises to increase his ability to breathe deeply into his lungs. This technique prolongs expiration, thereby decreasing respiratory rate. Abdominal muscles are strengthened so they can assist with breathing and the diaphragm is used instead of the accessory muscles. Have him practice while lying down or sitting up and then while walking. As the exercise becomes easier, he can perform it with any activity.

— Instruct Mr. Swenson to place one hand below his ribs and over his abdomen, the other on the middle of his chest. Tell him to push his abdomen out against his hand while he inhales through his nose slowly. Then ask him to exhale through pursed lips to the count of three while tightening his abdominal muscles (DaCunha 1991). When he is walking, teach him to count with his steps and to take two steps for inspiration and three to four steps for expiration.

❑ These procedures require concentration and practice of an activity that is usually accomplished without thought. Teaching too much at one time will increase his anxiety thereby increasing his breathing problems and discouraging him from trying. Monitor Mr. Swenson's activities and provide reminders or reinforcement when necessary. Gradually increase the distance he walks, being sensitive to any distress that he experiences. Decrease distance if necessary.

❑ Mr. Swenson's oxygen adequacy may be evaluated by arterial blood gas analysis and clinical examination.

TABLE 19–1	Oxygen Therapy
	Nasal Cannula 1–6 liters per minute (LPM). Rate should not exceed 2 LPM for persons with COPD or the stimulus to breathe is depressed. Mouth breathers achieve same oxygen delivery as nasal breathers. Cannot deliver concentrations greater than 40 percent. Keep water container filled above the add line with distilled water. Check flow rate and cannula frequently. Check nares for skin breakdown. Avoid applying elastic strap too tightly.
	Nasal Catheter O_2 should not be over 2–3 LPM for persons with COPD. Set flow rate before insertion. Measure from client's nose to earlobe for length of catheter to be inserted. Lubricate with water-soluble jelly. After insertion, the catheter should be visible on either side of the uvula — withdraw it so it is no longer visible. Secure catheter to nose and cheek with tape so that tape is not pulling on nose. Remove catheter, clean, and reinsert in opposite nares every eight hours.

Continues

	Simple Mask O_2 is set at 5–8 LPM. Concentrations of 40–60 percent can be delivered. Mask should fit snugly but should not press against skin. Room air dilutes O_2 unless mask fits firmly against cheeks, chin, and bridge of nose.
	Nonrebreathing Mask O_2 is set at 6–15 LPM. Delivers O_2 concentrations of 60–90 percent. One-way valve separates non-rebreather mask from bag. Valve opens during inhalation to allow O_2 to enter mask. One-way valve on mask closes to prevent mixing of room air. During exhalation, valve between mask and bag closes to prevent expired carbon dioxide from entering bag. Valves on mask open to release exhaled carbon dioxide. Marked or complete deflation of reservoir bag indicates flow rate is too low.
	Partial Rebreather Mask O_2 is set at 6–15 LPM. Delivers up to 60 percent O_2. The partial rebreather mask does not have the one-way valve between reservoir and mask. Marked or complete deflation of reservoir bag indicates flow rate is too low.
	Aerosol Mask O_2 concentrations can be adjusted from 25–100 percent. Use sterile water and remove condensed water from tubing at regular intervals. Mist must be constantly available during inhalation.
	IPPB (Intermittent Positive Pressure Breathing) Machine is plugged into a pressure source — oxygen or compressed air. Prescribed medication or saline is placed in nebulizer. Machine is regulated to deliver pressure on inhalation, assisting client to breathe deeply. Controls are adjusted according to directions for machine or physician's orders. Client must seal lips around mouthpiece and breathe only through mouth. The routine use of IPPB is controversial.

Collaboration: Interdisciplinary Team

☐ Consult with a respiratory therapist, if necessary, to assist in teaching Mr. Swenson.

Outcome

Mr. Swenson will
☐ Display self-help techniques by utilizing effective breathing techniques
☐ Experience effective breathing patterns evidenced by decreased respiratory rates during physical activity
☐ Exhibit decreased anxiety caused from ineffective breathing patterns

Interdisciplinary Assessment

Nursing.

Abnormal breath sounds are noted on auscultation. Mr. Swenson's attempts to cough are ineffective, seldom resulting in sputum production.

Nursing Diagnosis

Ineffective airway clearance related to ineffective cough and inability to remove airway secretions.

Nursing Interventions

❑ Coughing and clearing the airway
— Teach Mr. Swenson that coughing spells can make him tired and anxious, increasing his respiratory distress. The increased mucus production, loss of lung elasticity, and narrowed bronchial airways prevent him from coughing effectively. By learning to control his cough (not suppress it) and to cough deeply, there will be enough air pressure to move mucus from his lungs and clear his airway. The best time to use coughing techniques is upon arising in the morning. Advise him to avoid coughing on a full stomach because it may cause him to vomit.
— Instruct Mr. Swenson to sit upright with his head slightly forward and feet on the floor. Have him do pursed lip breathing once or twice. Then tell him to breathe in again, but only to the midinspiratory point, hold his breath for a few seconds, and then cough twice in rapid succession: once to loosen the mucus and the second time to bring it up (Swearingen 1992). Remind him not to take any quick breaths between coughs. Supply Mr. Swenson with tissues and ask him to dispose of them appropriately and promptly. Tell him to use this procedure anytime he coughs or feels like coughing. During a respiratory tract infection, the physician may order chest physical therapy to adequately clear the lungs.

❑ Chest physical therapy
Chest physical therapy consists of postural drainage done in conjunction with percussion and vibration. This procedure is ordered by the physician after an evaluation of the client's cardiac and respiratory status. Chest physical therapy is only done if there are secretions present in the lungs and is performed only by trained personnel. Postural drainage utilizes the force of gravity in removing retained secretions from the bronchioles. Coughing facilitates the movement of the secretions into the bronchi and trachea for expectoration. Percussion dislodges thick, tenacious secretions from the bronchial walls. Vibration can be used with percussion or as an alternate to percussion for clients who are frail, in pain, or recovering from surgery.
— Have Mr. Swenson lie on a bed or flat table. Specific positions are determined by the location of the mucus obstruction, Figure 19–1. The positions are maintained for ten to fifteen minutes. Do the exercises two to four times a day, before meals and before bedtime.
— Percussion is done by using a cupped hand to clap the chest wall in a rhythmical, painless manner. Instruct Mr. Swenson to breathe deeply and slowly, using the diaphragm. Alternate hands in a rhythmic manner. Perform this procedure over the involved areas, with Mr. Swenson in the appropriate position. Injury may occur if clapping is done over the scapula, clavicle, sternum, spine, breast, liver, kidneys, or spleen. Do the percussion for one or two minutes, alternating with vibration.
— To do vibration, place one hand flat on top of the other to apply manual compression and vibration over the chest wall, while Mr. Swenson exhales slowly through pursed lips. As he exhales, firmly press your fingers and palms of your hands against the chest wall. Vibrate during five exhalations over each chest segment (Schull 1992). After three or four vibrations, tell

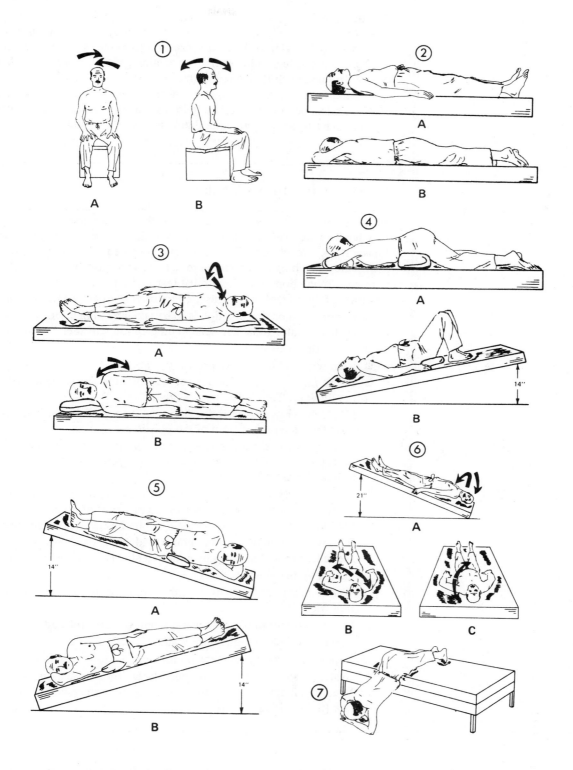

Figure 19–1 Positions for chest physical therapy *(From Hegner and Caldwell,* Geriatrics: A Study of Maturity, *5th ed. [Albany, NY: Delmar Publishers Inc., 1991].)*

him to cough, using the abdominal muscles. After he rests, repeat the percussion and vibration.

❑ Adequate fluid intake
  —Maintain a fluid intake of 2500 ml per day to liquify chest secretions, making it easier to clear the secretions from the lungs. Warm, clear liquids are preferable. Avoid beverages containing caffeine or alcohol. Milk should be avoided if it thickens the mucus.
  —Monitor for signs of congestive heart failure with the increased fluid load — rales, edema, and weight gain. Measure and record intake and output.

❑ Give expectorants or bronchodilators as ordered by physician.

TABLE 19–2	Using a Metered-Dose Inhaler
	Inhalers are used to disperse medication through an aerosol mist, spray, or powder. The medication is administered to dilate narrowed bronchioles or to loosen thick, mucus secretions. The drug is placed in a canister that fits into the inhaler. The inhaler is metered to deliver a specific amount of medication with each inhalation. The client must learn how to use the equipment and to be aware of the hazards of overuse. These directions are written for the client. ❑ If more than one medication is to be taken by inhalation, administer the bronchodilator first. The second medication will then be fully inhaled. ❑ Shake the canister. ❑ Remove mouthpiece and protective cap. ❑ Insert metal stem on bottle into small hole on flattened portion of mouthpiece. Turn bottle upside down. ❑ Hold inhaler with your index finger on the top of the metal canister and your thumb on the bottom of the plastic mouthpiece. ❑ Exhale, then place the inhaler in your mouth, just past your front teeth. Direct the opening toward the back of your throat. Close your lips around the mouthpiece. ❑ Inhale slowly and deeply while you are depressing the medication canister. Breathing deeply carries the particles of medication deep into the lungs. It is important to inhale while the spray is administered. ❑ Remove mouthpiece from mouth and hold your breath for several seconds. Empty the lungs by exhaling slowly through pursed lips. ❑ Cough up the mucus. ❑ Wait a few minutes between inhalations or as long as the directions indicate. ❑ Rinse your mouth out with water when you are finished. ❑ Rinse mouthpiece with warm water. ❑ Replace protective cap back on inhaler. ❑ Systemic side effects of bronchodilators include shakiness, dizziness, sweating, irritability, insomnia, feelings of anxiety, and increased heart rate (Schull 1992).

A humidifier puts moisture in the air and helps loosen secretions. Clean and disinfect the equipment regularly to avoid bacterial growth.

Collaboration: Interdisciplinary Team

❑ Consult with the physical therapist or respiratory therapist for additional information on chest physical therapy.
❑ Consult with the respiratory therapist for additional information on the use of inhalers.

Outcome

Mr. Swenson will
❑ Demonstrate ability to cough effectively, maintaining an open airway
❑ Expectorate fluid secretions. Lung sounds are improved.

Interdisciplinary Assessment

Nursing and Physical Therapy.

The niece states that Mr. Swenson spent most of his day at home sitting in a chair. In the nursing home, he is reluctant to get out of bed without a great deal of encouragement. His strength and endurance are greatly decreased. Joint pain and stiffness are increasing with the inactivity.

Nursing Diagnosis

Impaired physical mobility related to shortness of breath with exertion, and chronic joint pain and stiffness due to arthritis.

Nursing Interventions

❑ Teach Mr. Swenson that daily exercise will help alleviate joint discomfort and prevent other complications associated with inactivity. Advise him that walking every day will increase his strength and endurance. Without adequate activity, large muscles become deconditioned and consume more oxygen, placing an additional burden on the lungs.
❑ Set up a schedule for ambulation twice a day, gradually increasing the distance. Accompany him on his walks, reminding him to count steps — two steps for inspiration and four for expiration. Reinforce breathing techniques while walking with him. Provide encouragement and praise for his efforts. Monitor breathing and pulse rate.
❑ Carry out active assistive range-of-motion exercises twice a day. As his strength increases, have him do active exercises without your help. Add stretching activities to this routine as his endurance improves.
❑ Supplemental oxygen may be needed during periods of increased activity.
❑ Transport Mr. Swenson to the dining room and to other areas of the facility per wheelchair.
❑ Give pain medication for joint pain as ordered.

Collaboration: Interdisciplinary Team

❑ Consult with physical therapist and occupational therapist for suggestions for beneficial physical activities for Mr. Swenson that will not cause him shortness of breath.

Outcome

Mr. Swenson will
- Ambulate two times each day. Evidence of increasing strength and endurance will be noted by his ability to walk increasing distances without increased respiratory distress. Breathing and pulse rates will remain within acceptable parameters.
- Participate in the exercise plan twice each day. He will maintain joint mobility and experience less joint stiffness and pain.

Interdisciplinary Assessment

Nursing.

Inadequate ventilation due to COPD places Mr. Swenson at risk for respiratory infections. Insufficient fluid intake and physical inactivity increase the risk. The stresses associated with the recent loss of his wife and with his nursing home admission are contributing risk factors.

Nursing Diagnosis

High risk for respiratory tract infection related to compromised defenses.

Nursing Interventions

- Monitor Mr. Swenson for signs of infection — fever; increased pulse rate; increased shortness of breath; changes in the amount, consistency, color of mucus; and loss of appetite. Report changes to the physician promptly. Remember that older people do not always have elevated temperatures with infections.
- Consult with the physician for administration of flu and pneumonia vaccine.
- Restrict Mr. Swenson's outdoor activities during periods of increased air pollution and during cold weather. Instruct him to avoid the tobacco smoke of others and to avoid close contact with persons who have respiratory tract infections.
- Inhalation devices should be disinfected or sterilized at least daily as the manufacturer directs. Eliminate the use of perfumed lotions and bath powders that might irritate his respiratory tract. Ask the staff to avoid wearing perfume. Advise Mr. Swenson to stay away from areas of the building where paint or other fumes are present.

Outcome

Mr. Swenson will
- Remain free of respiratory tract infections

Interdisciplinary Assessment

Nursing and Dietary.

Mr. Swenson is five pounds lower than his usual body weight and ten pounds under his ideal body weight. Since admission to the hospital, he has consistently consumed less than 50 percent of his meals.

Nursing Diagnosis

Alterations in nutrition, less than body requirements, related to fatigue and shortness of breath while eating, and anorexia.

Nursing Interventions

❑ Transport Mr. Swenson to the dining room ten to fifteen minutes before the meal is served. This will allow him time to relax and "settle in" before eating.
❑ Serve Mr. Swenson his fluids thirty to sixty minutes before the meal. During the meal, advise him to drink just enough to facilitate swallowing the food. This routine may prevent abdominal distention and dyspnea.
❑ Help Mr. Swenson to a comfortable, upright position before meals. Monitor his progress and assist him when he starts to tire.
❑ If the physician orders a diuretic, include high-potassium foods in his diet — oranges, orange juice, bananas, dried fruits, fresh pineapple, apricots, peaches, whole grain breads, bran cereal, beef, and potatoes are good sources.
❑ Weigh Mr. Swenson weekly.

Collaboration: Interdisciplinary Team

❑ Mr. Swenson is on a 2-gram sodium diet. The dietician will meet with Mr. Swenson to discuss the use of salt substitutes and other spices for flavoring if he finds the food flat tasting. Avoid gas-forming foods that could increase his difficulty breathing. Avoid serving dry foods that may trigger coughing.
❑ Ask the dietician to divide his daily food intake into six small meals to prevent fatigue. If shortness of breath is a problem in the morning, liquid instant breakfast may be easier to ingest than solids. Easy-to-chew foods help preserve energy.

Outcome

Mr. Swenson will
❑ Consume at least 75 percent of each meal
❑ Regain one-half pound per week until his usual body weight is attained

Interdisciplinary Assessment

A total score of eight on the Pressure Ulcer Potential Assessment indicates a risk for skin breakdown.

Nursing Diagnosis

High risk for impaired skin integrity related to presence of risk factors for pressure-sore development — inactivity, poor nutritional status, chronic disease.

Nursing Interventions

❑ Implement Pressure Ulcer Prevention Protocol. (See chapter 4.)

Outcome

Mr. Swenson will
❑ Remain free of skin breakdown

Interdisciplinary Assessment

Nursing and Social Services.

Mr. Swenson verbalizes feelings of panic when he becomes short of breath with exertion. For this reason, he avoids physical activity when possible.

Nursing Diagnosis

Fear and anxiety related to shortness of breath secondary to COPD.

Nursing Interventions

❑ As Mr. Swenson gains control of his breathing by using the procedures he is learning, his anxiety and fear should decrease. In addition, he can be taught relaxation techniques to further alleviate his feelings of fright and apprehension. There are a number of stress-reducing activities, including audio tapes that provide step-by-step instructions. Relaxation techniques can be combined with pursed lip breathing to relieve tension.
❑ Have Mr. Swenson sit in a quiet room, in a comfortable chair, with his arms and legs supported. Tell him to close his eyes and to do pursed lip breathing. As he exhales, suggest that he imagine he is breathing the tension out of his body.
❑ After he does this a few times, have him tighten various sets of muscles and then relax them. He can start with his forehead, face, and neck muscles and progress down his body by shrugging his shoulders, tightening his arm muscles, and making fists with his hands. After he tenses each part have him relax the muscles and do pursed lip breathing before going on to the next part.
❑ Help him to imagine soft breezes, the roar of the ocean, or the birds singing to aid in relaxation. Tell Mr. Swenson to think "I am in control" as he goes through the exercises.

Collaboration: Interdisciplinary Team

❑ Consult with Social Services about evaluating Mr. Swenson further for the need for additional counseling in order to overcome his fear and anxiety. Ask them to arrange for a clergyperson to see Mr. Swenson as he has requested. He would also like to attend the weekly church services.
❑ Diversional activities may help Mr. Swenson by providing mental stimulation and fulfilling psychosocial needs. Talk with the activities staff about providing quiet activities until he regains some strength and control of his respiratory status. Utilize his enjoyment of listening to the radio.
❑ The social worker will serve as liaison for Mr. Swenson, his niece, and the admissions director if Mr. Swenson's condition improves sufficiently that he may be discharged to the retirement center.

Outcome

Mr. Swenson will
□ Control his feelings of anxiety and panic

COMMENTS

There are several factors to consider if Mr. Swenson is discharged. His ability to continue with the breathing procedures and relaxation techniques after discharge would need to be evaluated. If Mr. Swenson is discharged, he may benefit from attending a support group sponsored by the lung association to gain more information about COPD and to meet others with similar problems.

He will not be responsible for any household tasks at the retirement center. But he needs to know how to manage his energy for completing his personal care and for other activities that he chooses to undertake. Tell him to avoid standing if he can sit. He should find the easiest way to do things. Discuss with him how he can pace himself by moving slowly and calmly and resting often. Suggest that he space his activities, not planning too many for any one day and planning for rest periods in between his daily activities. Remind him to use the breathing techniques with all activities.

Assess his understanding of his care.
□ Does he understand his medications and when he is supposed to take them?
□ Does he know the signs of infection and when to call his physician?
□ If he uses breathing aids, will he be able to use and clean them correctly?
□ Will the retirement center be able to meet his nutritional needs? If he is unable to continue with six small meals a day, suggest that he take nonperishable leftovers back to his room for snacks.
□ Will there be appropriate diversional activities available?

All people need meaningful, interesting physical and mental activity. Friendships are also important. Mr. Swenson may need encouragement to invite old friends to his new home and to make new friends with the people that live there.

While Mr. Swenson has not manifested any objective signs, look for subtle cues that may indicate dysfunctional grieving related to Mrs. Swenson's death. These may include expressions of guilt or unresolved issues, denial of his wife's death, emotional lability, crying, or regression. Actively listen and encourage his verbalization and/or his need for privacy and acknowledge his feelings.

Mr. Swenson has not been sexually active for two or three years. He has not indicated a desire to resume sexual activity. Other clients with chronic airflow limitations may need additional teaching regarding sexuality. For couples in a permanent relationship, the need for role reversals may diminish self-esteem, resulting in feelings of guilt and shame. This can be a greater factor in sexual dysfunction than the disease process. A sensitive, understanding, and knowledgeable partner and the ability to communicate honestly with each other are prerequisites to a satisfying relationship. Sexual activity is possible in the early stages of COPD, especially if the client has effectively learned controlled breathing techniques. Planning ahead is necessary, avoiding activity after a full meal or after physical exertion, and allowing time for rest periods. Using an inhaler beforehand may be helpful. The partner can learn to take the more active role, assuming positions that minimize pressure on the chest. Prolonged kissing can cause panic due to feelings of suffocation. Activity may be interrupted by coughing, making it difficult for the male with COPD to regain an erection. It is important for the couple to avoid setting goals that, if unmet, lead to feelings of shame, frustration, or resentment. Intimacy and touching, especially for older adults, are often more satisfying than physical intercourse and eliminate the possibility of failure.

Mr. Swenson can experience enjoyment and reason for living if he remains in control of his disease. The sense of control alleviates some of the anxiety associated with COPD and decreases feelings of helplessness, dependency, and despair. Establishing a routine that includes interesting physical and mental activities will help prevent further deterioration.

QUESTIONS AND DISCUSSION

1. What programs are available to assist individuals to stop smoking?
2. What actions can nurses take to educate the public about the risks associated with smoking?
3. What are the systemic side effects of bronchodilators?
4. What suggestions can you give Mr. Swenson for maximizing his energy level?
5. Are there additional interventions that can be implemented by the interdisciplinary team to improve the quality of life for clients with COPD?

REFERENCES

DaCunha, J.P., ed. 1991. *Respiratory Support*. Springhouse, PA: Springhouse Corporation.

Dennison, R.D. 1991. In M. Shaw, ed. *Illustrated Manual of Nursing Practice*. Spring-house, PA: Springhouse Corporation.

Gyetvan, M.C. and J.A.S. McMann, eds. 1988. *Diseases and Disorders Handbook*. Springhouse, PA: Springhouse Corporation.

McCann, J.A.S., ed. 1991. *Diagnostic Test Implications*. Springhouse, PA: Springhouse Corporation.

National Institutes of Health. 1986. *Chronic Obstructive Pulmonary Disease*. Washington, DC: U.S. Department of Health and Human Services.

Schull, P.D. 1992. *Nursing Procedures*. Springhouse, PA: Springhouse Corporation.

Swearingen, P.L. 1992. *Pocket Guide to Medical-Surgical Nursing*. St. Louis: Mosby-Year Book, Inc.

SUGGESTED READINGS

Bolgiano, C.S., K. Bunting, and N.M. Shoenberger. 1990. Administering Oxygen Therapy: What You Need to Know. *Nursing 90* 20(6): 47–51.

Hahn, K. 1989. Sexuality and C.O.P.D. *Rehabilitation Nursing* 14(4): 191–95.

Janelli, L.M., Y.K. Scherer, and L.E. Schmieder. 1991. Can a Pulmonary Health Teaching Program Alter Patients' Ability to Cope with COPD? *Rehabilitation Nursing* 16(4): 199–202.

CHAPTER ■20■ A Restorative Approach to Caring for the Client with Sensory Impairments

CONTENT OUTLINE

I. Description of the problem
II. Hearing
   A. Diagnosis and treatment of hearing loss
III. Hearing aids
   A. Troubleshooting for hearing aids
IV. Vision impairments
V. Causes, descriptions, and treatments of severe visual impairments
   A. Cataract
   B. Glaucoma/Procedure for administration of eyedrops
   C. Age-related macular degeneration
   D. Diabetic retinopathy
VI. The sense of touch
VII. Case study
   A. Strengths
   B. Interdisciplinary assessment
   C. Nursing diagnoses
      1. Self-care deficit
      2. Diversional activity deficit
      3. Social isolation
VIII. Comments

OBJECTIVES

❑ Differentiate between conductive hearing loss and sensorineural hearing loss.
❑ Identify the different types of hearing aids.
❑ Describe the nurse's responsibility in the care and use of hearing aids.
❑ List techniques for communicating with hearing-impaired persons.
❑ Describe the causes and characteristics of pathological visual impairments.
❑ Discuss postoperative nursing care for a client recovering from cataract surgery.
❑ Plan nursing interventions for a client with severe visual impairment that will increase the level of function in performance of activities of daily living.
❑ Identify the role of the interdisciplinary health care team in the management of the client with a sensory impairment.

DESCRIPTION OF THE PROBLEM

Almost all individuals experience sensory alterations as they age. The visual, auditory, kinesthetic, olfactory, tactile, and gustatory senses all diminish to some extent. These changes may be so minor as to be only an irritation or so major that they severely affect the person's quality of life. Sensory impairments usually occur gradually, but in some cases may be abrupt. The degree to which each sense is impaired varies greatly within an individual. For example, the person with severe hearing loss may have adequate visual skills with corrective lenses. As individuals reach the seventh and eighth decades, the impairments become more noticeable often interfering with their performance of activities of daily living. Advanced age makes it more difficult for the person to adapt to his/her sensory changes.

Reactions to sensory changes are as varied as the persons experiencing them. Some individuals, particularly those with hearing loss, may try to ignore the deficits. They withdraw from contacts with others, avoiding conversations and social affairs, becoming more and more isolated. Because this is a hidden deficit, people may be mistakenly considered confused, mentally incapacitated, or stubborn. Most individuals compensate for their sensory losses by using corrective devices such as glasses and hearing aids. They are not ashamed of the changes and will ask for assistance if needed. When a sensory loss has been abrupt, the individual generally experiences all the reactions associated with grieving. Adaptation to sensory changes is a continual process. Tasks that were once completed automatically now require more attention, care, and energy.

The quality of life for the elderly can be enhanced greatly with appropriate environmental planning. Nursing homes and other residential buildings for the elderly are usually wheelchair accessible but are severely inadequate in meeting the sensory needs of the people living there. Few public places are designed with older people in mind. Education is greatly needed for people of all ages to increase public understanding and empathy for the normal changes of aging. People responsible for environmental planning and design, both interior and exterior, need specific information on sensory changes and how to adapt the environment to these alterations.

Education is needed for older people so they understand the aging process. Greater awareness reduces anxiety and increases acceptance. People will then be more willing to use adaptive devices and the resources available to them. The implications associated with impairments in taste, smell, and touch are sometimes overlooked by health care staff.

HEARING

D.A. Ramsdell describes three levels of hearing: primitive, signal, and social. The primitive level includes environmental sounds that facilitate interaction with the world. Hearing the sounds of nature, traffic noises, and voices are ways of connecting with the surrounding environment. Warning sounds are at the signal level. Sirens, fire alarms, a baby's cry, calls for help, and car horns provide a means of creating a safer environment. The social level is used for comfortable and satisfying conversational exchange (Washburn 1986).

Hearing loss affects an estimated 21 million people in this country. Hearing impairments can occur at any time, but the incidence increases dramatically with age. The degree of loss may range from mild to severe. This can place the individual at risk for injury, affect the ability to communicate, and reduce socialization (National Information Center on Deafness 1989). Conductive hearing loss occurs when some part of the conductive mechanism is disrupted. This may be caused by injury, disease, or obstruction in the outer or middle ear. Accumulation of wax in the outer ear obstructs hearing and is a temporary, easily rectified cause of hearing loss. Middle ear impairment may result from damage to the eardrum or from bony growths that prevent movement of the stapes, malleus, and incus. When either of these situations occurs, sound is not conducted into the inner ear. Persons with conductive hearing loss find that sounds are softer and muted. They can usually benefit from a hearing aid or medical or surgical treatment. Sensorineural hearing loss results from damage to the delicate nerve endings in the inner ear. The damage is caused by head or ear injuries, infectious diseases, or continued exposure to high noise levels. Presbycusis is a sensorineural cause of hearing loss most commonly associated with aging. It results from progressive deterioration of inner structures or degenerative changes in the acoustic nerve. Sounds may be heard but are distorted. A hearing aid may help, but may not eliminate the distortions (National Information Center on Deafness 1989).

A person experiencing hearing loss may talk loudly and complain that others are mumbling. The individual often confuses words with similar sounds and watches the speaker's face intently. Environmental sounds may be ignored completely. Signs of embarrassment, frustration, anger, or withdrawal are often noted. Persons with hearing loss frequently complain of ringing in the ears (tinnitus) (McFarland and Cox 1987).

Diagnosis and Treatment of Hearing Loss

The person with suspected hearing impairment should see an otologist or ear, nose, and throat specialist for detection of medical problems and recommendations for treatment.

The audiologist assesses the type and degree of loss and the ability to understand speech under various conditions. Testing may include an air conduction test to determine the degree of loss. A bone conduction test and impedance audiometry will pinpoint the type of loss. Speech reception threshold audiometry determines how loud speech must be to be understood. A speech discrimination test (word recognition test) is given to evaluate how well speech is understood once it is loud enough to hear.

After analyzing the test results, the audiologist recommends the services appropriate to the individual. Recommendations may include hearing aid evaluation and orientation, auditory training, training in lip-reading techniques, and speech conservation and counseling (McFarland and Cox 1987).

There are numerous communication and alerting devices available to ease the life of hearing-impaired persons. The quality of life experienced by the hearing-impaired elderly person also depends on the environment and the skill of other people in utilizing communication techniques.

TABLE 20–1	Techniques for Communicating with Hearing-Impaired Clients
	❏ If the client appears inattentive, confused, or slow, assess hearing and note whether hearing aid is in place.
	❏ Place yourself in good light. Face client and light. Client may read your lips or watch your facial expression.
	❏ Address client directly; do not turn your face and do not cover your mouth with your hand. Avoid talking with food or gum in your mouth. Use eye contact.
	❏ Eliminate distracting noises in the environment and turn off the TV. Lower the tone of your voice. It is easier to hear.

Continues

❑ Let the client see you first, then touch the client's hand or shoulder and call by name. Start with a key word or phrase. Repeat the same words if necessary.

❑ Do not be afraid to ask a hearing-impaired person if one ear is a "good" ear. If so, stand or sit on that side.

❑ Talk at a moderate rate and wait for a response. Speak clearly and distinctly without overarticulating. Keep your voice at the same volume throughout the conversation.

❑ Avoid complex, lengthy sentences. Ask only one question at a time. Too many may be difficult to sort out and follow.

❑ When changing to a new subject, slow your rate down and make sure the client is following the change before proceeding. Watch the client's face for understanding.

HEARING AIDS

The use of hearing aids by older adults is so common that the topic deserves additional attention. All types of aids have the same basic components. The microphone picks up the sound and the amplifier receives the sound from the microphone to make it louder. The battery provides the power for the hearing aid to work and is contained in a battery case. The volume control adjusts the level of sound. The receiver is a tiny speaker that conveys sound to the ear. The ear mold is attached to the hearing aid and channels the sound from the aid to the wearer's ear (Williams and Jacobs-Condit 1987). The behind-the-ear (BTE) aid fits over and behind the ear. The hearing aid case contains the battery and is connected to a plastic ear mold inserted into the ear canal. This type is suitable for individuals with mild to severe losses. The in-the-ear (ITE) aid contains a small battery and fits within the ear canal. This type is useful for people with mild to moderate loss. Eyeglass models utilize a hearing aid that fits in the ear canal and is attached by tubing to the eyeglass frame which holds the battery. These are designed for people with mild to severe losses. The body aid utilizes an ear mold that inserts into the ear and is connected by a cord to the case of the body aid. The body aid is enclosed in a case that is carried in a pocket or attached to clothing. This type helps people with severe loss (Williams and Jacobs-Condit 1987).

The client should insert and care for the hearing aid. If this is not possible, follow these steps. Remember, hearing aids are delicate and expensive.

❑ Before inserting a hearing aid, check the battery. Each type of aid requires a specific type of battery and these are not interchangeable. To check, turn the control to "M" or "on."

❑ Some models have a "T." This is a telephone switch that activates a telecoil. Telecoil circuitry is built into some hearing aids to facilitate hearing over the telephone. The telephone must be compatible with the telecoil circuitry in order to work.

❑ After turning the hearing aid on, test the battery by cupping your hand over the battery enclosure. A constant whistle indicates a functioning battery. If there is no whistle, replace the battery. Match the positive markings on the battery and battery case.

❑ Turn the aid off and the volume down. Place the ear mold in the external ear canal, turn it on and adjust the volume. The hearing aid should fit snugly but comfortably, flush with the ear. The upper extension fits into the upper earlobe.

❑ To adjust the volume, talk to the person as you increase the volume. Stop when the person can hear you.

Troubleshooting for Hearing Aids

- ❑ If the aid is making squealing noises, check the ear mold for placement and fit. Examine the plastic tubing on a BTE for cracking or splitting. Test the volume and if it is too high, turn it down until the squealing stops.
- ❑ If the hearing aid does not work, replace the battery. Check the battery terminals for correct position. If there is corrosion on the battery compartment, remove it with a pencil eraser.
- ❑ Examine the ear mold for wax. To remove wax, wash the ear mold in warm, soapy water and rinse. Make sure the switch is set on "M" and not on "T." If the sound on a body-type aid clicks on and off, check the wire between the receiver and hearing aid; listen to the hearing aid through the receiver and wiggle the wire. If it is broken or cracked, the sound will go on and off.
- ❑ If these techniques are not effective, consult the audiologist for repair, replacement, or suggestions. The average hearing aid lasts from two to five years.

Check the hearing aid daily. Keep a supply of extra batteries on hand and a spare cord for body aids. Keep the aid dry and avoid exposure to temperature extremes. If the aid becomes wet, remove the battery and drain the water. Place the aid in a plastic bag with silica gel to absorb excess moisture.Do not use solvents or lubricants on the hearing aid. Turn the aid off before removing it. Open the battery door to help dry any body moisture that seeps in. Store the aid in its case. Avoid hairspray because it can clog the aid, causing excessive damage. To wash the ear mold, detach it from the battery compartment and use warm, soapy water. Rinse with clear water and let it dry before reconnecting. Use a pipe cleaner for the plastic connecting tube.

Assistive listening devices may be used by people who wear or do not wear hearing aids. These devices are defined as any non-hearing aid device designed to improve the hearing-impaired person's ability to communicate. A "hard-wire system" amplifies the sender's voice into earphones worn by the hearing-impaired person. Amplification of background noises is eliminated and the device can be used with a radio or television. The device is connected to a wire that limits the use of the device. Infrared systems are another device that transmit signals consisting of light waves spread throughout the room. The light waves carry the message and are picked up by receivers worn by the user (Palumbo 1990). There are various alerting and alarm systems that signal hearing-impaired persons. The signal may be a flashing light or an increase in amplified sound. These are used for doorbells, paging devices, smoke alarm systems, security alarms, and wake-up alarms. Telecommunication devices for deaf people (TDDs) permit conversations in print (DiPietro, Williams, and Kaplan 1987). Amplification devices for telephone use include telephone handsets, portable amplifiers, and telephone adapters.

VISION IMPAIRMENTS

Vision occurs when rays of light from an object pass through the cornea, aqueous humor, lens, and vitreous humor to the retina and the cerebral cortex. Vision is normal (emmetropia) when the rays coming from the object at a distance of twenty feet or more are brought to focus on the retina by the lens. Myopia, or nearsightedness, occurs when rays of light from twenty feet or more are brought to focus in front of the retina. This condition is corrected with concave lenses. Hyperopia, or farsightedness, results when rays of light coming from the object at twenty feet or more are brought to focus behind the retina. Convex lenses correct hyperopia.

Accommodation is a process that allows the eye to adjust to objects at different distances. This is caused by increasing convexity of the lens by contraction of the ciliary muscles. As people age, the lens gradually loses elasticity. The lens becomes progressively less able to increase its curvature in order to focus on near objects. This results in presbyopia and is correctable with prescription eyeglasses. There are numerous other age-related visual alterations. (See chapter 2, "The Restorative Nursing Process.") These changes are universal in nature, affecting almost everyone. Although they are annoying and require adaptation, they seldom interfere with daily living activities. The impact of these changes can be reduced considerably with eyeglasses, contact lenses, or magnifying hand lenses and by altering the environment.

TABLE 20–2	Creative Environments for Persons with Impaired Vision
	□ Use bright, diffuse, consistent lighting without shadows and glare.
	□ Avoid lighting changes in adjacent areas.
	□ Avoid barriers in traffic patterns by placing furniture appropriately.
	□ Use large, broad print for signs. Leave extra space between letters and words. White letters on black or black letters on yellow are easier to read. Use a matte finish for signs and pictures rather than glossy.
	□ Place signs, pictures, and wall hangings at a low height so people in wheelchairs can see them. As people age, they lose "upward gaze."
	□ Cooler colors (shades of green and blue) tend to appear faded to elderly eyes. The institutional use of these colors creates a dull, gray, unstimulating environment. Use eye-pleasing shades of red, yellow, orange, pink, and brown.
	□ Long halls appear as endless tunnels. Make use of color, contrast, and design to alter this.
	□ Edges and boundaries are difficult to visualize. Delineate edges of tables, counter tops, stairs, and curbs. Paint doors to contrast with adjacent walls. Use contrasting table coverings and dishes. Avoid white plates — white and light-colored foods cannot be identified.
	□ Avoid glare and shiny surfaces. Note placement of mirrors and use nonglare glass for pictures and paintings. Use dull finish paint rather than glossy. Use sheer curtains over windows that bring in outside glare from the sun. Shiny floors are particularly dangerous.
	□ Use large-numbered telephone dials and digital clocks.
	□ Obtain large-print editions of books and magazines.

Severe vision impairments can be very disabling. The person with normal vision has 20/20 vision. The normal eye can see letters at twenty feet when tested with the Snellen Chart. Legal blindness is a term used for purposes of establishing qualifications for disability benefits. It is defined as central visual acuity in the better eye of 20/200 or less when using a corrective lens or a visual field of twenty degrees or less at the widest diameter. It is important for health care staff to know how the visually-impaired individual functions in the environment.

CAUSES, DESCRIPTIONS, AND TREATMENTS OF SEVERE VISUAL IMPAIRMENTS

Cataract

A cataract is a cloudy or opaque area in the lens of the eye. The lens is normally clear. But when a cataract forms, the passage of light is obstructed and vision is impaired. Cataracts can develop over a period of years or within just a few months. They can vary from very small opacities to large cloudy areas and can start in the nucleus of the lens or in the cortex. One or both eyes can be affected. The most common form of cataract is related to aging. Congenital cataracts are present at birth or develop within the first year. Traumatic cataracts result from a blow, penetration of a foreign body, or exposure to harmful chemicals. Radiation, intense heat, or intense light and the toxic effects of certain drugs, such as cortisone derivatives, can also cause cataract formation.

The effect of the cataract on vision depends on the size, density, and location. Signs of a developing cataract include:

❑ hazy, fuzzy, or blurred vision
❑ dark spots in the field of vision that remain fixed as the eye moves
❑ a need for frequent changes in eyeglass prescriptions
❑ changes in pupil color and problems with light
❑ complaints of having a film over the eye
❑ frequent blinking in an effort to see better

(National Institutes of Health 1983)

Surgery is the only method at this time proven effective for treating cataracts. It is estimated that over 2 million surgeries are done per year. Most of these are done on an outpatient basis. The lens is surgically removed, using one of two methods. Mydriatic and/or cycloplegic drops are instilled into the affected eye preoperatively and prophylactic antibiotic eyedrops may be ordered. A facial scrub with antiseptic solution may be done by the client at home or immediately prior to surgery (Carver 1987). During intracapsular extraction, the entire lens and its capsule are removed. Cryoextraction is done with a cold probe inserted through the dilated pupil to freeze a portion of the lens. This adheres to the probe, allowing the surgeon to lift the lens out of the eye.

Extracapsular extraction leaves the posterior part of the lens capsule intact while most of the front lens capsule, the cortex, and nucleus are removed. The posterior portion of the lens is not removed, to allow for implantation of an intraocular lens. Phacoemulsification (emulsification of the cataract) uses ultrasound vibrations to soften and liquify the lens so it can be aspirated through a hollow needle placed in a tiny incision. An intraocular lens (IOL) is then implanted. If this procedure is not used, the person will require thick cataract glasses or contact lenses. It is possible to have secondary implant surgery several years after cataract surgery (Stinger 1991).

After surgery, the operated eye is treated with antibiotic drops or ointment and covered with a dressing. The surgeon may remove the dressing the next day. For two weeks, an eye shield is worn over the eye during sleep and removed while the client is awake. Antibiotic eyedrops are administered to prevent infection and steroid eyedrops may be ordered to decrease inflammation (Carver 1987). Because of the microsurgery techniques and methods of wound closure, there are few postoperative restrictions. The client may be instructed to avoid strenuous physical activity, heavy lifting, straining, and bending over. These activities increase pressure in the eye and place stress on the incision. The client returns to the surgeon one or two weeks after surgery and in five to six weeks for glasses.

Cataract surgery is one of the most successful operations done today. Serious complications are rare, but can occur. Among the possible complications are macular edema, intraocular hemorrhage, corneal edema, retinal attachment, secondary glaucoma, uveitis, and infection. Postoperative assessment of the client's visual acuity is performed by asking the client how many fingers are being held up. Check the eye for bulging or deviation and inspect the lids, conjunctiva, and sclera for inflammation or discharge. Any redness and swelling from the surgery should subside within seventy-two hours. The cornea should be clear, the iris visible, and the pupil round. Unless there is some coexisting condition that causes visual impairment, surgical removal of a cataract followed by a substitute lens should restore useful vision.

Glaucoma

Glaucoma is a general term for diseases of the eye caused by an increase in intraocular pressure. Excessive pressure results when the input of aqueous humor through the pupil is greater than the outflow. The outflow takes place through the meshwork located at the juncture of the iris and cornea. There are two primary types of glaucoma. Acute narrow-angle glaucoma (closed angle) develops rapidly and is characterized by pain, blurring of vision, nausea, and vomiting. Open-angle glaucoma is chronic, progressive, and painless, especially in the early stages. Symptoms include clouding and blurring of vision and the appearance of halos around lights. Open-angle glaucoma affects 90 percent of all persons with glaucoma. Secondary glaucoma is associated with other ocular diseases that impair the circulation of aqueous humor. Without treatment, blindness will occur with all types as a result of the increasing pressure on the optic nerve (Stinger 1991).

Treatment is directed toward reducing intraocular pressure which is usually accomplished with eyedrops. The drug prescribed depends on whether the client also has a cataract, whether the glaucoma is resistant, or whether it is emergency treatment for narrow-angle glaucoma. Pilocarpine is generally the drug of choice for both chronic and acute glaucoma. There are sustained-release forms of Pilocarpine available. A unit is inserted into the upper or lower cul-de-sac and replaced weekly. If this treatment is inadequate, a drainage or fistulizing operation may be performed. An accessory channel is established through which the aqueous humor drains, reducing the intraocular pressure. Glaucoma is usually successfully managed with compliant use of the prescribed medication. Everyone over age thirty should have regular eye examinations for glaucoma detection.

Procedure

Administration of Eyedrops
1. Review physician's order, check medication, check client's identification.
2. Wash your hands.
3. Explain the procedure to the client.
4. Ask the client to lie in the supine position with neck slightly hyperextended.
5. Hold a clean tissue in your nondominant hand just below client's lower eyelid. Use your thumb or finger to gently retract the lower lid downward, pressing against the bony orbit, with the tissue resting against the lower lid margin. Do not press against the eyeball, which would increase pressure within the eye.
6. Ask the client to look up toward the ceiling. Use your dominant hand to hold the dropper about one-half inch above the conjunctival sac. Instill the prescribed number of drops. Ask the client to gently close the eye. After blinking several times to disperse the medication, have the eye remain closed for one to two minutes.
7. Wash your hands. Record the procedure.

Age-Related Macular Degeneration

Age-related macular degeneration (AMD) affects the macula, the yellow spot in the middle of the retina. The macula provides the sharp, straight-ahead vision that is needed for driving and reading small print. AMD is a leading cause of visual loss and affects 165,000 elderly people each year (Stinger 1991).

The dry form of AMD develops very slowly. Tiny yellowish deposits called drusen develop beneath the macula. The layer of light-sensitive cells in the macula becomes thinner as some cells break down. These changes cause a dimming or distortion of vision. The dry form of AMD usually affects both eyes eventually, but rarely causes total loss of reading vision. The dry form may give way to the wet or neovascular form of AMD. In the wet form, new blood vessels form beneath the macula, leaking fluid and blood, damaging the light-sensitive cells. The client may notice that straight lines look wavy and later there may be blank spots in the field of vision. If the leakage and bleeding continue, the macula may be destroyed within a few weeks or months.

Most people with the wet or neovascular form of AMD can usually be successfully treated with laser photocoagulation. Powerful light rays from a laser are focused on a tiny spot on the macula, destroying the abnormal blood vessels. This treatment is best applied before the abnormal blood vessels reach and damage the fovea, the central part of the macula. There is no evidence that laser photocoagulation is effective for the dry form nor does it restore vision already lost from AMD. Changes associated with AMD can only be detected through an eye examination. At present, there is no method for preventing either form of the disease. Although it is a leading cause of visual loss, the majority of people with AMD continue to have almost normal vision throughout their lives (National Institutes of Health).

Diabetic Retinopathy

Diabetic retinopathy is a deterioration of the small blood vessels that nourish the retina. It begins as a mild condition when the retinal blood vessels enlarge, balloon outward, and leak fluid, causing the retina to swell. When fluid collects in the macula, it may cause blurring of central vision. In about 80 percent of diabetics, the disorder never progresses beyond this stage and vision is not seriously impaired. If it does progress to the proliferative stage, neovascularization occurs. The abnormal blood vessels sprout and grow along the surface of the retina. These vessels rupture and bleed into the vitreous humor, interfering with the passage of light to the retina. Scar tissue may form, detaching the retina. In either case, severe visual loss or permanent blindness may result.

Laser coagulation is used to interrupt the disease process and prevent the development of additional retinal abnormalities. The decision to begin treatment is determined by the ophthalmologist, based on the presence or absence of certain changes in the retina. Laser photocoagulation cannot be used if bleeding inside the eye makes it difficult for the physician to see the areas that require treatment.

There are few symptoms of diabetic retinopathy, particularly in the early stages. Diabetics should have an annual eye examination by a physician trained to diagnose diseases of the retina and to determine when treatment is needed (National Institutes of Health 1983).

THE SENSE OF TOUCH

The sense of touch diminishes less than other senses. There is, however, an increased threshold for pain, touch, and the ability to feel pressure. Touching, like hearing and seeing, is a powerful method for communication. When caring for elderly clients, it may be the most successful method of communication.

TABLE 20–3	Touch and Touching
	□ Many older adults suffer sensory deprivation because of a lack of touching from others.
	□ Touching often gives the most pleasure of all the senses and yet is sometimes the least appreciated.
	□ Touch comforts.
	□ Touch expresses affection.
	□ Touch is the stimulus for the passion of sexual ecstasy.
	□ Touch can also be an act of violence.
	□ Touch can be misinterpreted by a confused client or by the person whose only experience with touching is with sexual activity.
	□ Touch can be condescending when we pat someone on the head.
	□ Touch may be the only method of communication left to the person with dementia who scratches and bites as a way of saying "I don't like what you are doing."
	□ Touch is acceptance. It says "I think you are an attractive, kindly person."
	□ Nurses use touch to assess clients.
	□ Nurses provide care and caring with touch.
	□ Nurses touch with their voices, eyes, and facial expressions.
	□ Nurses use the healing power of touch. Gently rubbing a client's temples or giving a back massage has a calming influence.

CASE STUDY

Miss Roberts, an eighty-five-year-old female, was admitted to the nursing home because of severe visual impairment related to macular degeneration. She lived in an apartment with her sister and beloved pet Frisky, a dog of undetermined origin. Miss Roberts's sister managed the household and assisted Miss Roberts with her personal care. Six months ago, the sister died suddenly from a massive stroke. Miss Roberts was an administrative secretary for several years, retiring at the age of sixty-seven. She has few close friends and her only relatives are a few nieces and nephews scattered around the country. In spite of her visual impairment, she is able to crochet and play the piano. Miss Roberts is having increasing difficulty maintaining her home. She was afraid she would fall and not be able to summon help. A young couple in her building looked in on her frequently and ran her errands. They both worked during the day and were frequently out in the evening. Miss Roberts and her sister were accustomed to going out often, but since the sister's death, she has felt confined and lonesome. Miss Roberts decided to enter the long-term-care facility.

Strengths

- □ General health status adequate; history of mild hypertension managed with medication and low-sodium diet
- □ Adequate communication skills
- □ Has relinquished roles as phases of life require

❑ Participates in self-care by making decisions and accepting responsibility for decisions
❑ Accepts what cannot be changed

Interdisciplinary Assessment

Nursing.

Although Miss Roberts is able to make responsible decisions, she is lacking in self-care skills. She has the physical ability to complete these tasks with guidance from staff. She will adjust to the change in her life-style more readily if she increases her independence. Interventions are directed to teaching Miss Roberts the skills she needs to carry out activities of daily living with minimal assistance. The staff also needs instruction to ensure that techniques and routines are consistent.

Nursing Diagnosis

Self-care deficit related to visual impairment and lack of opportunity to develop new self-care skills.

Nursing Interventions

❑ Communications
 — When you walk into Miss Roberts's room, call her name, touch her lightly, and identify yourself. You may need to give her additional information, such as "I'm your nurse on the day shift." Tell her when you leave her presence.
 — Be specific when giving directions, e.g., "I will put the pill in your right hand" or "I am setting a glass of water on the table to your left."
 — If Miss Roberts needs to sign her name, teach her to place her index finger at the start of the line. She can locate that finger with her pen and begin writing.
❑ Eating
 — After Miss Roberts is at the table, teach her to place one hand on the back of the chair and slide it out. Then tell her to make sure the seat is clear by using her free hand to brush back and forth. Ask her to move to the front of the chair, line the back of her knees against the front of the chair, anchor the chair with one hand, and sit down. After she is seated, have her feel for the edge of the table and adjust her position.
 — To find her plate, teach her to reach forward with both hands and place her fingertips on the top edge of the table. Ask her to flex her fingers and move her hands straight ahead until she finds her plate. Suggest she use a trailing technique when reaching for objects to avoid upsetting glasses and cups. Have her flex her fingers slightly and keep her fingertips in continuous contact with the table surface as she moves her hand gently forward or laterally on the table.
 — Ask Miss Roberts how she likes her food arranged. Describe her plate like a clock, with meat at 6:00, potatoes at 3:00, vegetable at 9:00. Describe the food that is served and the position and contents of any side dishes. Items such as condiments, cream, and sugar should be placed in the same spot on the table at every meal.
 — Teach her to bend her trunk (not her head) forward over the plate as she eats in case something falls from her fork. She can learn to judge the amount

of food on her fork by sensing the weight. When she is cutting with a fork and knife, tell her to anchor the plate by pressing down with the knife.

— Teach her to use a pusher to pick up food like peas or corn. This can be a piece of bread or her knife. If the dish has sides, have her push the food toward the side.

— Teach her to shake salt and pepper into her hand first rather than directly on the food to prevent overuse.

— To pour liquids, tell her to determine the size, shape, and weight of the container. Then with one hand, have her hold the cup with the thumb and middle finger close to the top, with the cup handle close to the tip of her thumb. Teach her to use her index finger as a point of reference to center the pouring container spout. Have her take the pouring container in her other hand and bring the tip of the spout to the side of the cup. With her index finger as guide, the spout is centered over the cup. To determine when the cup is full, tell her to bend the first joint of her index finger over the edge of the cup and to stop pouring when she feels the liquid.

— To handle serving dishes, suggest she take the serving dish in her right hand, transfer it to her left hand, and hold it over her plate. Have her locate the serving utensil by following the rim of the serving dish.

— It will take time for Miss Roberts to learn these procedures, so avoid expecting too much too soon. The caregivers may need to help her at first, by cutting her meat, pouring liquids, and buttering bread.

❑ Mobility

— When walking with Miss Roberts, have her grasp the caregiver's arm just above the elbow and have the caregiver remain about two steps ahead of her. This enables her to pick up cues about changes in the walking pattern. Tell her if there are steps or curbs or if the incline changes or remains flat. Pause before going up or down. When she walks in the hall, suggest she put one hand on the rail. When walking with her, describe landmarks like doors and windows. Suggest that she trail the wall with her hand and count doorways to facilitate her orientation. As she becomes more independent, give her directions by telling her how many doors to pass before she turns right or left.

— If she is in a strange area, describe the surroundings. Never take Miss Roberts to another area of the building and leave her without telling her when someone will help her back to her room.

— Help her become oriented to her room by telling her where the bathroom, bed, chairs, dressers, and closet are in relation to the door. Do not rearrange furniture unless it is necessary, and then reorient her to the change. Orient her to the bathroom by describing the location of the toilet, sink, toilet paper, and towel racks. Describe the environment to Miss Roberts, using multiple adjectives for colors, textures, and shapes.

— Monitor the halls and floors frequently for clutter or unnecessary and unexpected items. Never leave doors or drawers partially open.

❑ Bathing, grooming, hygiene

— Teach Miss Roberts to develop a system of organization in her room. Have her decide where she wants to put her belongings and personal care items. Once this is done, make sure the system is maintained.

— Remain with Miss Roberts while she bathes and encourage her to do what she can. Provide the assistance that she needs.

— If you help her with daily hair care, ask her how she likes to wear it. Even though she cannot see it, she can "feel" if it is right or not. Ask her if she wants to go to the hair dresser on a regular basis. It is important that Miss Roberts be well groomed. Encourage her to wear makeup, perfume, and jewelry. Compliment her appearance.

—When Miss Roberts is ready to dress, have her choose what she wants to wear. If she prefers, her clothes can be labeled so she can identify them by "feel." Tactfully inform her if her clothing is soiled, she has a run in her stocking, or her slip is showing.

Collaboration: Interdisciplinary Team

❑ Inform all staff of Miss Roberts's visual impairment and the interventions that have been established. It is important that these be implemented consistently.
❑ The skills of a rehabilitation teacher for the visually impaired or a vocational counselor may be needed to help establish the self-care program.

Outcome

Miss Roberts will
❑ Perform activities of daily living at her optimal level

Interdisciplinary Assessment

Nursing, Activities, and Social Services.

Miss Roberts rarely leaves her room except for meals. She spends most of the day sitting in the chair dozing and occasionally listening to the radio. She states, "I wish there was more to do here." When Miss Roberts was at home, her sister planned outings and other activities they both enjoyed.

Nursing Diagnosis

Diversional activity deficit related to visual impairment and past life-style.

Nursing Interventions

❑ Consult with activities staff for developing activities of Miss Roberts's choice.

Collaboration: Interdisciplinary Team

❑ Ask the activities aide to read Miss Roberts the weekly schedule of events every Monday so she can choose the ones she would like to attend. Have the aide circle these so that the staff can remind her to go.
❑ Activities staff may capitalize on her previous interests by providing her with supplies for crocheting. Let her know that she can sell or donate these items to the gift shop if she desires.
❑ Miss Roberts enjoys playing the piano. Offer to have someone escort her to the piano until she is able to get there by herself. After she becomes adjusted to her new environment, she may enjoy playing for others.
❑ Social Services may be able to supply Miss Roberts with talking books. The equipment can be obtained through the local library. She may also enjoy a radio unit that broadcasts daily the contents of the daily local newspaper.
❑ Ask Miss Roberts if she would like to purchase a clock that announces the time. By pressing a button, she can hear the current time.

Outcome

Miss Roberts will
- Participate in the activities of her choice
- Express satisfaction with her routine in the long-term-care facility

Interdisciplinary Assessment

Nursing and Social Services.

Miss Roberts's sister was her major source of socialization. She frequently verbalizes how much she misses her sister and her beloved pet. The young couple from the apartment building visit her weekly, but otherwise she has few outside contacts. For many elderly people, pets are a valuable source of love and affection. Miss Roberts may be feeling guilty because she had to place her pet in the animal shelter. Losing an animal companion due to nursing home admission is traumatic and triggers a number of emotions associated with grieving. Clients may not verbalize their feelings because they fear others will think them crazy for mourning an animal's loss. If this is true in Miss Roberts's situation, she needs assurance that what she is feeling is normal.

Nursing Diagnosis

Social isolation related to sister's recent death and the loss of her pet.

Nursing Interventions

- Encourage Miss Roberts to verbalize her feelings regarding her sister's death and the loss of her dog. She will need to complete the grieving process before she is able to go on with her life.
- Arrange for Miss Roberts to meet other residents on her nursing unit with whom she can visit. Many rewarding relationships are established between nursing home clients.

Collaboration: Interdisciplinary Team

- Assign Miss Roberts a dependable volunteer to visit her regularly.
- Ask the activities department to invite Miss Roberts when community outings are planned. She may find it rewarding to rekindle her interests in cultural and sports events.
- Invite Miss Roberts to become involved in the nursing home's pet therapy program. This may help her recapture some of the satisfaction that she received from her own pet.
- Arrange for the social worker to meet with her regularly to provide additional support and guidance.

Outcome

Miss Roberts will
- Express her feelings to the nurse and/or social worker concerning her recent losses.

❏ Verbalize satisfaction in her involvements with other people and with the pet therapy program.

COMMENTS

Miss Roberts has lost her sole sources of support, love, and companionship. The decision to enter the nursing home was her own, and with adequate help from the staff, she will probably be able to make a satisfactory adjustment to her current status. As she gains competence in self-care, she may also increase her self-confidence.

If ongoing assessment reveals changes in her health status, it may be necessary for the staff to take over more of her care. Restorative nursing involves the ability to know when to intervene as well as knowing when to encourage independence.

QUESTIONS AND DISCUSSION

1. Evaluate the environment of your facility. Does it take into consideration the sensory losses of older adults?
2. What can the dietary department do to enhance the taste of food for clients with diminished taste sensation?
3. Sensory stimulation is an enjoyable activity for clients with altered thought processes. What foods would be appropriate for the sense of smell and taste?
4. What items could you use for sensory stimulation that would be appropriate for the sense of touch?

REFERENCES

Carver, J.A. 1987. Cataract Care Made Plain. *American Journal of Nursing* 87(5): 626–30.

DiPietro, L., P. Williams, and H. Kaplan. 1987. Alerting and Communication Devices for Hearing Impaired People: What's Available Now. *National Information Center on Deafness/American-Speech-Language-Hearing Association*. Washington, DC: Gallaudet University.

McFarland, W. and B.P. Cox. 1987. Aging and Hearing Loss. *National Information Center on Deafness/American-Speech-Language-Hearing Association*. Washington, DC: Gallaudet University.

National Information Center On Deafness. 1989. *Deafness: A Fact Sheet*. Washington, DC: Gallaudet University.

National Institutes of Health. 1983. *Cataracts*. Washington, DC: U.S. Department of Health and Human Services.

National Institutes of Health. 1983. *Diabetes and Your Eyes*. Washington, DC: U.S. Department of Health and Human Services.

National Institutes of Health. (no date). *Age-Related Macular Degeneration*. Washington, DC: U.S. Department of Health and Human Services.

Palumbo, M.V. 1990. Hearing Access 2000: Increasing Awareness of the Hearing Impaired. *Journal of Gerontological Nursing* 16(9): 26–31.

Stinger, K.A. In M. Shaw. 1991. *Illustrated Manual of Nursing Practice*. Springhouse, PA: Springhouse Corporation.

Washburn, A.D. 1986. Hearing Disorders and the Aged. *Topics in Geriatric Rehabilitation* 1(4):61–70.

Williams, P.S. and L. Jacobs-Condit. 1987. Hearing Aides: What Are They? *National Information Center on Deafness/American-Speech-Language-Hearing Association*. Washington, DC: Gallaudet University.

SUGGESTED READINGS

Barto, C.P. 1990. What Are TDDs? *Fact Sheet, National Information Center on Deafness*. Washington, DC: Gallaudet University.

Brady, B.A. and S.N. Nesbitt. 1991. Using the Right Touch. *Nursing 91* 21(5): 46–47.

Stanlis, I. 1990. Let's Hear It for Hearing Aids! *Nursing Homes* 39(5 and 6): 27, 36.

Wax, T. and L. DiPietro. 1987. Managing Hearing Loss in Later Life. *National*

Information Center on Deafness/American-Speech-Language-Hearing Association. Washington, DC: Gallaudet University.

CHAPTER 21

A Restorative Approach to Caring for the Client with Left Hemiplegia

OBJECTIVES

- Identify characteristics of the individual with left hemiplegia.
- Describe how to assess a client with left hemiplegia for the presence of sensory-perceptual-spatial deficits.
- Discuss nursing interventions to assist the client to compensate for the deficits.
- Create a care plan to teach self-care skills to a client with left hemiplegia.
- Evaluate a client with left hemiplegia for discharge potential.
- Identify the role of the interdisciplinary health care team in the management of the client with hemiplegia.

DESCRIPTION OF THE PROBLEM

Hemiplegia generally occurs as a result of a cerebral vascular accident (stroke). A stroke occurs when a cerebral artery is blocked, preventing the flow of blood to specific areas of the brain. The consequences may be devastating, with symptoms dependent on the location and extent of the brain damage. Stroke is usually a manifestation of an underlying disease process, such as hypertension, blood vessel disease, impaired cardiac function, or a disturbance in the blood-clotting mechanism. Five hundred thousand strokes occur each year. There are three million individuals in this country living with the after affect of stroke. Seventy-two percent of all strokes occur in persons over sixty-five years of age (Chipps, et al. 1992).

The risk of stroke can be reduced by avoiding known risk factors. Elevated cholesterol levels, the use of tobacco, obesity, and a lack of exercise are associated with cardiovascular disease. A history of hypertension or diabetes increases the risk. People with these diagnoses require close monitoring. Progress is being made in the effort to reduce the numbers of strokes. Between 1968 and 1985, deaths from stroke in this country declined from 72.8 to 33.8 per 100,000 population (American Heart News 1991).

One of three mechanisms causes the disruption in circulation that results in a stroke. Sixty percent of all strokes are caused by cerebral thrombosis, embolism accounts for twenty percent, and hemorrhage twenty percent (National Stroke Association 1989). A thrombus is formed after atherosclerotic deposits cause the inner walls of the artery to become thick and rough. Stroke due to thrombus results in progressive neurological deficits with symptoms gradually worsening over a period of minutes or a few hours. An embolus causes a sudden blockage of cerebral blood flow when a clot originating in another part of the body breaks loose and is carried by the bloodstream to the brain. The onset of stroke due to an embolus is usually rapid, with no warning signs. The third mechanism causing a stroke is hemorrhage that occurs when a cerebral artery ruptures, spilling blood into the brain tissue or the surrounding area. A subarachnoid hemorrhage is usually caused by a ruptured aneurysm, causing bleeding into the fluid-filled space around the brain and spinal cord. Intracerebral hemorrhages are usually caused by hypertension, and vessels bleed directly into the substance of the brain. This type of stroke has a sudden onset of excruciating headache. It advances from weakness to paralysis within a few minutes (Mitiguy 1991).

Transient ischemic attack (TIA) is a temporary interruption in cerebral blood flow. A focal neurological deficit, such as loss of speech or hemiplegia, occurs. Complete recovery takes place within twenty-four hours, leaving no residual effects. TIA is not a stroke, but four out of five survivors of thrombotic stroke have a history of TIAs. The physician should be notified immediately of symptoms suggestive of TIA. Complaints of blacking out or dizziness are generally not associated with TIA.

Prognosis after a stroke depends on the extent of spontaneous recovery. This occurs when cerebral edema decreases, healthy cells in the brain take over the functions of the damaged cells, and revascularization takes place. If the client begins to recover control over lost functions within three to four days, the outlook is good. If, after four to five weeks, there is no evidence of spontaneous recovery, the prognosis is much less positive. Most functional improvements occur within the first three months after the stroke; in some cases, improvements may be noted as long as a year afterward.

Ninety-seven percent of the population has a dominant cerebral hemisphere — usually the left — that contains the speech centers (Adkins 1991). For this reason, symptoms associated with left brain damage usually include aphasia as well as some degree of hemiplegia on the right side. Right brain damage results in left hemiplegia and perceptual deficits. Major differences exist in the deficits seen in right and left damage. Nursing care is planned according to the assessment of each individual. Deficits in motor and intellectual functions may affect persons with either right or left brain damage. This chapter presents a client with right brain damage, left hemiplegia and the nursing diagnoses commonly associated with this type of stroke. Aphasia and consequences of left brain damage are presented in chapter 12.

Hospital discharge planning after a stroke depends less on the age of the individual than on the functional abilities of the client, existing support systems, and availability of community resources. Rehabilitation is started in the hospital as soon as the client's condition stabilizes but is usually not completed by discharge. If outpatient therapy is not appropriate, transfer to a rehabilitation center will provide the client with opportunity to reach an optimal potential. If this is not possible, or if the client "peaks out" at the rehabilitation center, transfer to a skilled nursing facility may be necessary. Upon admission to the facility, thorough assessment will identify the client's potential for further improvement. Placement may be viewed as permanent or temporary depending on assessment findings and the progress made by the client. In all cases, preventing complications and maintaining current levels of function are major goals. It is important for clients with stroke — as it is for all clients — to utilize their strengths and to stress ability rather than disability.

CASE STUDY

Mrs. Mary Peters, a sixty-nine-year-old female, was in good health until she had a stroke two weeks ago. At that time, she was admitted to Community Hospital for care and treatment. Rehabilitation was initiated and although some progress was made, she is unable to carry out activities of daily living without assistance. Nursing home placement is deemed advisable at this time. Mr. Peters wants to take his wife home and plans to do so if she can learn to transfer independently and regain some self-care skills. Mrs. Peters's admitting diagnoses are: CVA with left hemiplegia, generalized degenerative arthritis, and iron deficiency anemia. The admission assessment identified a stage 2 pressure ulcer on the left heel.

Strengths

- Appetite is good; no problems associated with eating
- Weight is within acceptable range.
- Oriented to place and person and usually to time
- Communicates verbally, although comprehension is questionable at times
- Hearing is adequate.
- Right hand has always been dominant hand.
- Husband expresses willingness to do whatever he can to assist in Mrs. Peters's recovery.
- Successful career as a social worker before retirement eight years ago; has numerous friends in the community
- Has always been active and independent
- Strong spiritual faith and beliefs

Interdisciplinary Assessment

Nursing and Occupational Therapy.

Mrs. Peters has deficits in visual, tactile, and kinesthetic senses. She is unable to record visual stimuli from the left side because of left homonymous hemianopsia. This means the left side of each eye is affected and she is blind to objects on that side. This is noted when she eats only the food on the right side of her plate and does not respond to people approaching from the left. When she is wheeled around the building, she becomes confused because she sees one side of a room or hall going and sees the other side coming back. Hemianopsia is permanent. There is no medical treatment and glasses will not change this visual impairment (National Stroke Association 1986).

Impairment of the tactile sense is reflected in the lack of pain and temperature sensation (hemianesthesia) experienced by Mrs. Peters when stimuli are applied to the left side of her body. In some clients, a distorted quality of sensation may return with an over response to stimuli characterized by poorly localized pain sensations. This is referred to as thalamic syndrome and is the result of damage to the thalamus. It is characterized by intractable, persistent pain on the affected side of the body. The pain has been described as stabbing, crushing, burning, gnawing, and shocklike. The pain may be provoked or agitated by external factors such as rubbing, scraping, or a change in room temperature. Even sounds, emotional disturbances, or sudden fright can trigger the sensation. Thalamic syndrome is difficult to treat and outcomes are unpredictable (Tikare 1990).

The loss of position sense (proprioception) occurs with alteration of the kinesthetic sense. The proprioceptors (specialized sensory nerve endings), located in the muscles, transfer information used to coordinate muscle activity. The tension and stretch of muscles change to accommodate movement and maintain position. This is done without conscious attention. The loss of this sense means that Mrs. Peters is unable to determine where her left arm and leg are without looking at them. This increases the risk for falling.

Spatial deficits are reflected in the inability to judge distance, size, position, rate of movement, form, and relation of parts to wholes. These problems generally result from a disturbance in visual perceptual organization. Assessment of this alteration is made for Mrs. Peters by several observations. She has balance problems, noted by her tendency to slump to the left while she is sitting although she thinks she is upright. This is evident when she stands and leans to the left during transfers. She dislikes being assisted to an erect position, because it feels like she is being pushed over. This disturbance means Mrs. Peters is living in a world of "tilted space." As her mobility increases and she navigates her own wheelchair, she may bump into a door frame. She may also have problems setting objects back down, e.g., missing the saucer when putting a cup back. Mrs. Peters has difficulty judging distances. Staff needs to be aware of this when she learns to self-transfer. There may be more distance between her and the surface she is transferring to than she realizes, causing her to fall (Swearingen 1992). As Mrs. Peters begins to relearn the activities of daily living, it may become evident that she confuses the inside and outside of her clothes and that she is unable to distinguish right from left.

Aphasia is not usually a problem with left hemiplegia. Mrs. Peters has adequate verbal skills. However, she is unable to read because she loses her place on the page.

Assessment findings indicate that Mrs. Peters does not recognize familiar objects, such as a comb, toothbrush, or pencil. This is agnosia, another perceptual impairment. She is also unable to perform certain purposeful movements with her right arm, even though she has adequate strength and sensation. This deficit is due to a perceptual-cognitive impairment called apraxia (Chipps, Clanin, and Campbell 1992). Mrs. Peters cannot distinguish foreground from background, which is the loss of figure-ground skill.

A combination of sensory and perceptual deficits results in unilateral neglect of the left side of her body and of the environmental space on her left side (Chipps et al. 1992). Mrs. Peters does not recognize her left arm and leg as a part of her own body. This disturbance of body image is confirmed by looking at a self-portrait Mrs. Peters has drawn, which has body parts missing.

Mrs. Peters denies her disabilities, frequently displaying poor judgment and impulsive behavior. She attempts activities she is incapable of performing, such as getting up from her wheelchair unassisted. These personality changes dramatically increase her risk for accidental injury.

The nursing interventions for the specific problems described for Mrs. Peters often overlap. General directions are given here and additional suggestions are included for subsequent nursing diagnoses. Both Mr. and Mrs. Peters need to attend the care plan conference so they are both aware of the identified problems and planned interventions. If Mrs. Peters is discharged, her husband will be better prepared to help her.

Nursing Diagnosis

Sensory-perceptual-spatial alterations related to neurological impairments due to stroke. (This nursing diagnosis is listed first because the characteristics of sensory-perceptual-spatial alteration affect every activity and increase the potential for injury.)

Nursing Interventions

❑ Because the left hemisphere of her brain is intact, Mrs. Peters will learn more successfully if she is given brief, simple, verbal cues. The use of touch with the verbal cues is often more effective than the cues alone. Give verbal encouragement and feedback instead of relying on your facial expressions. Demonstrations and the use of body language are distracting and ineffective, as are the use of pictures, signs, and written instructions. Since use of the terms right and left confuse her, give her frequent reminders of right and left. Teach Mrs. Peters to use verbal self-cuing as a way to increase focusing and attention. Do not assume she can safely complete an activity because she says she can. Rely on your observations to evaluate her abilities (Shah, Avidan, and Sine 1988).

❑ Because of the impulsivity and lack of judgment associated with right brain damage, Mrs. Peters needs clear limits on what is and what is not acceptable behavior. Consistency among staff helps to reinforce the instruction.

❑ To compensate for the hemianopsia, arrange the room so Mrs. Peters's right side is facing the door when she is in bed or a chair. Talk to her and present activities to her from the right side. When she is taken around the building in her wheelchair, point out landmarks on the left side so she learns to recognize both sides of the area. Place the call light and other objects Mrs. Peters may need on her right side. Some people with hemianopsia learn to scan. Try this with Mrs. Peters, teaching her to move her head to increase her field of vision (National Stroke Association 1986).

❑ Prevention of injuries is a concern related to lack of sensation, unilateral neglect, and loss of proprioception. Because feeling is diminished on her left side, check it frequently for signs of injury, pressure ulcers, or infection. Avoid situations that could result in thermal injuries. Before moving Mrs. Peters in the wheelchair or before transferring her, check the position of her left leg and foot. She would not notice if her foot was doubled over or dragged along the floor. Give as much feedback as possible about the neglected left side. Place her arm on a lapboard when she is up, placing it in her line of vision. Therapeutic activities are sometimes presented on the impaired side to increase awareness of that side.

❑ Agnosia can also cause injuries. The lack of recognition of familiar objects can result, for example, in drinking liquids not meant for ingestion. Check Mrs. Peters's room frequently for potentially dangerous objects or poisonous substances.

❑ Tell Mrs. Peters the name of objects used for activities of daily living. Because of the apraxia, Mrs. Peters may not be able to carry out a task when asked, but may be able to do it without thinking, as a learned habit. Lengthy instructions will be ineffective. For example, placing a bowl of cereal in front of her and then handing her the spoon and saying "This is your spoon and this is your cereal" works better than saying "Here is a spoon. Now put it in your cereal and try to eat as much as you can."

❑ Compensate for the figure-ground impairment by arranging items so they are on surfaces of contrasting colors. Avoid clutter, which increases difficulty in distinguishing objects.

TABLE 21–1	Guidelines for Teaching the Person with Left Hemiplegia
	❑ Adapt your teaching to the impairments resulting from right brain damage. Assess client for excessive verbalization, emotional lability, unilateral neglect, easy distractibility, impaired short-term memory, impulsivity, lack of judgment, left hemianopsia, and time disorientation. The presence of apraxia, agnosia, perseveration, and latency increase the challenge.
	❑ Sit on client's right side. Choose a time and place when interruptions and visual or auditory distractions are eliminated.
	❑ Minimize clutter and avoid rapid movement around client.
	❑ Give brief and simple verbal instructions.
	❑ Break procedures down into small steps and then present in sequence.
	❑ Give verbal feedback. Avoid using facial expressions or other forms of body language when communicating. Brief touching with verbal feedback may increase its effectiveness.
	❑ The use of verbal self-cuing helps client to concentrate on the task and compensates for deficits associated with left hemiplegia.
	❑ Encourage the use of both hands if possible. This stimulation increases client's awareness of left side of body and increases tactile feedback to right side.
	❑ You can guide by standing behind or to the side of the client. Place the client's hand(s) on the object and your hands over the client's hands. This technique gets the client started if latency is a problem and it tactfully interrupts perseveration.
	❑ The client with apraxia may perform whole tasks better than individual steps. The client may respond better with no instruction at all for automatic activities.

Outcome

Mrs. Peters will
❑ Remain free of injury
❑ Use compensatory techniques to attain higher levels of ability in completing activities of daily living
(Perceptual problems may or may not improve with time.)

Interdisciplinary Assessment

Nursing and Physical Therapy.

Mrs. Peters is unable to move herself in bed. She can transfer and ambulate a short distance with the assistance of two people. Observation of gait pattern reveals a lack of hip flexion on her affected side, a vaulting movement on the right side and uneven step lengths. Resistance is noted during passive movement of the affected limbs, confirming the presence of spasticity. The left upper extremity assumes a flexion synergy pattern — the shoulder is retracted, internally rotated and adducted, with the elbow, wrist, and fingers in flexion.

Initially after a stroke, the limbs on the affected side are flaccid and nonfunctional due to the absence of muscle tone. Muscle tone is the degree of tension or "readiness" in a muscle at rest as determined by messages from the brain. During the flaccid stage, attention is given to prevention of injury to the affected limbs and to maintaining full range of motion. Within a few days or weeks, some degree of spasticity occurs in the affected limbs. Spasticity is an increased state of tension in the muscle and is a result of hyperactivity of the stretch reflex. Stretch reflex refers to the muscle contraction that occurs when a pull is exerted upon the tendon of the muscle. Impulses are sent to the spinal cord through sensory nerves. Motor nerves send messages to make the necessary changes in the muscle. In the presence of central nervous system damage, the balance between stimuli that increase muscle sensitivity and those that decrease muscle sensitivity is altered. The stretch reflex, which is normally inhibited by the central nervous system, becomes overactive. The muscles are more sensitive to stimuli and this causes the formation of synergies. A synergy is an abnormal pattern of movement seen with increased levels of spasticity (Loeper, Flinn, Irrgang, and Weightman 1986). The muscles tend to move together; voluntary movement of one joint is not possible. For example, an attempt to move the affected elbow would result in movement of all joints of that arm (National Stroke Association 1986). The effects of central nervous system damage are also observed in the presence of clonus, a rhythmical contraction of a muscle. It occurs in response to a suddenly applied and then sustained stretch stimulus. This can be noted when the affected foot is bent sharply upward in a position of dorsiflexion with upward pressure maintained on the sole of the foot. Eventually, spasticity decreases and reflexes become less hyperactive. Spasticity of the affected limbs triggers a number of complications. In the absence of intervention, contractures will eventually form. In the presence of spasticity, predictable movement is not possible and balance is precarious when weight is placed on the paralyzed leg. If the foot is plantar flexed as a result of spasticity, gait is affected, inhibiting ambulation.

Interventions for impaired mobility are planned to prevent contractures, to promote healing of the pressure ulcer, and to increase mobility, thereby increasing independence. (See chapter 3, "Exercise and Activity," for further information on all procedures discussed for impaired mobility.) After a stroke, the leg generally retains more strength than the arm does. The leg extensors return earlier and remain stronger than the flexors, thus facilitating walking. The flexors dominate in the upper extremity. Function is seldom regained in the upper extremity if volitional movement is not present by the third week after the stroke. It is therefore often more beneficial to the client to work on skills for the strong arm, rather than investing too much time and energy in the arm that will not improve (Sine 1988). Mrs. Peters was admitted with an indwelling catheter in place. Seek a physician's order for removal as soon as possible to facilitate independent movement.

Nursing Diagnosis

Impaired physical mobility related to hemiplegia and spasticity of the left extremities, loss of endurance, and perceptual deficits related to right brain damage.

Nursing Interventions

Positioning Devices.

A variety of devices is available to help compensate for lack of muscle tone or to counteract spasticity. These may require a physician's order and need to be properly fitted.

❑ *Resting hand splint* — A resting hand splint maintains functional position of the hand and prevents contracture formation during the spastic stage. The thumb is slightly abducted, fingers and thumb slightly flexed, and wrist extended. Remove the splint for cleaning and to maintain cleanliness of the hand. There is lack of universal agreement on the use of splints.

❑ *Fingerspreader* — A fingerspreader maintains a relaxed position of the affected hand and prevents contractures of the fingers and wrist. The fingers are slightly abducted and the wrist is extended.

❑ *Slings* — The weight of a flaccid, unsupported arm can cause subluxation (partial dislocation) of the shoulder joint, a painful and serious complication associated with stroke. A hemisling worn during the flaccid stage supports the entire arm and hand close to the body, preventing injury. A shoulder girdle sling maintains the shoulder joint in normal position and alignment, leaving the elbow and forearm free to move. Slings are usually removed when the client is in bed. A sling must be applied correctly and checked periodically for adjustment. The use of slings is controversial. However, evidence exists to show that a sling does not promote contractures or retard the return of normal functioning (Shah et al. 1988).

❑ *Arm trough* — The arm trough protects and supports the affected upper extremity when the client is sitting in a wheelchair. The device attaches to the arm of the chair, supporting and maintaining proper position of the paralyzed arm.

❑ *Lapboard* — The lapboard attaches to both arms of the wheelchair, supporting the affected arm. It also provides a convenient surface for eating or working. Using a lapboard places the affected arm within the range of vision of the user, stimulating the client to use it more frequently. For this reason, the lapboard is better than the arm trough for the person with perceptual or visual deficits. Encourage Mrs. Peters to interact with her affected side by holding the left arm with her strong arm and to use the left arm when possible.

Supine Positioning:

❑ The key to positioning Mrs. Peters is to place her extremities "out of synergy" to avoid contracture formation.

❑ With Mrs. Peters in the supine position, place a small, firm pillow under her head and far enough under her shoulders to avoid flexion of the neck.

❑ The affected shoulder should be protracted (place a folded towel underneath) and abducted with the elbow, wrist, and fingers in extension, as these joints tend to assume a flexion synergy pattern. Do not place folded washcloths in the hand. This increases spasticity and flexion of the wrist and fingers, thereby contributing to contracture formation. The physician may order a resting splint, which, if properly fitted and applied, will maintain the fingers in the correct position.

❑ Position the lower extremity so the hip is protracted, with hip and knee extended, Figure 21–1. Avoid external rotation of the hip by using a trochanter roll if necessary. Pillows properly placed under the lower extremity prevent pressure under the heel and promote healing of the pressure ulcer. The use of a footboard may increase extensor spasticity. Plantar flexion contractures of

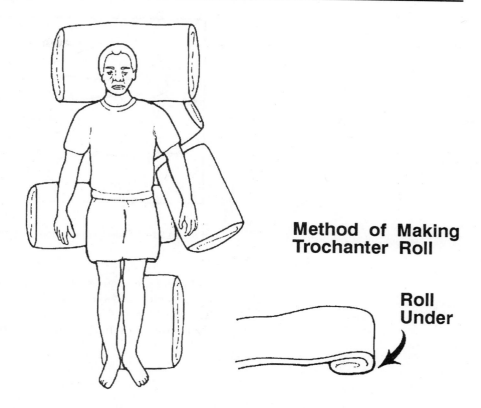

Method of Making Trochanter Roll

Roll Under

Figure 21-1 Alternate supine position with trochanter roll to prevent external rotation of the affected hip

the foot can be prevented by using a bed cradle to relieve pressure from the bed covers and by performing range-of-motion exercises at least twice a day.

Positioning on Unaffected Side:

❑ Use the same guidelines for positioning Mrs. Peters on her unaffected side. The affected shoulder is protracted, with elbow, wrist, and fingers extended.

❑ The affected hip is protracted and slightly flexed, with knee slightly flexed and foot in neutral position. When the pillows are correctly placed, the affected shoulder, elbow, and hand are elevated to the same height. The hip, knee, and foot on the affected side are also level. A small pillow placed between the rib cage and pelvic crest under the unaffected side offsets shortening of the trunk on the affected side, which is caused by the sag of the mattress, Figure 21-2.

Positioning on Affected Side:

❑ When positioning Mrs. Peters on her affected side, remember that lack of sensation on this side requires special care to avoid problems caused by pressure of body weight on the paralyzed limbs. Place the shoulder in protraction, with elbow and wrist extended.

❑ The hip is protracted, with hip and knee slightly flexed. The pillow between the rib cage and pelvic crest is not necessary as the sag of the mattress will lengthen the affected side of the body when Mrs. Peters is lying on that side.

Prone Position:

❑ Prone position is beneficial because it is the only position in which the hips

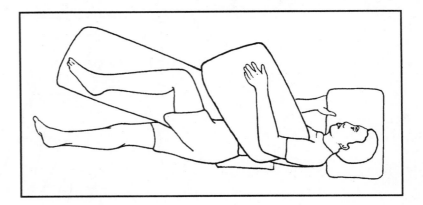

Figure 21–2 Side-lying position on right (unaffected) side

and knees are completely extended. Body alignment is adequate if the chin, sternal notch, and symphysis pubis form a straight line (Alexander 1990).
❑ The shoulders need to be supported and the feet should hang over the end of the mattress to avoid plantar flexion of the ankle, Figure 21–3.

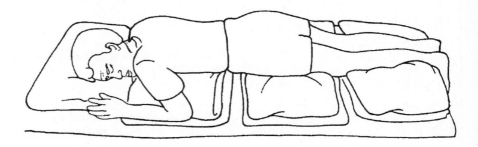

Figure 21–3 Prone position

❑ Three-quarter prone position is beneficial for the client who is unable to tolerate full prone position.

Range-of-Motion Exercises:

❑ Carry out passive range-of-motion exercises at least twice each day on the affected side. Instruct Mrs. Peters to do active exercises on her strong side. She can be taught to do self range of motion, thus exercising both sides at the same time (see chapter 3).

Bed Mobility:

❑ Review chapter 3 for bed mobility programs. Because Mrs. Peters has a pressure ulcer, support the left heel during bed movement to prevent friction between the heel and bed. There are alternative methods that may be used for the client with hemiplegia.

The reader is advised to investigate the literature to learn the Bobath approach (Bobath 1978). With this approach, care is planned to help the client regain awareness of the affected side. The objective is to improve function on the affected side so that the affected side and unaffected side will ultimately function together in harmony (Passarella and Gee 1987).

Transfer Techniques:

❑ Once Mrs. Peters is able to move herself in bed, self-transfer techniques can be initiated. Because of her spatial-perceptual deficits, safety is an issue to be considered with all procedures. Persons with left hemiplegia tend to lack judgment and impulse control. Denial of disability is also common. This combination of factors may lead Mrs. Peters to overestimate her abilities, causing her to fall.

❑ The use of a trapeze may be detrimental for the client who is attempting to regain mobility skills. This activity strengthens the biceps muscles but does little for the triceps. The triceps muscles are needed for such actions as pushing off of the bed or chair to come to a standing position.

❑ Follow the guidelines in chapter 3 for teaching Mrs. Peters a standing transfer. Continue to use the transfer belt until she demonstrates adequate ability to transfer independently.

❑ Remember that getting out of bed requires a number of activities and Mrs. Peters may never accomplish all of them. For example, unless she learns to walk unassisted, you will need to position the wheelchair next to the bed before she transfers out of bed into the wheelchair. Shoes are worn for transfers and Mrs. Peters may need assistance with this. Do not expect her to learn the entire transfer procedure at once. Break down the procedure into individual steps.

— First, teach her to get to a sitting position on the side of the bed. Apply the transfer belt and assist her in the transfer. When you judge her sitting balance to be adequate, proceed with the next step. (See chapter 3.) Mrs. Peters has suffered a loss of proprioception, which means she is unable to determine the position of her legs and feet without looking at them. Be sure that her feet are flat on the floor (with shoes on) and in alignment before standing.

— Teach her to push off the bed to come to a standing position. Allow her to stand, lengthening the time she stands, as she gains endurance and balance. Eventually decrease the amount of assistance you give until she can come to a standing position and remain standing without any assistance. This is a necessary preliminary measure for toilet transfers, which require a period of standing.

— When she is able to do this by herself, then teach her to pivot around to the chair, to place her hands on the chair arms, and to seat herself. Remember to instruct her to move toward her strong (right) side. Give simple, brief, verbal instructions for each step.

— Once she is seated, teach her to unlock the brakes on the wheelchair with her strong right hand. Removal of the footrest on the strong side allows Mrs. Peters to use her right foot to move the wheelchair, increasing her freedom. Before she attempts this, teach her to safely operate the wheelchair. Continue to apply the transfer belt as a precautionary measure until she has proven that she can safely complete the transfer procedure.

❑ When Mrs. Peters has conquered the basics, she can learn to get back into bed by reversing the procedure. Teach her to wheel up to the bed so she transfers toward her strong (right) side. The wheelchair will be facing in the opposite direction from what it was when she got out of bed. Be sure she understands the importance of locking both brakes on the wheelchair before attempting to stand.

❑ After she completes the transfer and is sitting on the edge of the bed, she may need assistance in removing her shoes and getting her left leg up onto the bed.

Toilet Transfer:

❑ The next step is learning to transfer to and from the toilet. Include Mr. Peters when teaching the self-transfer techniques. If discharge to home becomes possible, he will be ready and able to provide the assistance his wife needs. After Mrs. Peters is competent in these procedures, continue to increase her independence by teaching her to transfer in and out of the car with her husband's help.

Ambulation:

❑ Walking is a complex motor act that depends on several other skills before it can be mastered. Mrs. Peters must be able to carry out all previous mobility techniques competently before learning to walk. She needs sufficient strength and weight bearing in her right (unaffected) leg to compensate for the paralysis in her left leg. The ankle-foot orthosis compensates for weakness but does not improve muscle strength. Sufficient trunk stability and balance are required to remain upright and prevent falling while ambulating.

❑ She should be able to sit without back or arm support and to stand on both feet without falling. The unaffected arm must have enough strength to hold and bear down on a walking device.

❑ Mrs. Peters is going to be taught to use a broad-based quad cane and a three-point gait. This will provide her with stability and compensation for the loss of strength in her left leg. Eventually she may be able to change to a narrower-based cane that is less cumbersome.

❑ Put a gait belt on Mrs. Peters when she ambulates. Stand on her left side and a little behind her, with your right hand on the gait belt and your left hand in front of her left shoulder. Standing and moving with her on the affected side is not only safer, but helps her attend to that side of her body.

❑ Assume a wide base of support and coordinate your steps with hers. Mrs. Peters's gait pattern is affected by uneven step lengths, a lack of flexion in her left hip, and vaulting on the right. As you walk with her, monitor her progress and strive for continued improvement.

Collaboration: Interdisciplinary Team

❑ Passive stretching exercises are beneficial but should be done by or under the supervision of the physical therapist.

❑ The physical therapist may have suggestions for additional exercises to prepare Mrs. Peters for transferring and ambulation.

❑ An orthotist will need to be consulted if the physician orders an ankle-foot orthosis.

Outcome

Mrs. Peters will
❑ Maintain current levels of range of motion in all joints
❑ Remain free of contractures
❑ Transfer independently with only stand-by assistance
❑ Ambulate with the assistance of one person and a quad cane

Interdisciplinary Assessment _____

Nursing.

There is a stage 2, yellow pressure ulcer on the heel of the left foot, probably caused by friction between the heel and sheet as a result of the spasticity. The pressure ulcer risk assessment score is 8.

Nursing Diagnosis _____

Impaired skin integrity related to impaired mobility and spasticity.

Nursing Interventions _____

❑ Initiate the pressure ulcer prevention protocol immediately. Range-of-motion exercises and positioning procedures are already being implemented as interventions for impaired mobility.
❑ Apply heel and elbow protectors and place a water mattress on the bed. Clean the pressure ulcer with normal saline. Apply a transparent, semiocclusive dressing. Change as needed or according to facility protocol. Assess and record status of pressure ulcer daily.
(See chapter 4, "Maintaining Skin Integrity.")

Collaboration: Interdisciplinary Team _____

❑ Ask the dietician to complete a nutritional assessment.

Outcome _____

Mrs. Peters will
❑ Be free of any new pressure ulcers
❑ Have intact skin within three months

Interdisciplinary Assessment _____

Nursing and Dietary.

Mrs. Peters has lost four pounds since her stroke, although her weight is still within normal limits. Iron deficiency anemia is a secondary admission diagnosis; hemoglobin is 11 g/dl and hematocrit is 36 percent. All other laboratory findings are within normal range.

Mrs. Peters has no problems with swallowing. She eats poorly due to fatigue and a dislike of being fed. It takes her a long time to complete a meal and she has a tendency to pocket food on the left side of her mouth. Mrs. Peters frequently leaves food on her tray because of the impaired vision on the left side. She is on a 2-gram sodium diet.

Nursing Diagnosis _____

Alterations in nutrition, less than body requirements, related to anorexia.

Nursing Interventions

❑ See section of this chapter under self-care deficit, eating.
❑ Arrange Mrs. Peters's schedule so she can have a rest period before meals to avoid fatigue.
❑ Weigh weekly, until appetite has improved.
❑ The physician has ordered an iron supplement to correct the anemia.

Collaboration: Interdisciplinary Team

❑ The dietician will meet with Mrs. Peters to discuss food choices that are allowed on the low-sodium diet.

Outcome

Mrs. Peters will
❑ Maintain weight within normal limits
❑ Attain normal hemoglobin and hematocrit levels

Interdisciplinary Assessment

Nursing and Occupational Therapy.

At the time of admission, Mrs. Peters required almost complete assistance with all activities of daily living. She was convinced that having a stroke meant she would be an invalid the rest of her life. Her husband encouraged her helplessness by doing everything for her and expecting the staff to do the same. Mrs. Peters's performance during the functional assessment indicated she had potential for increasing abilities. (See chapter 2, "The Restorative Nursing Process.") Mrs. Peters has always been an independent, active person. With instruction and encouragement, it is highly probable that she will succeed in maximizing her potential. Her husband is willing to cooperate, since he is anxious for his wife to return home. Assessment findings include the presence of agnosia, apraxia, left homonymous hemianopsia, and figure-ground impairment.

Nursing Diagnosis

Self-care deficits (total) related to hemiplegia of left arm and spatial-perceptual alterations.

Nursing Interventions

❑ Relearning activities of daily living is usually directed toward learning to carry out tasks one handed with the unaffected hand. If some neurological recovery has occurred, the affected upper extremity can be used to stabilize objects. With additional recovery, the extremity can be used for gross motor skills that require little dexterity or coordination. Relearning should begin quickly; to wait for recovery of the affected arm is unwise as it may not recover at all. In the meantime, the client is sinking into acceptance of helplessness and diminishing self-worth.
❑ A sense of normalcy helps reestablish motivation for relearning activities of daily living. This requires a structured routine in which the client gets up in

the morning, is fully clothed, and remains up except for intermittent rest periods if necessary. Meals are eaten at the table in a dining area rather than in bed.

❑ When planning interventions, consider the spatial-perceptual deficits identified on the assessment. Remember that all activities of daily living consist of many small tasks. Mrs. Peters may never be able to complete all the steps of an activity.

❑ Plan small goals, concentrating on what she can learn at the present time. As each step is accomplished, revise the goal to include another step of the procedure. Refer to the functional assessment when establishing goals and interventions for self-care deficits. Begin with the simplest steps and progress to the more complicated ones. Remember that Mrs. Peters may never accomplish every step in a task. The goal is optimal potential, whatever it may be for Mrs. Peters.

Eating:

❑ Position Mrs. Peters so her trunk is erect with head in midline and slightly flexed. Place her chair close enough to the table to facilitate hand-to-mouth movements. A quiet room without distractions helps Mrs. Peters focus on the task at hand. Give verbal cues and feedback as you help her, but avoid unnecessary conversation and movements that may interrupt her attention span. Sit on her right side and take your time.

❑ Prepare the items on the tray for Mrs. Peters before she starts eating. She can then use her attention and energies for hand-to-mouth actions. Use hand-over-hand techniques if necessary. For example, place a glass in her hand with your hand over hers. Then lift it to her mouth and ask her to drink, providing only the assistance that she really needs. Continue with these procedures until Mrs. Peters is able to eat her meal by herself.

❑ Remind her to concentrate on keeping the food in the middle and the right side of her mouth. This will avoid pocketing of food on the weak, left side. When Mrs. Peters finishes eating, take her to her room and teach her to place her right index finger in her left cheek to remove any food that is remaining in her mouth. Help her with oral hygiene. Aspiration can occur during sleep from food left in the mouth.

❑ To compensate for the hemianopsia, teach her to scan by turning her head to the left so that side of her tray will be within her line of vision.

❑ Because of the agnosia, she does not recognize eating utensils; as a result of the apraxia, she is unable to use them. Place the appropriate utensil in her hand and say, "This is your fork. Please eat your dinner with it." She may need hand-over-hand assistance at first. Once she is successful in self-feeding, she can learn more difficult tasks associated with eating.

—*Spreading bread.* Use soft butter or other spread and place the slice of bread on a plate. Ask Mrs. Peters to pick up the knife and place the butter on the bread. Have her place her index finger on the side of the blade while she holds the knife with her thumb, middle, and ring finger. Her little finger is used to stabilize the bread.

—*Cutting food.* To cut meat with a knife, ask Mrs. Peters to place the tip of the knife in the meat, press down, lower the blade, and use a rocking motion to cut. As one section is cut, have her place the tip of the blade in another section of meat and repeat until a bite-size piece is separated.

—Fruits, vegetables, and tender meats can be cut with a fork. Tell Mrs. Peters to grasp the handle with the eating surface facing her so the fork is against the food. Have her insert the fork tip into the food, with her index finger on the top tine, and use a rocking motion to cut the food. A rocker knife facilitates cutting of food.

— *Opening milk cartons.* Place the carton so the opening side is facing Mrs. Peters. Instruct her to use her thumb to bend each flap back while she holds the carton in the palm of her hand with her other fingers. Then have her bend both flaps back together. Now tell her to push the outer edges together to form the spout. An alternate method is to place the carton of milk between her knees to stabilize it.

— There are a variety of adaptive devices available to simplify eating. A plate guard prevents spills and a heavy bottom cup will not tip over. A combination fork and spoon eliminate the need to change utensils while eating. Place dycem or another nonslip product under the plate or tray for stability.

Bathing:

❏ Have Mrs. Peters sit in a chair in the tub or shower. Self-bathing begins by giving the washcloth to Mrs. Peters and asking her to wash her face. Then progress to the chest and affected arm. Continue through all the steps she is able to complete. Unless she regains considerable use of her left arm, she will not be able to wash her right arm. Whether she will be able to wash her lower extremities depends on whether she can maintain her balance while bending forward.

❏ Soap on a rope simplifies bathing. A wash mitt is easier to manipulate than a washcloth and a long-handled brush allows Mrs. Peters to extend her reach. Either spray or roll-on deodorant can be applied with her right hand under both arms. Complete the steps Mrs. Peters cannot do, giving verbal praise for her accomplishments.

Hair Care, Makeup, and Nail Care:

❏ Place Mrs. Peters in front of a mirror, give her the comb or brush, and ask her to comb (brush) her hair. She may have trouble reaching all the areas without help. Remember that because of the apraxia and agnosia, she may not know what the comb or brush is for and how it is used. If verbal cues are not successful, use a hand-over-hand technique.

❏ Makeup, particularly lipstick, is very difficult to apply in the presence of perceptual deficits. It may be better to continue to do this for Mrs. Peters until she has mastered some of the simpler skills.

❏ Mrs. Peters can use her strong hand to place her left forearm and hand on a stable surface for nail care. Instruct her to use her right hand to file the nails on her left hand. She can also apply nail polish with some practice. You will have to do this on her right hand. Nail brushes with suction cups that attach to the sink are available for scrubbing the nails.

Oral Care:

❏ Arrange the needed items on the work surface. This task can be completed at the sink while Mrs. Peters is seated in the wheelchair or in her room with the items laid out on table or lapboard.

❏ Instruct Mrs. Peters to pick up the toothpaste with her right hand, using her thumb and index finger to unscrew the cap. Then have her squeeze paste onto the brush, set the paste down, and pick up the brush.

❏ Remind her to brush on the affected side of her mouth. Have her rinse the brush and her mouth, spitting the water out. If Mrs. Peters had dentures, she would need a denture brush that attaches to the sink with suction. This enables the user to clean the dentures by moving them against the brush.

Dressing:

❏ Dressing independently requires balance, adequate range of motion, endurance, and time. Wait with the dressing procedure until Mrs. Peters has mastered some of the other self-care activities. In the meantime, give her choices of clothing and allow her to do what she can. Ask Mr. Peters to bring in clothing that is washable, loose-fitting, and easily fastened in front. Large buttons are easier to manipulate than small ones. Button hooks can facilitate this task. Buttons on blouse sleeves can be resewn with elastic thread to eliminate the need for buttoning. Rings added to zipper tabs make them easier to grasp. Lay out items in the order they are put on. Labels help Mrs. Peters distinguish between inside and outside of clothing. Directions are given here in the order in which clothing is usually put on. For most clients, it is better to start a dressing program with one upper body item at a time.

Procedure: Dressing

Putting On Underwear and Slacks

1. Have Mrs. Peters put on her underpants while she is still in bed. Ask her to sit up in bed and use her right hand to place the left leg opening up over her left foot.
2. Have her repeat this step with the right foot and then move the underpants up both legs as far as she can. Ask her to lie back down and work the underpants up over her hips by bending the right knee and hip, pushing the strong foot against the bed to raise her hips.
3. Instruct Mrs. Peters to reverse the procedure to remove the underpants.
4. The same procedure is used for putting on slacks. If Mrs. Peters regains adequate balance, she can put on these items while sitting on the edge of the bed.

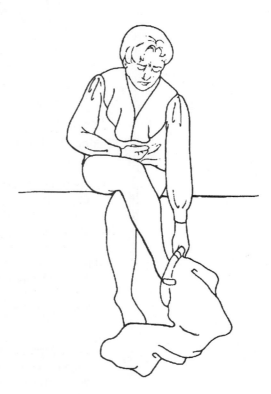

Figure 21–4 Pull left slacks leg over the weak foot.

5. Tell her to use her right hand to grasp her left leg under the knee, lift it, and cross it over the right leg. Have her grasp the center front of the waistband, bring the slacks down toward her left foot, and then pull the slack leg up over her foot, Figure 21–4. Now tell her to place her left foot back on the floor and put her right foot into the other slack leg, pulling the slacks up over her knees.

6. You can help Mrs. Peters to stand to finish pulling her slacks up.

7. If Mrs. Peters has difficulty standing, have her lie down. Ask her to bend her strong knee and hip, pushing the strong foot against the bed to raise her hips and pull pants up over hips, Figure 21–5.

8. The pants can be fastened while she is lying down.

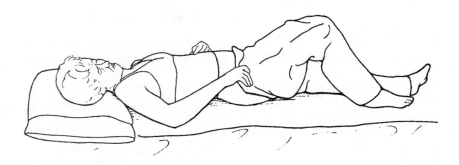

Figure 21–5 Alternate method for client with unstable balance

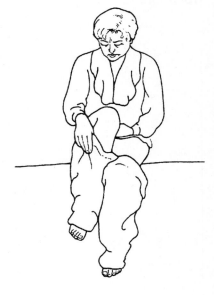

Figure 21–6 Use right arm to push slacks off the right leg.

Taking Off Slacks

1. Help Mrs. Peters stand with her right leg against the bed, using her right arm to pull the slacks down over her hips.

2. Then tell her to sit on the side of the bed and use her right arm to push her slacks off the right leg, Figure 21–6.

3. Now have her cross her left leg over her right one and pull the slacks off the left leg.

   Note: This procedure requires adequate balance.

Putting On a Bra

1. Have Mrs. Peters place the bra around her waist with the back in front and then fasten the hooks, Figure 21–7. Now tell her to turn the bra around into position, with her right hand.

2. Then instruct her to place her left hand inside the left strap and pull the strap up her left arm, Figure 21–8. Next, have her insert her right hand in the right

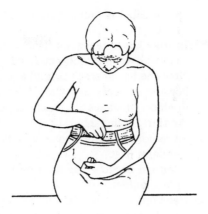

Figure 21–7 Fasten bra with the back of the bra in front.

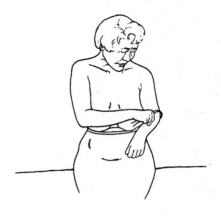

Figure 21–8 Pull straps up the left arm.

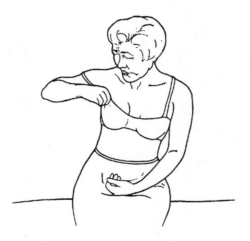

Figure 21–9 Pull straps up the right arm.

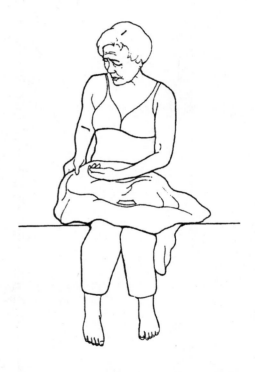

Figure 21–10 Begin with the shirt lying on the lap.

strap, pull the strap up her arm to the shoulder, and then push the left strap up arm to the shoulder and adjust for fit, Figure 21–9.

3. Adjust this procedure for putting on a front-closing bra. To remove the bra, reverse the procedure.

Putting On and Taking Off a Button-Front Dress, Shirt, or Jacket_____

1. Place the shirt on Mrs. Peters's lap. Have her open the front so the inside is

up, the label is facing her, and the collar or neck is away from her, Figure 21–10.

2. Instruct her to place her hand in the left armhole. Then tell her to bring the sleeve up over her left hand and arm, up to her shoulder.

3. Now she has to reach behind and place her right hand in the sleeve, moving her arm as necessary. Once the sleeve is in place, she can arrange the shirt in place. Mistakes are less likely if she begins buttoning from the bottom of the shirt, Figure 21–11.

4. To remove the shirt, have Mrs. Peters reverse the procedure, removing her right arm first.

5. Then tell her to grasp the front edge of the shirt and pull it out and off the right shoulder.

6. Have her work her right arm out of the sleeve and then use her right arm to pull the left sleeve off her left arm, Figure 21–12.

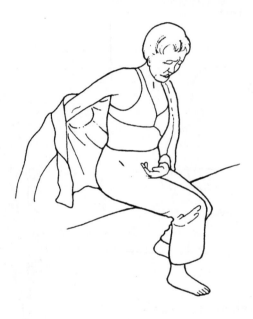

Figure 21–11 Reach behind and place the right hand and arm in the sleeve.

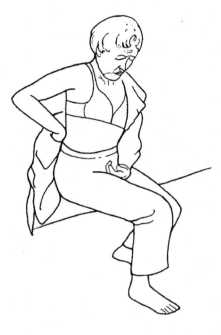

Figure 21–12 Work the right arm out of the sleeve.

Slipover Blouse or Dress

1. Place the shirt on Mrs. Peters's lap with the back up and the neck away from her. The label is facing down.

2. Tell her to gather up the back of the shirt with her right hand, exposing the left armhole. Now have her use her right hand to place her left hand in the armhole, bringing the shirt midway up her forearm. Then tell her to put her right hand in the other armhole up to her elbow.

3. Instruct Mrs. Peters to gather up the back of the shirt, bring it up toward her shoulders and place her head through the neck of the shirt. Now she can use her right hand to adjust the fit.

4. To remove the shirt, tell her to reverse the procedure, removing her right arm first.

Socks

1. Tell Mrs. Peters to use her right hand to lift her weak leg over her strong (right) leg. Have her use her right hand to pull the sock up over her weak foot, Figure 21–13.

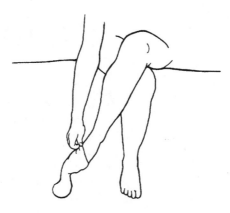

Figure 21–13 Use the right hand to lift the weak (left) leg over the right leg.

2. Then tell her to place her left leg back in position with the foot on the floor and to repeat the procedure with her strong leg, crossing it over the left leg, pulling the sock onto her right foot. To remove the sock, tell her to reverse the procedure.
3. Pantyhose are more difficult to put on and require an alteration in the procedure. Tell Mrs Peters to bring the hose up over the first foot and leave the second foot on the floor while working the hose up over the right foot. Then have her gather up the hose in the middle and work them up over her legs to her hips. She will have to stand to finish bringing the hose up over her hips.
4. Stocking aids are available for putting on nylon hosiery and are helpful for people who cannot bend over far enough to reach the foot.

Shoes

1. The procedure for putting on shoes is essentially the same as for putting on socks. Tell Mrs. Peters to cross the left leg over the right leg and to place the shoe on the left foot. Then have her slip her right leg into the right shoe while it is on the floor.
2. Mrs. Peters has an ankle-foot orthosis on her left shoe. Instruct her to handle the shoe by the top of the brace. After her foot is in the shoe, have her buckle the calf strap on the brace if she is able.
3. For shoes with tongues, sew the tongue to the top of the shoe at one side to prevent it from doubling under. Placing a footstool under the affected foot may make it easier to reach. Long-handled shoehorns also reduce the need to bend so far forward. If slip-on shoes are not practical, consider elastic laces or wrap-a-lace, which enables the client to tie and untie with one hand.

Collaboration: Interdisciplinary Team

❑ The occupational therapist may need to further assess the severity of Mrs. Peters's spatial-perceptual alterations.

Outcome

It may be unwise to set long-range goals for the nursing diagnosis of self-care deficit. While an optimistic approach is helpful, a tendency to become overly ambitious may be self-defeating. Set small goals and continue to increase these until Mrs. Peters reaches her maximal performance. Then establish maintenance goals to ensure that she does not lose these abilities. Discharge planning involves an evaluation of self-care skills, the extent to which her husband can and will provide assistance, the accessibility of their home, and the availability of community resources.

Dressing oneself, especially the lower body, requires considerable endurance, balance, and range of motion. Encourage Mrs. Peters to do as much as she can, but provide assistance when necessary.

Interdisciplinary Assessment

Nursing.

The indwelling catheter was removed two days after admission. Mrs. Peters expresses the need to void, but wets before assistance is provided.

Nursing Diagnosis

Alterations in bladder elimination (urge incontinence) related to stroke and recent removal of indwelling catheter.

Nursing Interventions

❑ Complete a bladder training assessment. (See chapter 7, "Alterations in Bladder Elimination.") Assessment results will determine further planning. Regardless of the method used, the major objective is to avoid incontinence, thereby preventing skin breakdown and enhancing Mrs. Peters's self-esteem.
❑ The success of the program is interdependent on Mrs. Peters's mobility skills. As she becomes more skillful in transferring to the toilet or commode, either with or without assistance, the greater her chances for avoiding incontinence.
❑ In the meantime, maintain adequate fluid intake and provide meticulous skin care when she is incontinent. Instruct staff to toilet Mrs. Peters promptly when she indicates the need to void.

Outcome

Mrs. Peters will
❑ Remain continent

Interdisciplinary Assessment

Nursing and Social Services.

Mrs. Peters has always been an active person, taking pride in her ability to be successfully involved in many projects simultaneously. She and Mr. Peters shared the responsibility for household tasks throughout their marriage. She has always enjoyed her role as Mrs. Peters, sharing many mutually enjoyable activities with her husband.

She displays the characteristic behavioral style of a person with right brain damage — denial of disability, overestimation of abilities, quick, and impulsive. Although her husband is very protective, he is eager to do whatever is necessary to facilitate Mrs. Peters's recovery.

Nursing Diagnosis

Coping: Potential for family growth related to husband's expressed desire to learn how to assist Mrs. Peters to reach her optimal level of functioning and well-being.

Nursing Interventions

- ❑ Invite and encourage both Mr. and Mrs. Peters to attend the care plan conference so they will have the opportunity to discuss her care, treatment, and progress.
- ❑ Invite Mr. Peters to observe and learn assistive techniques used by the staff for mobility and self-care.
- ❑ Discuss with Mrs. Peters her perceptions of the current situation. Discuss with her and Mr. Peters their thoughts for the future and how they perceive their roles if Mrs. Peters is discharged. Provide an open environment for Mrs. Peters to express concerns about sexuality and her feelings about herself as a woman. Establish an atmosphere conducive to the discussion of sexual issues by both her and her husband.
- ❑ Give Mrs. Peters opportunities to make decisions regarding her care and routine. Encourage Mr. Peters to discuss events of home and community with her.

Talk with Mr. Peters about taking his wife out for rides in the car. As her transfer abilities improve, encourage longer outings, then overnights, as rehearsals for possible discharge. Discuss with Mr. Peters how he can best help his wife regain some independence without compromising her safety.

Collaboration: Interdisciplinary Team

- ❑ The social worker will meet regularly with both Mr. and Mrs. Peters and will begin arrangements for discharge when it is appropriate.
- ❑ Refer Mr. Peters to a support group, if an appropriate one is available, or introduce him to a spouse who is successfully coping with a similar situation. Since both Mr. and Mrs. Peters have indicated strong spiritual beliefs, ask the chaplain to visit with them. This can be an important additional source of support and strength for them both.
- ❑ Provide opportunities for Mrs. Peters to participate in activities that she finds satisfying. These need to be challenging enough to interest her without causing

her frustration. Invite her husband to join her in some of the activities when possible.

❑ Ask the occupational therapist and physical therapist to talk with Mr. Peters to evaluate his need for additional instructions in assisting with Mrs. Peters's care when she returns home.

Outcome

Mr. Peters will

❑ Participate in the care plan conference and express willingness to assist in implementation of the plan.

❑ Express positive feelings regarding his wife's progress.

❑ Develop realistic plans with his wife for adapting to the role changes experienced by them both.

TABLE 21–2	Wheelchair Accessibility in the Home

Steps

❑ Maximum height of six inches, minimum width of thirty inches, minimum depth of fourteen inches

Ramps

❑ For self-propelling, ratio of eight inches length per one inch of height; made of nonskid material that does not become slippery when wet

Doors

❑ Twenty-nine inches minimum width; thirty-two inches needed for self-propelling to allow room for user's hands on wheels

❑ To widen door for extrawide wheelchair: remove door frame molding or change to offset door hinges or swing-free hinges. These move door out of opening as they swing, providing two more inches of width.

❑ A width reducer for wheelchair is operated by a crank that narrows the chair by squeezing hips three to four inches just long enough to get through door.

❑ Door thresholds can be removed and replaced with strip of polyethylene tubing.

❑ Loop handle installed on pull side eases door opening. Add-on lever handles are available for doors.

❑ Kick plates attached to bottom of door prevent marring by wheels.

Windows

❑ Windowsills no higher than thirty-six inches are necessary for wheelchair viewing.

Floors

❑ Plastic runners placed over thick carpeting facilitate wheelchair movement. Remove loose rugs, cords, and wires from floors.

Furniture

❑ Most chairs are about fifteen inches high. A height of nineteen to twenty inches is easier to get out of. Blocks can be placed under the legs of sturdy chairs. Firm cushions can be placed on the seat.

❑ Place furniture around periphery of room, removing all unnecessary objects from tables.

Continues

Bedroom

❑ Twenty-two inches is best height for bed. Stabilize by placing one side against wall. Stable, firm mattress eases bed movement.

❑ Armless chair on wheels (with brakes) can be used for dressing and for moving from bedroom to bathroom.

❑ Closet rods should be thirty-six inches from floor.

Bathroom

❑ Add raised toilet seat for height of nineteen inches. Install wall handrail at forty-five-degree angle and thirty-three to thirty-five inches long, with lower part of bar placed two inches behind leading edge of toilet. If there is no wall beside the toilet, a right angle handrail can be fastened to floor and wall to extend six inches in front of toilet.

❑ Recommended sink height is twenty-four inches from floor with space underneath for wheelchair. Bottom of mirror should be thirty-six inches from floor.

❑ Place grab bars on wall next to tub or attach guard rail to tub. Use tub seat nineteen inches high. Place slip-proof mats on tub floor.

❑ Attach one-handed shower hose.

❑ Use unbreakable shower doors.

Kitchen

❑ Use lapboard for wheelchair or cart on wheels.

COMMENTS

A stroke abruptly disrupts one's life and is a devastating experience for the client as well as the family. The losses associated with stroke must be mourned by both the survivor and the loved ones. During this grieving process, a number of stages are worked through, which, if successfully resolved, result in the ability to cope with the situation. The client and family adapt and live with the changes brought about by the stroke. Anger, frustration, guilt, and resentment are all natural and common feelings. These feelings must be acknowledged so that healing can take place.

Mr. and Mrs. Peters communicate effectively with each other and the staff, are eager to learn, and look forward to their future life together. This would indicate they are successfully coping. Listen to their comments to pick up any clues of distress from either of them. It is not uncommon for persons who have had a stroke to become depressed. Monitor Mrs. Peters for symptoms of anxiety, insomnia, loss of appetite, and loss of energy.

In preparing for discharge, discuss with Mr. Peters the role of the caregiver. It is important that he plan for regular respite from his responsibilities to avoid caregiver burnout. The local Family Service Agency may provide a homemaker a few hours a week to assist with some of the household chores. While the evidence suggests they are coping well in the nursing home, a number of adjustments will have to be made again when Mrs. Peters returns home.

Mr. and Mrs. Peters have many strengths and a mutually satisfying marital relationship. With appropriate education, counseling, and support, it is highly probable they will function well at home, enabling them to enjoy the next phase of their life together.

QUESTIONS AND DISCUSSION

1. What examples of sensory-perceptual-spatial deficits have you observed in clients who have had a stroke?
2. What other interventions would be appropriate for a client with the deficits described in this chapter?

3. Which community resources will Mrs. Peters require when she returns home?
4. How would you approach the subject of sexuality with Mr. and Mrs. Peters?
5. What suggestions would you give Mr. Peters so that he will avoid overprotecting his wife when she returns home?
6. Are there additional safety issues concerning Mrs. Peters's behavior that were not addressed in the case study?
7. What additional interventions by the interdisciplinary health care team would be beneficial to Mrs. Peters?

REFERENCES

Adkins, E.R.H. 1991. Nursing Care of Clients with Impaired Communication. *Rehabilitation Nursing* 16(2): 74–76.

Alexander, T.T. 1990. In C.E. Carlson, W.P. Griggs, and R.B. King, eds. *Rehabilitation Nursing Procedures Manual*. Rockville, MD: Aspen Publishers, Inc.

Bobath, B. 1978. *Adult Hemiplegia: Evaluation and Treatment*. 2d ed. London: Heinemann Medical.

Chipps, E., N. Clanin, and V. Campbell. 1992. *Neurologic Disorders*. St. Louis: Mosby-Year Book, Inc.

Loeper, J.M., N.A. Flinn, S.J. Irrgang, and M.M. Weightman. 1986. *Therapeutic Positioning and Skin Care*. Minneapolis: Sister Kenny Institute.

Mitiguy, J. 1991. The Brain under Attack. *Headlines* 2(3): 2.

Passarella, P. and Z. Gee. 1987. Starting Right after Stroke. *American Journal of Nursing* 87(6): 802–7.

Shah, M., R. Avidan, and R.D. Sine. 1988. In R.D. Sine, S.E. Liss, R.E. Roush, J.D. Holcomb, and G. Wilson, eds. *Basic Rehabilitation Techniques*. Rockville, MD: Aspen Publishers, Inc.

Sine, R.D. 1988. In R.D. Sine, S.E. Liss, R.E. Roush, J.D. Holcomb, and G. Wilson, eds. *Basic Rehabilitation Techniques*. Rockville, MD: Aspen Publishers, Inc.

Staff. 1989. *Stroke: Reducing Your Risk*. National Stroke Association.

Staff. 1986. *The Road Ahead: A Stroke Recovery Guide*. Denver: The National Stroke Association.

Staff. 1986. *Stroke: Why Do They Behave That Way?* Dallas: American Heart Association.

Staff. 1991. Stopping Stroke. *American Heart News* 8(2).

Swearingen, P.L. 1992. *Pocket Guide to Medical-Surgical Nursing*. St. Louis: Mosby-Year Book, Inc.

Tikare, S.K. 1990. Thalamic Pain — An Uncommon Complication with Stroke. *Be Stroke Smart* 7(1): 9, 11.

SUGGESTED READINGS

Behren, R.V. 1990. After the Stroke — Adult Day Care. *Be Stroke Smart* 7(2): 7, 14.

Brannon, M. 1989. A Hands-On Rehab Technique That Really Works. *RN* 52(11): 65–67.

Butler, M.E. 1985. Spasticity: A Consideration in Rehabilitation of the Elderly. *Rehabilitation Nursing* 10(3): 14–15.

Frye-Pierson, J. and J.F. Toole. 1987. *Stroke*. New York: Raven Press.

A Restorative Approach to Caring for the Client with Spinal Cord Injury

---

OBJECTIVES

- ❏ Describe the differences between complete and incomplete spinal cord injury.
- ❏ Identify the nursing diagnoses commonly associated with spinal cord injury.
- ❏ Describe nursing interventions that will prevent the onset of complications associated with spinal cord injury.
- ❏ Discuss the psychosocial implications of spinal cord injury.
- ❏ Describe how the level of injury affects activities of daily living.
- ❏ Recognize the causes and symptoms of autonomic dysreflexia.
- ❏ Describe the immediate nursing care following the onset of autonomic dysreflexia.
- ❏ Identify the role of the interdisciplinary health care team in the management of the client with spinal cord injury.

DESCRIPTION OF THE PROBLEM

Spinal cord injury is a catastrophic event, disrupting all aspects of the individual's previous life-style. Fifteen thousand to 20,000 persons each year suffer a spinal cord injury (Chipps, Clanin, and Campbell 1992). Five percent of these are over the age of sixty. Falls are the primary cause of injury for this age group, with vehicular accidents the major cause within all age groups (Gokbudak 1985). Unlike the slow-onset disability caused by chronic illness, the person with spinal cord injury has not had time to adapt and compensate to a situation that will be lifelong.

The elderly person with spinal cord injury is more likely to require admission to a long-term-care facility than is a younger person. The combined effects of the injury, the aging process, and inadequate support systems create a situation that often precludes independent living. The client may be transferred to the nursing home from the rehabilitation center, from the hospital, or after a trial period of living at home.

Classifications and Types of Spinal Cord Injuries

There are three classifications of spinal cord injuries. A concussion of the spinal cord can occur with or without damage to the vertebra. It is manifested by generalized paralysis with usually complete recovery in twenty-four hours. A contusion results from a blow to the spinal cord, producing hemorrhage and swelling within the cord. The symptoms depend on the severity of the contusion. Laceration causes edema and hemorrhage, with interruption of the spinal cord.

There are two types of spinal cord injury; complete and incomplete. The outcome depends on the level of injury and the degree of completeness. Bowel, bladder, and sexual functions are affected to some degree in all spinal cord injuries, because these activities are controlled by the lower level of the spinal cord. A complete spinal cord injury occurs when there is complete interruption of ascending and descending tracts below the level of lesion. This results in total paralysis and loss of sensation. There is no measurable neurological function more than three segments below the level of injury. Most complete injuries occur at the lower level of the spinal cord.

There are several types of incomplete injury. These are categorized according to the area of damage. With these injuries, some sensation is retained below the level of injury and some function may be recovered. However, this is difficult to predict. Most incomplete injuries are the result of damage to the cervical area.

Spinal Shock

The quality of care rendered immediately after injury is critical in terms of stabilizing the client's condition and preserving as much function as possible. Within thirty to sixty minutes after injury, spinal shock occurs and the body shuts down normal activities below the level of injury. There is a flaccid paralysis of the muscles; muscle tone and reflex activity are absent. An indwelling catheter is usually inserted to compensate for the client's inability to void. Paralytic ileus is common and resolves as the spinal shock subsides. This condition may last for just a few hours or from several days to several months (Chipps et al. 1992).

Immediate Postinjury Care

After assessing the extent of neurological and orthopedic injury, healing is initiated by reducing pressure on the spinal cord. How this is accomplished depends on the level and extent of injury to the spinal cord and vertebra. Surgery may be necessary to decompress the spinal cord at the site of injury. There are various types of jackets, braces, collars, and traction available to immobilize the involved part of the body. A halo frame is frequently used for cervical injuries. This is a steel ring that fits around the head, secured with two occipital and two temporal screws. Steel bars connect the ring to a plastic or plaster vest. The apparatus remains in place for three or four months but does not restrict general mobility.

Sequelae of Spinal Cord Injury

Spastic paralysis occurs in injuries at or above the T12 level. Messages from the brain get only as far as the injury. Messages from the body below the injury also stop at the site of injury. This interruption results in a loop of nerve impulses, causing spasticity with intensified muscle tone and heightened reflex activity. Spasticity is an exaggerated reaction to a stimulus below the level of injury. Injury at or below T12 is more accurately described as injury to the cauda equina rather than as spinal cord injury. All reflex activity is absent, with complete interruption of all messages. These injuries result in flaccid paralysis with total loss of muscle tone and atrophy of the leg muscles. Pain is experienced by most individuals with spinal cord injury. Initially, the client may complain of intense, sharp pain, which disappears in a few weeks. Mechanical pain is sharp, intermittent, and localized. This may be an indication of an underlying neurological or orthopedic process at the site of injury and requires medical investigation. Phantom sensations or spinal cord dysesthesia are experienced by 95 percent of people with spinal cord injuries. These sensations are described as burning, painful, tickling, creeping, itching, and shivering. They begin distally and spread up the lower extremities, stopping at the hips. Medication is generally not effective in relieving these feelings. As time goes on, the phantom sensations usually diminish (Phillips, Ozer, Axelson, and Chizick 1987).

A number of emotional responses occur after the injury. The degree of adaptation is influenced by the attitudes and abilities of the health care staff, the client's personality, family support system, and availability of community and financial resources. The client experiences shock and panic in the first few weeks following injury. For the next three or four months, the individual may appear indifferent, denying the situation and the implications of injury. Eventually, anger occurs as the person acknowledges the reality of what has happened. Depression follows acknowledgement and may last as long as several months. As these emotions are worked through and resolved, adaptation takes place. Self-esteem is regained and the individual is ready to get on with life (Harmarville 1983).

Long-Term Care

The long-term care of the client with spinal cord injury is based on prevention of complications, maintaining the existing abilities of the client, and assisting the client to create a life of quality and meaning. The care plan is therefore directed toward maintaining skin integrity, managing bowel and bladder functions, preventing respiratory and urinary tract infections, and implementation of an exercise program. Psychosocial care is ongoing with nursing intervention dependent on the needs of the particular client.

CASE STUDY

Mrs. Jackson, seventy-seven years old, fell down the stairs as she was leaving her apartment. The neighbor called an ambulance and Mrs. Jackson was transported to the hospital. The emergency room examination revealed a T7 spinal cord injury. She was admitted to the hospital and after the acute phase of the injury was resolved, was transferred to a regional rehabilitation center where she regained some functional abilities.

Previous to injury, Mrs. Jackson was independent, drove her own car, was active in her church, and frequently took over the care of her grandchildren. Her health history is uneventful. She is moderately obese and has had generalized osteoarthritis for several years. On days when her arthritis was particularly bothersome, she used a cane to get around. Mrs. Jackson was divorced several years ago and since that time has lived alone in an upstairs apartment. After discharge from the rehabilitation center, she went to live with her daughter. The daughter is a single parent and works to support her three children. She is no longer able to provide the care that Mrs. Jackson needs. The demands of three young children, a job, and household management leave the daughter with little time and energy for her mother's care. Mrs. Jackson is not happy about moving to the nursing home but realizes that it is the only recourse.

Strengths

- ❏ Physical health adequate
- ❏ Free of cognitive impairment
- ❏ Loving daughter and grandchildren
- ❏ Has successfully dealt with many crises in her life
- ❏ Strong spiritual beliefs and ties with church

Interdisciplinary Assessment

Nursing, Physical Therapy, Occupational Therapy.

Mrs. Jackson is a paraplegic as a result of the T7 injury. Before her accident, she walked up and down the steps of her apartment building at least twice each day. This was the extent of her exercise, other than occasional walks. She indicates that the arthritis prevented her from being as active as she would have liked to have been. During her rehabilitation, Mrs. Jackson learned mobility skills but after discharge, spent most of her day in a chair.

Physical activity is an essential component of Mrs. Jackson's care. She is at high risk for all complications associated with immobility. Exercise reduces the risk of these complications and increases general health and well-being. Strengthening upper body muscles will help compensate for the loss of function in the lower extremities. For Mrs. Jackson, exercise will alleviate the pain and stiffness associated with arthritis and will help prevent weight gain. Persons with T7 spinal cord injuries usually have normal upper extremity muscle function and partial to good trunk stability.

Nursing Diagnosis

Impaired physical mobility related to paralysis, spasticity, osteoarthritis, and obesity.

Nursing Interventions

- ❏ Mrs. Jackson's physician has ordered support stockings to decrease the risk of deep vein thrombosis due to immobility of her legs. Elevate her legs periodically and inspect them for asymmetry and other indications of thrombosis. Measure and document the circumference of her feet, ankles, calves, and thighs weekly.
- ❏ Teach Mrs. Jackson bed mobility skills. This activity not only provides exercise but decreases the risk of pressure-ulcer formation. A trapeze applied

to the bed frame will facilitate her ability to move herself in bed, thereby alleviating pressure on the buttocks.

❏ Remember that Mrs. Jackson has a spastic paralysis. Muscle spasms, causing flexion or extension of the lower extremities, increase the risk for injury during mobility procedures.

❏ Participation in wheelchair exercises can benefit her heart and lung functions. These are held three times a week and provide opportunity for socialization as well as exercise. Explain this program to Mrs. Jackson and encourage her to join.

Collaboration: Interdisciplinary Team

The following mobility plan was established in consultation with the physical therapist.

❏ Carry out passive range-of-motion exercises at least twice a day on Mrs. Jackson's lower extremities. You can teach her to do self-range-of-motion exercises with her legs, if she has adequate flexibility of her trunk and range of motion in her upper extremity joints.

❏ Active range-of-motion and stretching exercises will improve circulation, maintain joint flexibility, and prevent contractures of the upper extremities. Teach her to do these at least twice each day. Explain the health and fitness trail to Mrs. Jackson and show her where it is. Suggest that she go through the trail every day for additional exercise.

❏ Independent transfer and wheelchair mobility are realistic goals for most individuals with a T7 injury. In Mrs. Jackson's case, obesity, arthritis, and bone and joint changes related to aging are additional factors to consider. Following the exercise plan will increase her abilities for these activities.

❏ A sliding-board transfer is appropriate for Mrs. Jackson. Place the wheelchair and board in position and then evaluate her ability to complete the transfer by herself. If she is unable to do this, assist her in sliding across the board into the wheelchair. She may never be able to complete all the steps for a totally independent transfer, but if she is able to move herself from bed to chair, she will benefit from the movement involved in this procedure.

❏ Standing enhances many body functions. It improves respiratory and digestive function, facilitates drainage of urine from the bladder, relieves pressure on the hips and buttocks, and stretches the muscles of the legs and back. Standing increases visual access to the environment and makes arm movements more efficient. A stand-up wheelchair can allow Mrs. Jackson to receive these benefits. If this is not practical, a tilt table can be used several minutes a day.

❏ For the paraplegic, a wheelchair is an extension of the body. It allows a measure of independence that would not otherwise be possible. Even though Mrs. Jackson is living in a nursing home, a wheelchair will enable her to get around the building and go outside in nice weather when she wants to. Propelling the wheelchair increases the muscle strength in her arms. Ideally, Mrs. Jackson will have a wheelchair that is made to fit her measurements and needs. Place a high-quality seat cushion in the chair to alleviate pressure on the bony prominences.

❏ The occupational therapist may have additional ideas for upper body activities to strengthen the muscles of Mrs. Jackson's arms and trunk. (See chapter 3.)

Outcome

Mrs. Jackson will

❏ Maintain joint flexibility in the upper extremities

- ❑ Remain free of contractures
- ❑ Remain free of circulatory complications of the lower extremities
- ❑ Increase her upper body strength and endurance to enable her to retain her functional abilities for activities of daily living
- ❑ Transfer with a sliding board and minimal assistance

Interdisciplinary Assessment

Nursing.

Lesions above the S2–S4 segment may cause reflex neurogenic bladder. In this instance, voiding is reflexive but involuntary. Mrs. Jackson has no sensation of bladder fullness or urge to void. Urological evaluation at the rehabilitation center revealed the presence of uninhibited bladder contractions and moderate postvoid residual. Management of a reflex neurogenic bladder may include a retraining program to establish regular bladder emptying. Anal stretch may be used with clients with complete spinal cord lesions above the sacral segments or with a reflex neurogenic bladder. This procedure requires a physician's order. Gloves are worn and lubricant applied to the index and middle fingers. First one finger is inserted and then two fingers inserted into the rectum. The fingers are then gently spread apart. The fingers are withdrawn once voiding is finished. The client should do the Valsalva or Credé maneuver to increase intra-abdominal pressure to facilitate emptying. The Credé maneuver also requires a physician's order. Hands are placed flat against the client's abdomen, lateral to and below the umbilicus. Firm downward and medial strokes are applied toward the bladder and then both hands press directly over the bladder. This is repeated several times. For the Valsalva maneuver, the client is instructed to hold the breath while straining to urinate and move the bowels. This is repeated several times. After these procedures, the client is catheterized for residual urine, if ordered by the physician. Suprapubic tapping (fifty taps with the fingers) is another procedure used as a triggering technique to initiate voiding and to empty the bladder. Gently pulling the pubic hair for two to three minutes or stroking the medial thigh are other techniques that may facilitate voiding (Kubalanza-Sipp and French 1990). Other interventions for management of a neurogenic bladder include intermittent catheterization, indwelling catheter, or incontinent pads.

In Mrs. Jackson's case, the retraining program was not a success at the rehabilitation center. The nurse at the rehabilitation center attempted to teach her self intermittent catheterization but Mrs. Jackson was unsuccessful in her efforts to complete the procedure. The use of incontinent pads increases the risk of pressure-ulcer formation and does not eliminate the problem of residual. Although the use of an indwelling catheter is not usually the best choice, it seems the only choice for Mrs. Jackson. A catheter was inserted while she was at the rehabilitation center.

Nursing Diagnosis

Alterations in urinary elimination related to spinal cord injury (reflex neurogenic bladder).

Nursing Interventions

- ❑ The indwelling catheter places Mrs. Jackson at risk for urinary tract infection. Changing to a leg bag during the day frees her from the encumbrance of the large drainage bag and tubing, thereby facilitating her exercise and transfer programs. However, opening the urinary drainage system further increases the risk of bacterial contamination. Review with the staff correct techniques for the care of indwelling catheters and drainage systems (see chapter 7).

❑ Help Mrs. Jackson consume a daily fluid intake of at least 2500 ml. Offer her liquids that maintain a urinary pH of 6 or less to acidify the urine, decreasing the risk of infection. Cranberry juice and prune juice are good choices. Citrus fruits, including tomatoes and milk products, tend to make the urine alkaline and are best avoided.

❑ Autonomic dysreflexia is a life-threatening medical emergency for Mrs. Jackson, as it is for all persons with spinal cord injuries at level T6–T8 or higher.

Outcome

Mrs. Jackson will
❑ Remain free of urinary tract infection

Interdisciplinary Assessment

Nursing.

Mrs. Jackson is unaware of the need to defecate. In spinal-cord-injured persons, the signs of rectal fullness are not perceived. When the injury is above S2, as it is with Mrs. Jackson, the external sphincter remains closed all the time, preventing the passing of stool.

Nursing Diagnosis

Alterations in bowel elimination related to spinal cord injury (neurogenic bowel).

Nursing Interventions

❑ Although the ability to voluntarily defecate is lost, the bowel still responds when certain gastrointestinal reflexes are stimulated. Assist Mrs. Jackson to establish a bowel program for regular evacuation.

❑ Offer Mrs. Jackson a warm beverage to stimulate the gastrocolic reflex. Then insert a bisacodyl suppository to stimulate peristalsis. Digital stimulation may be needed to facilitate the moving of the bowels. Apply an anesthetic ointment to a gloved finger and insert the finger in the rectum (Chadwick and Oesting 1989). Stimulate the rectum by moving the finger in a circular motion. If these procedures are unsuccessful, a small enema can be administered. After several months, the digital stimulation may be enough to trigger the reflexes for evacuation and the suppositories can be omitted (Harmarville 1983).

❑ Assist Mrs. Jackson to a bedside commode for this procedure or position her on her left side in bed with an incontinent pad to protect the sheet. Avoid the use of a bedpan since the pressure may impair the skin integrity of the buttocks.

❑ Schedule this procedure for the same time each day. Regularity assures success. Maintain semisoft, formed stool with diet and fluid intake. (Refer to chapter 6.)

Outcome

Mrs. Jackson will
❑ Evacuate semisoft, formed stool daily

Interdisciplinary Assessment

Nursing.

Dysreflexia is a life-threatening, uninhibited sympathetic response of the nervous system to a noxious stimulus. Individuals with spinal cord injuries at T7 or above are at risk for dysreflexia (Gordon 1991). There are a number of causes for this emergency situation. A full bladder, constipation, or something as trivial as an ingrown toenail can be the stimulus that triggers the response. Signs and symptoms of dysreflexia include
❑ severe headache
❑ severe hypertension
❑ visual disturbances
❑ bradycardia
❑ chills, hot flashes, diaphoreses
❑ nasal congestion
❑ tinnitus
❑ flushing above the level of injury and pale skin below the level of injury

Nursing Diagnosis

High risk for dysreflexia related to spinal cord injury at T7 level.

Nursing Interventions

❑ Monitor for signs and symptoms of dysreflexia. *If dysreflexia is suspected, the stimulus must be identified and removed immediately. An untreated episode can lead to myocardial infarction, ruptured aneurysms, internal bleeding, and even death.*
❑ Raise head of bed ninety degrees.
❑ Stay with client; try to find and remove the noxious stimulus. Call someone to notify physician. *Stay with the client.*
❑ Monitor B/P every three to five minutes during the hypertensive episode.
❑ Assess for distended bladder. If catheter is in place, irrigate with no more than 30 ml normal saline. If catheterization is necessary, use anesthetic jelly. Obtain urine specimen for culture and sensitivities.
❑ Assess for constipation. Anesthetize rectal sphincter with anesthetic jelly before attempting rectal examination. Use large amounts of anesthetic jelly in the anus and rectum before removing stool.
❑ Assess for skin injuries. Check skin surface below level of injury for pressure areas, infection, lacerations, or ingrown toenails.
❑ Administer medications and treatments as prescribed.

(Swearingen 1992)

Collaboration: Interdisciplinary Team

❑ Alert all staff who have direct contact with Mrs. Jackson to the causes and symptoms of dysreflexia. Ask them to immediately report any signs or symptoms of noxious stimuli or of dysreflexia.
❑ Consult with a podiatrist for regular care of Mrs. Jackson's toenails to avoid ingrown toenails or infections.

Interdisciplinary Assessment

Nursing.

An assessment for pressure-ulcer potential places Mrs. Jackson at risk for skin impairment. Maintaining skin integrity is a high priority in her care. A pressure ulcer may require prolonged bedrest, increasing the risk of other complications associated with immobility. An infected pressure ulcer increases spasticity and can trigger autonomic dysreflexia.

Nursing Diagnosis

High risk for impaired skin integrity related to paralysis, spasticity, loss of skin sensation, and skin changes associated with aging.

Nursing Interventions

❑ Institute the preventive protocol (see chapter 4). Remind staff that skin inspection for Mrs. Jackson includes the feet. Her heels are especially prone to breakdown; ingrown toenails can trigger autonomic dysreflexia.
❑ Check the position of her feet and legs before and after she is transferred or moved in bed.
❑ Monitor for signs of infection if spasticity increases.
❑ In addition to the exercise and activity previously described, teach Mrs. Jackson to perform pressure releases at least hourly while she is in the wheelchair. (See chapter 3.)

Outcome

Mrs. Jackson will
❑ Remain free of skin impairments

Interdisciplinary Assessment

Nursing.

Thoracic nerves 6 through 12 control the abdominal muscles used for forceful exhalation of air and secretions. Mrs. Jackson's diaphragm is functioning normally and she has not lost her ability to inhale. The partial paralysis of the chest and abdominal muscles interferes with deep breathing and coughing, predisposing her to respiratory tract infection. The lung changes resulting from the aging process increase her risk. Respiratory complications are the leading cause of death for persons with spinal cord injuries.

Nursing Diagnosis

High risk for infection (respiratory tract) related to level of spinal cord injury.

Nursing Interventions

- ❏ Advise Mrs. Jackson to take pneumonia vaccine if she has not already been immunized. Recommend that she receive annual influenza immunizations.
- ❏ Help Mrs. Jackson maintain her exercise and activity regime and daily fluid intake as additional preventive measures. Monitor her closely for signs of respiratory infection and report them to the physician immediately.

Collaboration: Interdisciplinary Team

- ❏ Respiratory care is also high-priority for Mrs. Jackson. Consultation with the physical therapist for chest physical therapy and with the respiratory therapist may be advisable. Postural drainage, percussion, coughing, and deep breathing exercises may be ordered by the physician (see chapter 18).
- ❏ Blow bottles can be used to increase the inspiration and expiration of air. Mrs. Jackson can monitor her improvement by observing the amount of water displaced with each breath.
- ❏ If the physician orders incentive spirometry, you will have to teach Mrs. Jackson how to use the equipment. Do this while she is seated in an upright position and have her hold the spirometer upright. Ask her to exhale and then have her place her lips tightly around the mouthpiece and inhale deeply. Encourage her to try and raise the ball to the top of the chamber. Then instruct her to hold her breath for a few seconds. (The ball will drop.) Next, tell her to remove the mouthpiece and exhale normally. Repeat this exercise several times with rest periods in between.

Outcome

Mrs. Jackson will
- ❏ Remain free of respiratory tract infections

Interdisciplinary Assessment

Nursing and Dietary.

Mrs. Jackson is twenty-five pounds over her ideal body weight. She states this has been her usual body weight for several years. Her food selection habits are healthy, but she frequently snacks throughout the day as well as eating three full meals. Mrs. Jackson's daughter frequently brings food when she visits her mother.

Nursing Diagnosis

Alterations in nutrition, more than body requirements, related to lack of physical exercise and over eating.

Nursing Interventions

❑ A loss of weight will benefit Mrs. Jackson by facilitating her mobility and decreasing the discomfort of arthritis.
❑ Discuss the benefits of weight loss with Mrs. Jackson. Provide her with a diary in which she can record her intake and weekly weights, thus assuming some responsibility for the program.
❑ When Mrs. Jackson's daughter visits, give her suggestions for appropriate snacks and seek her cooperation in helping her mother lose weight.
❑ Weigh Mrs. Jackson weekly.

Collaboration: Interdisciplinary Team

❑ The physician has ordered a low-calorie diet. Ask the dietician to talk with Mrs. Jackson so her intake can be arranged to allow for nourishing, low-calorie snacks.

Outcome

Mrs. Jackson will
❑ Lose one-half pound per week

Interdisciplinary Assessment

Nursing, Social Services, and Activities.

Mrs. Jackson often makes comments about getting better and returning to her apartment to live. She is generally cooperative and will carry out her exercise regime and mobility plan if she is frequently reminded and encouraged. However, she expresses little interest in participating in planning her care. She rarely attends activities, preferring to spend most of the day in her room. Nursing home placement is viewed as permanent for Mrs. Jackson. Her apartment is not accessible for anyone with a mobility impairment. She does not have the financial resources for other living arrangements or for long-term home health care. Her nursing home care is reimbursed by Medicaid.

Mrs. Jackson has experienced the loss of her mobility, her home, and life-style within a short period of time. Her place of residence has changed four times in four months — the hospital, rehabilitation center, her daughter's home, and the nursing home. She has weathered many crises in her life and it is probable that, with time, she will successfully deal with this one. Mrs. Jackson can then move on, establishing for herself a life with meaning and quality.

Nursing Diagnosis

Impaired adjustment related to difficulty adapting to health change status and admission to nursing home.

Nursing Interventions

❑ Continue to involve Mrs. Jackson in planning her care. Take her to the care plan conference and include her by asking her questions and inviting her suggestions for interventions.

□ Use a positive approach in implementing her daily routine. Often times, the approach of the caregiver influences the client's response to participation.

□ Take Mrs. Jackson on a tour of the nursing home. Point out to her places she can go in the building for a change of scene. Encourage her to use her mobility skills for propelling the wheelchair around the building.

□ Mrs. Jackson's daughter visits regularly, but she seldom brings the children, since she is afraid they "will be a nuisance." Mrs. Jackson misses caring for them. Ask the daughter if she could bring one child each time she visits, allowing Mrs. Jackson to maintain her relationship with the children.

□ Encourage Mrs. Jackson to personalize her room with items from home that are important to her, such as family pictures, plants, afghans, or, if there is space, a favorite desk, dresser, or small table.

Collaboration: Interdisciplinary Team

□ The social worker will visit Mrs. Jackson three times a week, allowing her to express her feelings concerning her injury and nursing home placement. The social worker will discuss with Mrs. Jackson the coping mechanisms she has used in past situations.

□ Mrs. Jackson's care plan includes a number of physical activities already. It is possible she does not have the energy to attend those sponsored by the activities department. Find out if this is the reason for her refusal to participate. If so, rearrange her schedule so she can attend those of her choice two or three times a week.

□ Mrs. Jackson was very involved with her church before her injury. Inquire as to whether she would enjoy doing volunteer work for the church, such as preparing mailings or folding bulletins. If the church tapes Sunday services, get a tape recorder for Mrs. Jackson so she can listen to these every week. Be sure she knows about the weekly services held at the nursing home.

□ If her pastor has not visited Mrs. Jackson yet, ask him/her to do so. If it is agreeable to Mrs. Jackson, invite her pastor to the care plan conference. Because of her previous church connections, the pastor may be able to provide her with additional support.

Outcome

Mrs. Jackson will
□ Express her feelings openly and appropriately
□ Express understanding of her injury and the implications for her life-style
□ Actively participate in the planning of her care.
□ Be involved in activities of her choice.

COMMENTS

Health care professionals may view a sudden disruption of life-style as being less traumatic to the elderly client than it would be to a younger person. While it is true that the elderly person has "lived his/her life," each stage of life, including old age, has its developmental tasks that must be accomplished. The aging process requires physical and psychosocial adaptation. The onset of a chronic health problem and permanent disability demands additional adaptation and adjustment. Successful development in old age enables one to look ahead without fearing death. Mrs. Jackson has a strong spiritual faith that can facilitate her adaptation. With the encouragement and support of the staff, her daughter, and grandchildren, Mrs. Jackson will reestablish for herself a life with hope and meaning.

QUESTIONS AND DISCUSSION

1. How would you go about setting up a health and fitness trail that could be used by both ambulatory clients and those in wheelchairs?
2. Consult with a physical therapist or occupational therapist to determine if there are additional exercises for Mrs. Jackson that will strengthen her trunk and upper extremity muscles.
3. Plan some activities within the facility that Mrs. Jackson and her grandchildren could do together.
4. How would you communicate to staff the symptoms and need for urgent intervention for dysreflexia?
5. What interventions can you implement that will utilize Mrs. Jackson's strong spiritual beliefs?
6. What topics would you include in an in-service for staff?
7. What additional interventions by the interdisciplinary team may be beneficial to Mrs. Jackson?

REFERENCES

Chadwick, A.T. and H.H. Oesting. 1989. Caring for Patients with Spinal Cord Injury. *Nursing 89* 19(11): 53–56.

Chipps, E., N. Clanin, and V. Campbell. 1992. *Neurologic Disorders*. St. Louis: Mosby-Year Book, Inc.

Gokbudak, H.J. 1985. Maximizing Rehabilitation for the Elderly Patient with Spinal Cord Injury. *Rehabilitation Nursing* 10(1): 16–19.

Gordon, M. 1991. *Manual of Nursing Diagnosis 1991–1992*. St. Louis: Mosby-Year Book, Inc.

Kubalanza-Sipp, D. and E.T. French. 1990. In C. Carlson, W.P. Griggs, and R.B. King, eds. *Rehabilitation Nursing Procedures Manual*. Rockville, MD: Aspen Publishers, Inc.

Phillips, L., M.N. Ozer, P. Axelson, and H. Chizick. 1987. *Spinal Cord Injury*. New York: Raven Press.

Staff. 1983. *Learning and Living after Your Spinal Cord Injury*. Pittsburgh: Harmarville Rehabilitation Center, Inc.

Swearingen, P.L. 1992. *Pocket Guide to Medical Surgical Nursing*. St. Louis: Mosby-Year Book, Inc.

APPENDIX A Resources

These groups have literature available for public and professional education, some free and others with a minimal charge. Some of the groups have audiovisuals for free loan or with a user's fee.

Action
806 Connecticut Avenue NW
Washington, DC 20525

(202) 634-9380

Administration on Aging
330 Independence Avenue SW
Washington, DC 20201

(202)245-0641

Alzheimer's Association
70 East Lake Street
Chicago, IL 60601

(312)853-3060

American Cancer Society
1599 Clifton Road
Atlanta, GA 30329

(404)320-3333

American Council of the Blind
1010 Vermont Avenue NW, Suite 1100
Washington, DC 20005

(202)393-3666

American Dental Association
211 East Chicago Avenue
Chicago, IL 60611

(312)440-2860

American Diabetes Association
660 Duke Street
Alexandria, VA 22314

(703)549-1500

American Dietetic Association
216 West Jackson Boulevard, Suite 800
Chicago, Illinois 60606

(312)899-0040

American Foundation for the Blind
15 West 16th Street
New York, NY 10011

(212)620-2147

American Geriatrics Society
770 Lexington Avenue, Suite 400
New York, NY 10021

(212)308-1414

American Heart Association
7320 Greenville Avenue
Dallas, TX 75231

(214)750-5397

American Hospital Association
840 North Lake Shore Drive
Chicago, IL 60611

(312) 280-6000

American Lung Association
1740 Broadway
New York, NY 10019-4374

(212)314-8700

American Medical Association
535 North Dearborn Street
Chicago, IL 60610

(312)645-5000

American Nurses Association
2420 Pershing Road
Kansas City, MO 64108

(816)474-5720

American Occupational Therapy Association, Inc.
P.O. Box 1725
1383 Piccard Drive
Rockville, MD 20850-4375

(301)948-9626

American Optometric Association
243 North Lindbergh Boulevard
St. Louis, MO 63141

(314)991-4100

American Parkinson's Disease Association, Inc.
60 Bay Street, Suite 401
Staten Island, NY 10301

(800)223-2732

American Pharmaceutical Association
2215 Constitution Avenue NW
Washington, DC 20077-6718

(202)628-4410

American Physical Therapy Association
1111 North Fairfax Street
Alexandria, VA 22314

(703)684-2782

American Podiatric Medical Association
9312 Old Georgetown Road
Bethesda, MD 20814

(201)571-9200

American Psychiatric Association
1400 K Street NW
Washington, DC 20005

(202)682-6239

American Psychological Association
1200 17th Street NW
Washington, DC 20036

(202)955-7600

American Red Cross
17th and D Streets, NW
Washington, DC 20006

(202)737-8300

American Society on Aging
833 Market Street, Suite 512
San Francisco, CA 94103

(415)543-2617

American Speech-Language-Hearing Association
10801 Rockville Pike
Rockville, MD 20852

(301)897-5700

Arthritis Foundation
1314 Spring Street NW
Atlanta, GA 30309

(404)872-7100

Association for Gerontology in Higher Education
600 Maryland Avenue SW, West Wing 204
Washington, DC 20024

(202)484-7505

Center for the Study of Aging
706 Madison Avenue
Albany, NY 12208

(518)465-6927

Children of Aging Parents
2761 Trenton Road
Levittown, PA 19056

(215)945-6900

Consumer Information Center
P.O. Box 100
Pueblo, Colorado 81009

Consumer Product Safety Commission
5401 Westbard Avenue
Bethesda, MD 20207

(301)504-0580

Council of Better Business Bureaus
1515 Wilson Boulevard, Suite 300
Arlington, VA 22209

(703)276-0133

Department of Labor
200 Constitution Avenue NW, Room S3032
Washington, DC 20210

(202)523-6060

Environmental Protection Agency
401 M Street SW
Washington, DC 20460

(202)382-2080

Food and Nutrition Information Center
National Agricultural Library Building, Room 304
Beltsville, MD 20705

(301)344-3719

Foundation for Hospice and Home Care
519 C Street NE
Washington, DC 20002

(202)547-7424

Gerontological Society of America
1275 K Street NW, Suite 350
Washington, DC 20005-4006

(202)842-1275

Gray Panthers
1311 South Juniper Street, Suite 601
Philadelphia, PA 19107

(215)545-6555

Health Care Financing Administration
6325 Security Boulevard
Baltimore, MD 21207

(410)594-9086

Help for Incontinent People
P.O. Box 544
Union, SC 29379

(803)585-8789

Huntington's Disease Society of America
140 West 22nd Street, 6th Floor
New York, NY 10011

(212)242-1968

Legal Services for the Elderly
132 West 43rd Street, 3rd Floor
New York, NY 10036

(212)391-0120

Make Today Count
101½ South Union Street
Alexandria, VA 22314-3323

(703)548-9674

Medic Alert Foundation
P.O. Box 1009
Turlock, CA 95381-1009

(209)668-3333

National Alliance of Senior Citizens
2525 Wilson Boulevard
Arlington, VA 22201

(703)528-4380

National Arthritis and Musculoskeletal and Skin Diseases
    Information Clearinghouse
P.O. Box AMS
Bethesda, MD 20892

(301)468-3235

National Association for Home Care
519 C Street NE
Washington, DC 20002

(202)547-7424

National Association for the Deaf
814 Thayer Avenue
Silver Spring, MD 20910

(301)587-1788

National Association for Practical Nurse Education
    and Services
1400 Spring Street, Suite 310
Silver Spring, MD 20910

(301)588-2491

National Association of Area Agencies on Aging
600 Maryland Avenue SW, Suite 208
Washington, DC 20024

(202) 484-7520

National Association of Community Health Centers
1330 New Hampshire Avenue NW, Suite 122
Washington, DC 20036

(202)659-8008

National Association of Meal Programs
204 E Street NE
Washington, DC 20002

(202)547-6340

National Association of Social Workers
7981 Eastern Avenue
Silver Spring, MD 20910

(301)565-0333

National Association of State Units on Aging
2033 K Street NW, Suite 304
Washington, DC 20006

(202)785-0707

National Center for Health Services Research and Health Care
    Technology Assessment
Parklawn Building, Room 18-12
5600 Fishers Lane
Rockville, MD 20857

(301)443-4100

National Cholesterol Education Program
4733 Bethesda Avenue
Bethesda, MD 20814

(301)951-3260

National Citizens Coalition for Nursing Home Reform
1424 16th Street NW, Suite L2
Washington, DC 20005

(202)797-0657

National Council of Senior Citizens
925 15th Street NW
Washington, DC 20005

(202)347-8800

National Council on the Aging
600 Maryland Avenue SW, West Wing 100
Washington, DC 20024

(202)479-1200

National Diabetes Information Clearinghouse
Box NDIC
Bethesda, MD 20892

(301)468-2162

National Digestive Diseases Information Clearinghouse
Box NDDIC
Bethesda, MD 20892

(301)468-6344

National Eye Institute
Information Office
Building 31, Room 6A29
Bethesda, MD 20892

(301)496-5248

National Geriatric Society
212 West Wisconsin Avenue
Milwaukee, WI 53203

(414)272-4130

National Heart, Lung, and Blood Institute
    Information Office
Building 31, Room 4A21
9000 Rockville Pike
Bethesda, MD 20892

(301)486-4236

National Hospice Organization
1901 North Fort Myer Drive, Suite 307
Arlington, VA 22209

(703)243-5900

National Information Center on Deafness
Gallaudet University
800 Florida Avenue NE
Washington, DC 20002

(202)651-5051

National Institute on Aging
Public Information Office
Federal Building, Room 6C12
9000 Rockville Pike
Bethesda, MD 20892

(301)496-1752

National Institute of Mental Health
Public Inquiries Office, Room 15C-05
5600 Fishers Lane
Rockville, MD 20857

(301)443-4513

National Institute of Neurological Disorders and Stroke
    Information Office
Building 31, Room 8A06
9000 Rockville Pike
Bethesda, MD 20892

(301)496-5751

National Kidney and Urologic Diseases Information
    Clearinghouse
Box NKUDIC
Bethesda, MD 20892

(301)468-6345

National League for Nursing
10 Columbus Circle
New York, NY 10019-1350

(212)582-1022

National Multiple Sclerosis Society
738 Third Avenue
New York, NY 10017-3288

(212)986-3240

National Osteoporosis Foundation
1625 Eye Street NW, Suite 822
Washington, DC 20006

(202)223-2226

National Rehabilitation Association
633 South Washington Street
Alexandria, VA 22314

(703)836-0850

National Rehabilitation Information Center
8455 Colesville Road, Suite 935
Silver Spring, MD 20910-3319

(301)588-9284

National Rural Health Care Association
301 East Armour Boulevard, Suite 420
Kansas City, MO 64111

(816)756-3140

National Safety Council
444 North Michigan Avenue
Chicago, IL 60611-3991

(312)527-4800

National Society to Prevent Blindness
500 East Remington Road
Schaumburg, IL 60173

(312)843-2020

National Stroke Association
300 East Hampden Avenue, Suite 240
Englewood, CO 80110

(303)762-9922

Office of Disease Prevention and Health Promotion
Mary Switzer Building, Room 2132
330 C Street SW
Washington, DC 20201

(202)472-5660

Simon Foundation
Box 815
Wilmette, IL 60091

(708)864-3913

Social Security Administration
Office of Public Inquiries
6401 Security Boulevard
Baltimore, MD 21235

(410)594-1234

United Parkinson Foundation
360 West Superior Street
Chicago, IL 60610

(312)664-2344

Veterans Administration
Office of Public Affairs
810 Vermont Avenue NW
Washington, DC 20420

(202)233-2843

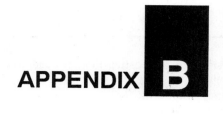

Residents' Rights as set forth in the Omnibus Budget Reconciliation Act of 1987

The resident has the right to an environment that
- ❑ Promotes maintenance or enhancement of quality of life
- ❑ Promotes dignity and respect in full recognition of each resident's individuality
- ❑ Is safe, clean, comfortable and homelike.
- ❑ Helps the resident maintain the highest practicable physical, mental, and psychological well-being.

1. **The resident has the right to free choice, including**
   - ❑ The right to choose an attending physician. If the attending physician refuses to comply with certain federal regulations regarding the resident's care, the facility may replace the physician after notifying the resident.
   - ❑ The right to full advance information about changes in care or treatment that affects the resident's well-being. This includes the right to refuse treatment. Treatment refers to procedures ordered by the physician. The resident must be consistent and persistent in indicating the wish to refuse treatment. The laws of each state govern the manner in which this right is implemented. For example, if a resident cannot take in food and fluids, the resident may refuse artificial nutrition. In this case, the specific laws of the state are followed.
   - ❑ The right to participate in the assessment and care planning process. The resident must be informed of the evaluations made by the members of the interdisciplinary team. The resident and the family are invited to the care plan conference so they may assist with the planning process.
   - ❑ The self-administration of medications, if the assessment demonstrates that this is feasible and the resident wishes to do so. The nurse is still responsible for overseeing this process.
   - ❑ The right to consent to participation in experimental research. Research that personally affects the resident cannot be carried out without the resident's consent.

2. **The resident has the right to freedom from abuse and restraints, including**
   - ❑ Freedom from physical, sexual, and mental abuse
   - ❑ Freedom from corporal punishment and involuntary seclusion. Corporal punishment is the use of painful treatment for correction of behavior. Involuntary seclusion is to isolate the resident without providing care.
   - ❑ Freedom from physical and chemical restraint, unless required to treat medical symptoms. Physical restraint refers to any device that limits the

resident's mobility. Chemical restraint is medication that influences behavior.

3. **The resident has the right to privacy, including**
   - ❑ Privacy during medical treatment and nursing care
   - ❑ Receiving and sending mail
   - ❑ Privacy during telephone calls
   - ❑ Privacy when visitors are present

4. **The resident has the right to confidentiality of personal and clinical records.**
   - ❑ Information about the resident is available only to those who need the information in order to provide care. This includes information on the resident's chart and care plan. It also includes any information about the resident's personal life and relationship with the family.
   - ❑ The caregivers who receive this information are obligated to keep the information confidential. They are not to talk about the resident outside the facility.

5. **The resident has the right to accommodation of needs, including**
   - ❑ Making choices about life that are significant to the resident. This includes activities, schedules, and health care that are consistent with the resident's interests and care plan.
   - ❑ Receiving assistance in maintaining independent functioning, dignity, and well-being. The staff must strive to meet the physical and psychosocial needs of the residents. The environment must be adapted to allow the residents to function as independently as possible.

6. **The resident has the right to voice grievances.**
   - ❑ The resident may voice grievances to the appropriate authority in the facility without fear of retaliation or discrimination. The facility must take prompt action to resolve the grievance.

7. **The resident has the right to organize and participate in family and resident groups.**
   - ❑ The facility must provide space for meetings.
   - ❑ A staff member from the facility will attend if invited.
   - ❑ The staff will address written recommendations from the meetings that concern decisions that affect the resident's care and life in the facility.

8. **The resident has the right to participate in social, religious, and community activities, including**
   - ❑ Activities that do not infringe on the rights of other residents
   - ❑ Activities consistent with the resident's interests, assessment, and plan of care
   - ❑ The right to vote
   - ❑ The right to keep religious items in the room
   - ❑ The right to attend religious services

9. **The resident has the right to examine survey results and correction plans.**
   - ❑ The resident may inspect these records during normal business hours or by special appointment.

10. **The resident has the right to manage personal funds.**
    - ❑ The resident may request the facility to manage the funds. The resident must give written authorization for this.
    - ❑ If the account exceeds fifty dollars, it must earn interest that is given to the resident.

11. **The resident has the right to information about eligibility for Medicare/Medicaid benefits.**
    - ❑ The resident has the right to receive these benefits if the facility participates in those programs.

12. **The resident has the right to file complaints about abuse, neglect, or misappropriation of property.**
    - ❑ If the resident believes there has been abuse, neglect, or property stolen, the resident can file a complaint with the state agency that inspects that facility.

13. **The resident has the right to information about advocacy groups.**
    - ❑ Each state has an ombudsman program.
    - ❑ Each facility also has agencies in the area that serve as advocates for the residents. An advocate serves as a spokesperson for residents to ensure that they are receiving appropriate care.
    - ❑ The telephone numbers of these groups must be available to residents.

14. **The resident has the right to immediate and unlimited access by immediate family or relatives, including**
    - ❑ The long-term care ombudsman
    - ❑ Government agency representatives
    - ❑ The attending physician
    - ❑ The right to withdraw consent to visit with any of these individuals

15. **The resident has the right to share a room with the spouse if they are both residents in the same facility.**

16. **The resident has the right to perform or not perform work for the facility if it is medically appropriate for the resident to work.**
    - ❑ The resident must formally agree to any work arrangement.
    - ❑ If the work is for pay, the resident is compensated at the prevailing rate for those services.

17. **The resident has the right to remain in the facility, *unless***
    - ❑ The resident no longer needs the care.
    - ❑ The resident's welfare requires transfer.
    - ❑ The facility can no longer meet the resident's needs.
    - ❑ The health or safety of others in the facility is endangered.
    - ❑ The resident fails to pay for services.
    - ❑ The facility ceases to operate.
    - ❑ In these cases, thirty days notice must be given, except where health is improved, there is an emergency, or there is danger to the health or safety of individuals in the facility.

18. **The resident has the right to use personal possessions, including**
    - ❑ Personal clothing
    - ❑ Personal furnishings to the extent these can be used in accordance with health and safety regulations.

19. **The resident has the right to notification of change in condition.** This means the facility will notify the resident's attending physician, legal representative, and family member within twenty-four hours of
    - ❑ An accident in which the resident was involved
    - ❑ A significant change in the resident's condition
    - ❑ A need to alter treatment significantly
    - ❑ A decision to transfer or discharge the resident

The members of the interdisciplinary team work together to provide the residents with the rights expressed in this document.

INDEX

Note: Page numbers in **bold type** refer to not-text materials.